D1477622

2005
YEAR BOOK OF
SPORTS MEDICINE®

The 2005 Year Book Series

Year Book of Allergy, Asthma, and Clinical Immunology™: Drs Rosenwasser, Boguniewicz, Milgrom, Routes, and Weber

Year Book of Anesthesiology and Pain Management™: Drs Chestnut, Abram, Black, Gravlee, Mathru, Lee, and Roizen

Year Book of Cardiology®: Drs Gersh, Cheitlin, Graham, Kaplan, Sundt, and Waldo

Year Book of Critical Care Medicine®: Drs Dellinger, Parrillo, Balk, Bekes, Dorman, and Dries

Year Book of Dentistry®: Drs Zakariasen, Horswell, McIntyre, Scott, and Zakariasen Victoroff

Year Book of Dermatology and Dermatologic Surgery™: Drs Thiers and Lang

Year Book of Diagnostic Radiology®: Drs Osborn, Birdwell, Dalinka, Gardiner, Levy, Maynard, Oestreich, and Rosado de Christenson

Year Book of Emergency Medicine®: Drs Burdick, Cydulka, Hamilton, Handly, Quintana, and Werner

Year Book of Endocrinology®: Drs Mazzaferri, Bessesen, Howard, Kannan, Kennedy, Leahy, Meikle, Molitch, Rogol, and Rubin

Year Book of Family Practice®: Drs Bowman, Apgar, Bouchard, Dexter, Miser, Neill, and Scherger

Year Book of Gastroenterology™: Drs Lichtenstein, Burke, Dempsey, Drebin, Ginsberg, Katzka, Kochman, Morris, Nunes, Shah, and Stein

Year Book of Hand Surgery and Upper Limb Surgery®: Drs Berger and Ladd

Year Book of Medicine®: Drs Barkin, Frishman, Klahr, Loehrer, Mazzaferri, Phillips, Pillinger, and Snydman

Year Book of Neonatal and Perinatal Medicine®: Drs Fanaroff, Maisels, and Stevenson

Year Book of Neurology and Neurosurgery®: Drs Gibbs and Verma

Year Book of Nuclear Medicine®: Drs Coleman, Blaufox, Royal, Strauss, and Zubal

Year Book of Obstetrics, Gynecology, and Women's Health®: Dr Shulman

Year Book of Oncology®: Drs Loehrer, Arceci, Glatstein, Gordon, Hanna, Morrow, and Thigpen

Year Book of Ophthalmology®: Drs Rapuano, Cohen, Eagle, Grossman, Hammersmith, Myers, Nelson, Penne, Sergott, Shields, Tipperman, and Vander

Year Book of Orthopedics®: Drs Morrey, Beauchamp, Peterson, Swiontkowski, Trigg, and Yaszemski

Year Book of Otolaryngology-Head and Neck Surgery®: Drs Paparella, Otto, and Keefe

Year Book of Pathology and Laboratory Medicine®: Drs Raab, Grzybicki, Bejarano, Bissell, and Stanley

Year Book of Pediatrics®: Dr Stockman

Year Book of Plastic and Aesthetic Surgery™: Drs Miller, Bartlett, Garner, McKinney, Ruberg, Salisbury, and Smith

Year Book of Psychiatry and Applied Mental Health®: Drs Talbott, Ballenger, Buckley, Frances, Jensen, and Markowitz

Year Book of Pulmonary Disease®: Drs Phillips, Barker, Dunlap, Lewis, Maurer, and Willsie

Year Book of Rheumatology, Arthritis, and Musculoskeletal Disease™: Drs Panush, Hadler, Hellmann, Hochberg, Lahita, and Seibold

Year Book of Sports Medicine®: Drs Shephard, Alexander, Cantu, Feldman, McCrory, Nieman, Rowland, Sanborn, and Shrier

Year Book of Surgery®: Drs Copeland, Bland, Cerfolio, Daly, Eberlein, Fahey, Mozingo, Pruett, and Seeger

Year Book of Urology®: Drs Andriole and Coplen

Year Book of Vascular Surgery®: Dr Moneta

2005

The Year Book of
SPORTS MEDICINE®

Editor-in-Chief
Roy J. Shephard, MD, PhD, DPE
Professor Emeritus of Applied Physiology, Faculty of Physical Education and Health and Department of Public Health Sciences, Faculty of Medicine, University of Toronto, Toronto, Ontario, Canada

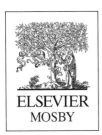

ELSEVIER
MOSBY

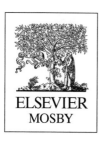

ELSEVIER
MOSBY

Vice President, Continuity Publishing: Timothy M. Griswold
Publishing Director, Continuity: J. Heather Cullen
Developmental Editor: Beth Martz
Senior Manager, Continuity Production: Idelle L. Winer
Senior Issue Manager: Pat Costigan
Illustrations and Permissions Coordinator: Dawn Vohsen

2005 EDITION

Printed in the United States of America
Composition by Thomas Technology Solutions, Inc
Printing/binding by Sheridan Books, Inc

Editorial Office:
Elsevier, Inc.
Suite 1800
1600 John F. Kennedy Boulevard
Philadelphia, PA 19103-2899

International Standard Serial Number: 0162-0908
International Standard Book Number: 0-323-02117-4

Editors

Marion J. L. Alexander, PhD
Professor, Research Associate, Faculty of Physical Education and Recreation Studies, University of Manitoba, Winnipeg, Manitoba, Canada

Robert C. Cantu, MD, MA
Chairman, Department of Surgery, Chief, Neurosurgery Service, and Director, Service Sports Medicine, Emerson Hospital, Concord, Massachusetts; Adjunct Professor, Exercise and Sport Science, University of North Carolina, and Medical Director, National Center for Catastrophic Sports Injury Research, Chapel Hill, North Carolina; and Co-Director, Neurological Sports Injury Center at Brigham and Women's Hospital and Neurosurgery Consultant, Boston College Eagles and Boston Cannon's, Boston, Massachusetts

Debbie Ehrmann Feldman, PhD, PT
Associate Professor, Faculty of Medicine, School of Rehabiliation, Université de Montréal; and Physiotherapist, Montreal Children's Hospital, McGill University Health Centre, Montreal, Quebec, Canada

Paul McCrory, MBBS, PhD
Associate Professor, Centre for Sports Medicine Research and Education, School of Physiotherapy, University of Melbourne, Parkville, Victoria, Australia

David C. Nieman, DrPH
Professor and Director of Human Performance Laboratory, Appalachian State University, Boone, North Carolina

Thomas Rowland, MD
Professor of Pediatrics, Tufts University School of Medicine, Boston; and Chief, Pediatric Cardiology, Baystate Medical Center, Springfield, Massachusetts

Charlotte F. Sanborn, PhD
Professor and Chair, Texas Woman's University, Denton, Texas

Ian Shrier, MD, PhD
Associate Member, Department of Epidemiology and Biostatistics, McGill University, Montreal, Quebec, Canada

American College of Sports Medicine Liaison Representative
Robert E. Sallis, MD
Assistant Clinical Professor, University of California Riverside/University of California Los Angeles Biomedical Sciences, Kaiser Permanente Medical Center, Fontana, California

Table of Contents

Journals Represented

Journal of the American Medical Association
Journal of the Canadian Chiropractic Association
Medical Journal of Australia
Medicine and Science in Sports and Exercise
Metabolism: Clinical and Experimental
Neurology
Neurosurgery
New England Journal of Medicine
Orthopedics
Pediatric Exercise Science
Pediatrics
Physician and Sportsmedicine
Preventive Medicine
Skeletal Radiology
Southern Medical Journal
Spine
Spine Journal
Sports Medicine
Stroke

STANDARD ABBREVIATIONS

The following terms are abbreviated in this edition: acquired immunodeficiency syndrome (AIDS), cardiopulmonary resuscitation (CPR), central nervous system (CNS), cerebrospinal fluid (CSF), computed tomography (CT), deoxyribonucleic acid (DNA), electrocardiography (ECG), health maintenance organization (HMO), human immunodeficiency virus (HIV), intensive care unit (ICU), intramuscular (IM), intravenous (IV), magnetic resonance (MR) imaging (MRI), and ribonucleic acid (RNA), and ultrasound (US).

NOTE

The YEAR BOOK OF SPORTS MEDICINE is a literature survey service providing abstracts of articles published in the professional literature. Every effort is made to assure the accuracy of the information presented in these pages. Neither the editors nor the publisher of the YEAR BOOK OF SPORTS MEDICINE can be responsible for errors in the original materials. The editors' comments are their own opinions. Mention of specific products within this publication does not constitute endorsement.

To facilitate the use of the YEAR BOOK OF SPORTS MEDICINE as a reference tool, all illustrations and tables included in this publication are now identified as they appear in the original article. This change is meant to help the reader recognize that any illustration or table appearing in the YEAR BOOK OF SPORTS MEDICINE may be only one of many in the original article. For this reason, figure and table numbers will often appear to be out of sequence within the YEAR BOOK OF SPORTS MEDICINE.

Introduction

These are exciting times for readers of the YEAR BOOK series. Elsevier Publishing is moving to a new electronic system that will allow the enormous number of journals that are reviewed each year to be delivered to individual editors in greater numbers and at a much faster rate. So, you can look forward to even more timely comments on new developments in Sports Medicine. One likely consequence of this shift will be that in general, the authors' own abstracts will be used. An advantage of this approach is that abstractors will no longer have the potential of introducing their own biases into the summaries of papers. At the same time, considerations of copyright could preclude alterations to abstracts, so that it may be necessary to accept minor differences in abstract structure, choice of units, and weaknesses of grammar such as the split infinitives that are missed by the less-vigilant of the original journal editors.

This year's volume retains the traditional format. It presents a stimulating mix of relevant new findings in preventive medicine, epidemiology, sports injuries, interactions between physical activity, environment and disease, and ergogenic aids and doping. For the orthopedic surgeon, many ethical issues remain to be resolved. Snowmobiling on roads increases the risk of injury to participants. Other surveys cover the hazards of top-level football, soccer, volleyball, baseball, rock and wall climbing, kite-surfing, alpine and cross-country skiing, prolonged road races, cycling on bicycles of inappropriate size, and the particular hazards of clipless pedals. Helmets are shown to reduce the risk of head injuries in skiers and snow-boarders, but information is needed concerning their impact on neck injuries in these same sports.

Trauma may contribute to the development of lipomas. The face accounts for a third of the injuries sustained in Rugby Union play. Revised criteria are suggested for determination of cognitive change in boxers; a prospective study found no deterioration of cognition among tournament participants. Spinal problems are prevalent in football linemen, wrestlers, golfers, and fast bowlers. Scintigraphy may help in revealing stress injuries of the spine. Snapping hip may result from overtraining. Acetabular labral injury can cause groin pain in soccer players. Laporoscopic repair is effective in treating groin pain. Early operation seems the best approach to rupture of the pectoralis major. Rotator cuff injuries are frequent in kayakers. Arthroscopic anterior shoulder stabilization works well in young athletes. The use of a trampoline can cause ulnar nerve injury in children. Long, smooth strokes reduces the risk of injury to median and ulnar nerves during wheelchair propulsion. Spiral fractures of the humerus occasionally develop in professional baseball pitchers. Subclinical injury of the medial collateral ligament is also common in baseball. Low-energy shock wave treatment is helpful in treating the lateral epicondylitis of tennis players.

The Ottawa rules are shown to be effective in avoiding unnecessary knee radiographs. In handball, valgus collapse near full extension of the knee contributes to injury of the anterior cruciate ligament. Lower-body positive pressure is suggested as a means of reducing the load on the lower limbs when exercising after knee surgery. Regular physiotherapy does not necessarily speed recovery after anterior cruciate reconstruction. Patello-femoral pain responds to a combination of exercise and taping. Pulsed ultrasound seems of no benefit in tibial stress fractures. Iliotibial band problems are helped by local corticosteroid administration. Stretching speeds recovery of hamstring injuries. Proprioceptive changes do not seem to contribute to instability of the ankle after injury of this joint. Ankle syndesmosis sprains are common in hockey players. Intra-articular hyaluronic acid is useful in treating "golfer's toe." Sesamoid mobilization seems a helpful treatment of Hallux Limitus.

Biomechanics continues to provide research insights applicable to the practice of sports medicine, with particular regard to the etiology of sports injuries and enhancement of the activities of daily living. Recent biomechanical analysis has also explored the causes and the most effective treatments of various sport injuries, including knee ligament replacements, as well as the treatment and repair of shoulder and elbow ligaments. Autologous serum is proving a promising treatment for muscle sprains. New information is available on gait mechanics in chronic anterior cruciate ligament deficiency and on methods of increasing quadriceps muscle activity. Proprioception of the shoulder joint has been studied in internal/external rotation, along with electromyograms of the rotator cuff during external shoulder rotation. Muscular efficiency has been reviewed in road cyclists, and the causes of training intolerance have been examined in various groups of elite athletes. Low back strength is noted in smokers, and techniques of patient education in low back pain are explored.

No difference of reliability is found between peak and average values for handgrip force. Values are largest if people select their own hand positions during testing. A reliable supine hip extensor test is described. Jump performance is greater from a soft surface. A golf-specific warm-up improves performance in this sport. Static stretching should be avoided to maximize force output. Further, stretching may impair balance. Muscle shows similar fatiguability in strength-matched men and women. Fatigue reduces position reproduction acuity. Massage may reduce fatigue, but it does not alter muscle blood flow or affect blood lactate after exercise. Neither preheating nor precooling of muscle seems to change the damage induced by eccentric exercise. Cryotherapy does not alter shoulder proprioception. The benefit of Swiss ball stability training is also questioned. However, progressive agility and trunk stabilization training reduce the risk of reinjury. Previous injury shortens optimum muscle length, influencing the risks associated with eccentric exercise. Ultrasound does not hasten recovery from blunt contusion.

Exercise prescriptions should be matched carefully with the patient's personality. A combination of exercise prescription and psychologically grounded counseling seems the most effective approach. Given adequate training, general practitioners can induce a cost-effective increase in the walking habits of sedentary patients. New research offers support to use of the talk test in exercise prescription. As little as 20 minutes of brisk walking per week appears to protect nursing assistants against occupational fatigue. However, 30 minutes of moderate aerobic activity per day may not be enough to control the obesity epidemic. Attempts to encourage active commuting by changing urban design have to date been discouraging. Moreover, commuting activity does not seem to have great influence on prognosis after allowing for the effects of other forms of physical activity.

Apparent longitudinal changes in the aerobic fitness of an individual arise in part because of methodological error and regression to the mean. Regular physical activity is usually associated with better health during the previous month, but excessive physical activity worsens recent health. A longitudinal study has demonstrated reduced hospital use among individuals who increase their personal fitness. Weekend warriors gain health benefit from infrequent bouts of activity, provided that they are free of cardiac risk factors. The European score provides a better assessment of cardiac risk than the Framingham score. Medical costs in patients with suspected coronary disease are inversely related to treadmill work capacity. Prolonged endurance events can cause temporary increases in traditional markers of cardiac damage and D-dimers. Moreover, highly specific tests for cardiac troponin confirm that triathlon participation can cause transient cardiac damage. Such damage does not seem more marked in older than in younger marathoners. Dobutamine stress tests predict a 10% higher ischemia threshold than exercise tests. Withdrawal of cardiac drugs to allow prognostic testing does not seem to carry excessive risk early after myocardial infarction. Patients with congestive heart failure seem at increased risk of ventricular overload during aqua exercises. In congestive heart failure, an 8-week training program apparently gives lower hospital usage over a 5-year follow-up. In claudicant patients, an intermittent shuttle run seems a better evaluation tool than a treadmill test.

Eucapnic hyperventilation is claimed to provide the best test for exercise-induced bronchospasm. Gains in muscle strength in chronic obstructive lung disease are augmented by administration of testosterone. Inspiratory muscle training substantially increases working capacity in patients with cystic fibrosis.

Television watching is associated with abnormal glucose metabolism after allowance for the effects of physical activity. A hand-held measure of oxygen consumption based on the fluorescent quenching of Ruthenium offers a novel approach to metabolic studies. Exercise sustains resting metabolism. Physical activity counts are much greater for patients who achieve weight loss than for their peers who have no success in a weight loss program. An increased participation in sports and exercise appears to limit menopausal weight accumulation. Those who report physical activity after gastric bypass are more successful in weight loss than those who do not. Excessive intakes of protein may work against the development of muscle strength. However, exercise-induced proteinuria does not seem of sufficient duration to worsen prognosis in patients with non-nephrotic renal disease. Gastrointestinal transit times do not differ between endurance competitors with and without athletic diarrhea.

The absence of heart rate drift is suggested as a method of screening for McArdle's disease. Exercise programs maintain an improved walking ability in fibromyalgia over at least 12 months of follow-up. The main abnormality in exercise response among those with chronic fatigue syndrome is an increased perception of effort. Kinesiophobia also contributes to limitation of physical activity in this condition. A program of progressive exercise enhances both physiological and psychological function in chronic fatigue syndrome. Muscle dysfunction seems an important cause of exercise-related osteoarthritis, Over the short term, manipulation gives better results than exercise in chronic osteoarthritis. Exercise seems to offer some protection against prostatic cancer. However, endurance cycling is associated with a deterioration in sperm morphology.

Grehlin levels are a useful indicator in menstrual disturbances. Puberty and menopause are important windows of opportunity for enhancing bone mass. Loss of bone mineral density is a potential complication of exercise-induced weight loss in older women. Weight cycling may cause redistribution of fat. Reported physical activity of children correlates only weakly with pedometer counts. Recent decreases in physical performance of children are not due simply to greater obesity. Physician advice increases the activity of adolescents. Increase of physical activity does not necessarily increase food intake. Physical activity is greater in children with well-developed movement skills. Run times over 1.6 km (1 mile) are best predicted by traditional units of aerobic power (mL/[kg·min]). A compendium of energy costs for children is developed. Constitution rather than training seems responsible for the short stature of gymnasts. Children have a good tolerance of dry heat, but cool quickly in the cold. Inappropriate use of ergogenic aids is associated with a high ego orientation. Boys recover from anaerobic exercise more rapidly than older individuals. Anaerobic exercise is helpful in children with cystic fibrosis. Leisure (but not occupational) activity reduces the risk of declining overall health and physical functioning in old age. The ability of elderly people to recall their level of physical activity 32 years earlier is shown to be quite limited. Those who are active as young adults have a much reduced risk of fractures at ages older than 60 years. Regular physical activity helps to sustain a vigorous response to novel antigenic challenge in old age. Exercise-induced increases in protein synthesis do not necessarily decrease with aging.

Resting and exercise-induced oxidized lipoprotein lipase platelet function are decreased by exercise training. A poor tolerance of endurance exercise is associated with low plasma levels of interleukin-6. Lymphocyte apoptosis is enhanced by high intensity exercise but is reduced by administration of antioxidants. Epinephrine infusion increases interleukin-6 mRNA in adipose tissue. Oral glycan reduces the risk of infection associated with stressful exercise, but vitamin E seems to increase the risk of lipid peroxidation and inflammation.

Some sports drinks cause a rapid erosion of dental enamel. Carbohydrate feeding serves to sustain CNS function during simulated team sport. A very high carbohydrate diet (65%) also seems to reduce the risk of overtraining during a bout of severe conditioning. Ingestion of mixtures of glucose and sucrose can increase the metabolism of exogenous carbohydrate. Adding protein to sports drinks helps to sustain protein balance and reduces muscle damage in ultra-endurance events. Because of poor regulation of the companies producing nutritional supplements, a high proportion of preparations are contaminated by unlisted materials, sometimes including sufficient anabolic steroids to disqualify an athlete. No increase in the excretion of endogenous steroids was found after 30 minutes of moderate laboratory exercise. Sperm counts can be maintained during abuse of steroids by simultaneous treatment with human chorionic gonadotrophin; nevertheless, the proportion of abnormal sperm increases with such therapy. The cardiac dangers of anabolic steroid abuse seem to persist for several years after doping has stopped. Suggestions that caffeine might be withdrawn from the list of prohibited substances have proven incorrect. Serum levels of soluble transferrin receptor offer a useful screening test for erythropoietin abuse. Gene doping may soon become a major challenge to fair competition.

Heat stress can develop under "green flag" conditions, particularly if the individual was heat stressed on the previous day. Despite significant differences in serum magnesium between athletes with and without muscle cramps, it is now argued that mineral loss is not responsible for cramping. Preliminary use of a cooling vest may enhance 5-km track performance under hot conditions. In victims of heat stroke, the best treatment seems immersion in cold water. Hypercapnia can accelerate the cooling of avalanche victims.

Acute mountain sickness is more likely in subjects who show early fluid retention. Sildenafil is suggested to control pulmonary hypertension in acute mountain sickness. A strenuous climb may help to reverse the potentially toxic activation of neutrophils at high altitude. A self-administered screening questionnaire for divers is described. Failure to equalize middle ear pressures in SCUBA diving may cause transient facial nerve paresis. Risks of decompression illness call for special precaution in SCUBA divers with patent foramen ovale.

This provides a brief survey of some of the exciting items in this year's edition. The completion of any book is essentially a team effort, and I pay tribute to all of my colleagues who have worked so hard to make this volume a success—both the co-editors, and Beth Martz and her team of professionals at Elsevier Publishing. We are extremely pleased to welcome new members to our editorial team this year. Our coverage has been strengthened by adding the experience of Dr Debbie Feldman in Sports Physiotherapy, Dr Paul McCrory in Sports Medicine, and Dr Tom Rowland in Pediatric Sports Medicine. We all hope that as readers you will find much to stimulate and enhance your practice of Sports Medicine.

Roy J. Shephard, MD, PhD, DPE

Preparticipation Screening of Young Athletes: An Effective Investment?

Roy J. Shephard, MD, PhD, DPE

Faculty of Physical Education and Health and Department of Public Health Sciences, Faculty of Medicine, University of Toronto, Toronto, Ontario

The Spectrum of Current Opinion

There is currently wide variation in both opinion and practice with regard to the preparticipation screening of young athletes. Physicians in many parts of the United States observe 4 or less of 13 American Heart Association recommendations for the preparticipation screening of high school athletes.[1] At one end of the spectrum, some exercise specialists regard the risk of a sudden, exercise-induced cardiovascular death in unscreened competitors as "unacceptable," and they maintain that it is unethical not to institute a comprehensive preparticipation screening program.[2] At the other end of the spectrum, there are sports physicians who argue that most of the apparent "abnormalities" detected by the application of noninvasive tests such as the ECG and the echocardiogram to healthy young athletes have no clinical significance, arising simply from a normal, training-induced physiologic hypertrophy of the left ventricle.[3] Believers in mass testing have frequently found it necessary to reset the boundaries between normal and supposedly abnormal records, but it has remained difficult if not impossible to reach an acceptable level of diagnostic accuracy when evaluating such items as the thickness of the posterior ventricular wall in young, healthy, and symptom-free athletes.[3] Moreover, far from being at an increased and "unacceptable" risk (as is commonly supposed), the endurance athlete enjoys a substantial advantage of life expectancy relative to his or her sedentary peers.[4]

In the context of this debate, the experience of Italian sports physicians has particular interest. Medical certification has been a condition of participation in both amateur and professional sport in Italy since 1950[5,6]; presently, requirements include a clinical examination, a 12-lead resting ECG, a simple bench-type stress test, and basic measurements of pulmonary function. Italian athletes undergo 5 million such tests every year[7]; the number of evaluations is so large that some competitors must be tested more than once per year. Further, a recent brief review of the Italian approach[7,8] continues to commend preparticipation screening as an appropriate means of avoiding incidents of sudden death among competitive athletes.

Nevertheless, before endorsing the Italian plan, it is important that we review critically its efficacy in terms of preventing cardiac catastrophes, the resulting costs to health insurance systems, possible adverse effects of universal cardiovascular screening on the athletes concerned, and implications for medical liability claims.

Efficacy of Preparticipatory Screening

The enormous numbers of Italian athletes who undergo annual preparticipation screening would seem to offer scope to conduct a unique epidemiological experiment.[9] If the screening process is indeed as effective as its proponents maintain, then it should be possible to demonstrate that Italian athletes suffer a much lower incidence of sudden, exercise-induced cardiac deaths than do competitors from other parts of the world where extensive preparticipation screening is a rarity. Despite repeated claims of efficacy,[1,10] there is no evidence that such a cross-national comparison has yet been attempted.

Pigozzi and associates[7,8] have argued that testing was useful, since a normal ECG had a high negative predictive value in their sample of competitors (96% of those with a normal ECG were free of cardiac disease, as judged by a combination of clinical examination and echocardiography). Several Italian reports have also claimed that it is possible to identify individuals with hypertrophic cardiomyopathy (HCM) from careful examination of a 12-lead ECG.[7,10,11] Finally, it has been argued that in those individuals where HCM was diagnosed, prospective studies have shown that the prohibition of sport prevented subsequent exercise-induced deaths.[1,10] Each of these suggestions will now be reviewed critically.

The claim that the ECG had a negative predictive value of 96% in young athletes[7] seems based on an article by Pelliccia et al.[12] The latter authors reported findings in a series of 1050 competitors who were tested at the Italian National Institute of Sports Science in Rome. It was necessary to exclude 45 individuals from the analysis because of technically unsatisfactory ECGs or echocardiograms, but a more important criticism of the report is that the apparent efficacy of the required test battery was augmented because 220 of the remaining 1005 competitors had been referred to the Institute for further investigation of a suspected cardiac anomaly. The diagnostic value of the ECGs was tested against a combination of clinical judgment and echocardiography. ECG tracings for the mixed sample (785 ostensibly healthy and 220 suspect) were rated as normal in 603 cases; this total included 26 false-negative reports (a negative predictive value of 577/603, or 95.7%). But despite the boosting of apparent test efficacy by the inclusion of 220 patients with suspected cardiac disease, the predictive value of a positive test was extremely weak. Only 27 of 402, or 6.7% of "abnormal" ECGs were judged to be true-positive tests relative to the criterion of clinical evaluation plus echocardiography, leaving a disturbingly large group of 375/1005 false-positive results (37.3%). One might wonder whether *all* of the true-positive results were drawn from the 220 clinical referrals, so that an "abnormal" test result had a positive predictive value of *zero* in the healthy athletic population.

Let us make the generous limiting assumption that true abnormalities were uniformly distributed between the general test sample of 785 and the 220 clinical referrals. At first inspection, the data seem to support the contention of Pigozzi et al of a useful dividend from a negative test.[7] But even if all of the ostensibly healthy adults were give reassurance, at most there would be 41/744, or 5.5% false-negatives, for a predictive value of 94.5%;

moreover, this result would be achieved without the unacceptably large burden of false-positive results. In line with this conclusion, Pelliccia et al[12] have shown that in an unselected sample of athletes, only 3% of "abnormal" ECG records are true-positive findings. It would remain possible to eliminate many of the 97% false-positive test results through additional costly investigations. But even then, the problem of false-negative results would not have been addressed, so that at best only about half of the individuals with true cardiac anomalies would have been identified. Application of Bayes theorem makes it clear[13] that such a conclusion is inherent in the stated sensitivity and specificity of testing in young and ostensibly healthy athletes (51% and 61%, respectively, in the sample of Pelliccia et al[12]).

The position statement of the American Heart Association on preparticipation screening[14] recognizes the major problem posed by false-positive diagnoses but continues with the ambivalent statement, "This viewpoint is not intended to discourage all efforts at population screening."

Given the lack of test sensitivity and specificity, it is not surprising that in one sample of 134 young athletes in the United States who died suddenly from cardiovascular diseases, 115 had undergone standard screening, but cardiovascular disease had been suspected in only 4 of these individuals. A correct diagnosis had been reached in only one instance, and none of those who died had been disqualified from sport as a result of their screening.[2] Nevertheless, there are still those who maintain that as many as 95% of athletes with HCM have an abnormal ECG,[15] and that many of this group can be identified using a simple 12-lead ECG. In support of this view, Corrado and associates[10] made an echocardiographic diagnosis of HCM in 22 of 33,735 athletes (a prevalence of 0.07%), and noted that 16 of the 22 individuals thus identified had an abnormal ECG. However, only 3 of the 22 individuals had a family history suggestive of HCM, and no other tests were performed to confirm the echocardiographic diagnosis, which is difficult to make with confidence.[16] The 33,735 athletes were drawn from the Veneto area of Italy. There is a total regional population of 2,009,600 people aged 35 years or less, and 90.4% of these are said to be "nonathletic." From 1979 to 1996, there were 220 sudden deaths among the 1,816,678 "nonathletes," (an incidence of 0.71 per 100,000 per year). There should have been 192,920 "athletes" (9.6% of 2,009,600), although data were presented for only 33,735, with 49 deaths (an incidence of 8.5 per 100,000 per year). Thus, despite mandatory screening, the incidence of sudden death was more than 10 times as high in the athletes as in the general population. At autopsy, 16 sudden deaths in the "nonathletic" group were reported as due to HCM, a disease-specific mortality rate of 0.052 per 100,000 per year. In the athletes, only 1 sudden death was attributed to HCM, a disease-specific mortality rate of 0.174 per 100,000 per year.

Sport participation was denied to 22 athletes where an echocardiographic diagnosis of HCM was reached, and none of these individuals died over a follow-up period averaging 8.2 years.[10] Does this prove the efficacy of preparticipatory cardiovascular screening? Given an 0.07% prevalence of HCM, there would have been some 1272 cases of HCM among the sample of 1,816,678 "nonathletes," giving an 8.2-year experience (1272 × 8.2, or

10,430 person-years) of HCM. By analogy with the 17-year study, 8 individuals would have died in the 8.2 years, so that 1303 person-years of HCM follow-up are needed to find a single death. The 22 athletes who were disqualified after an echocardiographic diagnosis of HCM provided a diagnosis-specific follow-up experience of only 180-person-years, far short of the figure needed to see even a single death. Plainly, it would be necessary to amass a much larger sample of HCM cases in order to establish clearly that the prohibition of sport participation avoided sudden death in cases where HCM was suspected.

Insurance Costs

The costs incurred by the prepartication screening of athletes inevitably differ from one country to another, depending on the type of screening that is recommended, fee schedules, and reimbursement procedures. However, the order of magnitude of costs associated with adoption of the Italian test protocol can be estimated by reference to approximate Canadian fee schedules. Figures are expressed in Canadian dollars, currently valued at about 0.80 US dollars.

Let us assume that all athletes meet the standards required in Italy since 1982: a detailed clinical examination ($120.00), a 12-lead ECG ($18.00), a stress test ($100.00), and simple measures of pulmonary function ($18.00); the total billing is Cdn$256.00. In many parts of the United States, the cost of a comparable noninvasive screening protocol would be 3 to 4 times larger than this.[1] But applying the Canadian estimate to the 5 million athletes who are tested annually in Italy, the total expenditure on first level screening is nearly Cdn$1.25 billion/year. Furthermore, this expense is associated with an enormous commitment of personnel and laboratory space.

Those athletes who have a positive test result need further evaluation; Maron suggested that 20% to 25% of athletes would need additional testing,[1] but in the Italian experience the proportion was 40%.[10] Potential additional investigations would certainly include echocardiography (about $210.00 per patient, or in a sample of 2 million individuals, an additional cost of Cdn$0.4 billion); some patients might also receive continuous ECG monitoring ($130.00 per patient, a total cost of up to Cdn$0.26 billion) and/or a more detailed stress test. The overall expenditure would thus be at least Cdn$1.65-2.0 billion per year. The total population of Italy is a little over 50 million, and since only 9.6% of those younger than 35 years are said to be athletes,[10] it appears that some of the athletes may have been tested at least twice during any given year. But assuming that there were 5 million athletes, with an HCM prevalence of 0.07%,[10] there would be 3500 potentially detectable cases of HCM; even on the unlikely assumption that screening was 100% effective, the cost would be around Cdn$470,000 to Cdn$570,000 per case of HCM detected.

Debate continues as to whether HCM is a significant concern when advising the young competitor. Some authors argue it is the most likely cause of sudden death in the young athlete,[1] but one recent analysis suggested that it accounted for only 7% of sudden deaths among young adults.[11] We do not know with any certainty the HCM mortality rate that would have occurred in Italian athletes in the absence of preparticipation screening, since at least some individuals would have been excluded from sport as a result of testing. Among 33,735 "athletes," HCM accounted for 1 sudden death in 17 years.[10] If the basic risk was the same among all 5 million athletes, and preparticipation screening was 100% effective in identifying the appropriate individuals and eliminating this risk, a maximum of 8 to 9 sudden HCM deaths would be avoided, at a cost of Cdn$190 million to Cdn$239 million for each premature death avoided. Plainly, the costs per life saved would rise progressively each year, as cases of HCM were eliminated from the pool of those tested.

In the Veneto study, a total of 621 out of 33,735 athletes (1.8%) were excluded from sport due to some perceived cardiovascular abnormality.[10] Assuming the athletes were tested annually for 17 years, the cumulative cost would be $28 billion to $34 billion, or $45 million to $55 million per exclusion. Further, even if all 621 exclusions were medically warranted, the majority must have been for some condition other than HCM. the cost was a more acceptable Cdn$18,000 per exclusion, but if indeed all exclusions were medically warranted, the majority must have been for some condition other than HCM. It thus appears to be almost impossible to make a fiscal case justifying the mandatory preparticipatory cardiovascular screening of athletes.

Adverse Effects of Screening on the Patient

Even in countries where the costs of medical investigations are paid by the state, mandatory preparticipation screening immediately imposes a barrier discouraging a person from adopting a physically active lifestyle. Given the small proportion of the population who currently take the recommended daily dose of physical activity,[17] it is important that such barriers be kept to a minimum compatible with patient health and safety.

In addition to those who themselves are dissuaded from becoming active because of demands for preparticipation screening, the data cited above suggest that the testing process causes a massive number of medical exclusions from sport. Corrado and associates[10] decided to prohibit exercise in 621 of their sample of 33,735 Italian athletes (1.8%). Assuming a similar rate of disqualification among a national population of 25 million under the age of 35 years, 9.6% of whom were athletes, this would imply that exercise was denied to a massive group of some 43,000 young Italians (25,000.000 × .096 × .018). There may have been good medical reasons why some of these people should not exercise, but at most 3500 of the those excluded would have had HCM. In the remaining individuals, the imposition of a sedentary lifestyle would have led to what was probably an unnecessary 2- to 3-fold worsening of long-term cardiovascular prognosis.[18]

The initial mandatory screening yielded false-positive diagnoses in some 37% of athletes,[12] some 900,000 young Italians. Further testing may have reassured many of these people that their hearts were in good condition, but there is increasing recognition that once fears have been aroused, they are difficult to dissipate. One study found a residual cardiac neurosis in about a third of patients, despite a subsequent normal test score.[19] This would imply that mass preparticipation screening may have left as many as 300,000 athletes with unresolved anxieties about their hearts.

Considerations of Medical Liability

In North America, the lack of consensus on the need for extensive screening of young athletes has as yet avoided establishing any dangerous legal precedents that could lead to claims of negligence through failure to perform such tests.[1,20] However, if we are to avoid the proliferation of costly and ineffective "defensive medicine," it seems important that we look very critically at reports suggesting that preparticipation cardiovascular screening has been effective in other jurisdictions.

Conclusions

Preparticipation cardiovascular screening of athletes has been mandatory in Italy for more than 30 years. The aim of this measure has been to avoid sudden, exercise-induced cardiac deaths. However, as might be predicted from Bayes theorem, there is little evidence that the mass screening of young and symptom-free individuals is effective. Italian authors have claimed that the finding of a normal ECG has a high negative predictive value, but the baseline assumption of normality in all of those who are screened also has a high negative predictive value. The finding of a supposedly abnormal ECG has a very low positive predictive value. A high proportion of positive reports are false-positives, which must then be refuted by further testing. The costs of mass screening are prohibitively high relative to any possible health dividend. Further, mandatory preparticipation screening imposes a barrier that discourages the young from exercising, and it has the potential to create a sedentary lifestyle and cardiac neuroses in a substantial group of previously healthy individuals, with a worsening of long-term cardiovascular prognosis. On present evidence, any claims of health benefit from mandatory screening must be regarded with considerable skepticism, and it is important to avoid statements that might lead to such testing becoming an element of defensive medical practice.

References

1. Maron BJ: Preparticipation screening in athletes. In: Shephard RJ, Åstrand P-O (eds): Endurance in Sport (2nd ed). Oxford, UK, Blackwell Scientific Publishers, 2000, pp 667-681.
2. Maron BJ, Shirani J, Poliac LC, et al: Sudden death in young competitive athletes: Clinical, demographic and pathological profiles. *JAMA* 276:199-204, 1996.
3. Shephard RJ: Cardiovascular risks of endurance sport. In: Shephard RJ, Åstrand P-O (eds): Endurance in Sport (2nd ed.). Oxford, UK, Blackwell Scientific Publishers, 2000, pp 708-717.
4. Sarna S, Sahi T, Koskwenvuo M, et al: Increased life expectancy of world class male athletes. *Med Sci Sports Exerc* 25:237-244, 1993.
5. Italian Ministry of Health: Norme per la tutela dell'attività agonistica. *Gazzetta Ufficiale* 5:63, 1982.6.
6. Pellicia A, Maron BJ: Preparticipation cardiovascular evaluation of the competitive athlete: perspectives from the 30-year Italian experience. *Am J Cardiol* 75:827-829, 1995.

7. Pigozzi F, Spataro A, Fagnani F, et al: Preparticipation screening for the detection of cardiovascular abnormalities that may cause sudden death in competitive athletes. *Br J Sports Med* 37:4-5, 2003.

8. Pigozzi F, Spataro A, Fagnani F, et al: Cardiovascular preparticipatory screening. In: *Br J Sports Med* 2003; e-letter, 27 February 2003.

9. Shephard RJ: Cardiovascular screening of athletes: A unique opportunity for an epidemiological experiment. In: *Br J Sports Med* 2003; e-letter, 12 February 2003.

10. Corrado D, Basso C, Schiavon M, et al: Screening for hypertrophic cardiomyopathy in young athletes. *N Engl J Med* 339:364-369, 1998.

11. Basso C, Thiene G, Corrado D, et al: Hypertrophic cardiomyopathy and sudden death in the young: Pathological evidence of myocardial ischemia. *Hum Pathol* 31:988-998, 2000.

12. Pelliccia A, Maron BJ, Culasso F, et al: Clinical significance of abnormal electrocardiographic patterns in trained athletes. *Circulation* 102:278-284, 2000.

13. Morise AP, Duval RD: Comparison of three Bayesian methods to estimate posttest probability in patients undergoing exercise stress testing. *Am J Cardiol* 64:1117-1122, 1989.

14. American Heart Association: Cardiovascular preparticipation screening of competitive athletes. *Med Sci Sports Exerc* 28:1445-1452, 1996.

15. Maron BJ, Wolfson JK, Ciró A, et al: Relation of electrocardiographic abnormalities and patterns of left ventricular hypertrophy identified by two-dimensional echocardiography in patients with hypertrophic cardiomyopathy. *Am J Cardiol* 51:189-194, 1983.

16. Shephard RJ: Exercise, hypertrophy, and cardiomyopathy in young and older athletes. In: Shephard RJ, Miller HS (eds): Exercise and the Heart in Health and Disease. New York, Marcel Dekker, 1999, pp 223-237.

17. U.S. Surgeon General: Physical Activity and Health. Atlanta, Ga, Centers for Disease Control, 1996.

18. Powell KE, Thompson PD, Caspersen CJ, et al: Physical activity and the incidence of coronary heart disease. *Ann Rev Publ Health* 8:253-287, 1997.

19. McDonald IG, Daly J, Jelinek VM, et al: Opening Pandora's Box: The unpredictability of reassurance by a normal test result. *Br Med J* 1996;313:329-332, 1996.

20. Mitten MJ: Team physicians and competitive athletes: Allocating responsibility for athletic injuries. *University of Pittsburgh Literary Review* 55:129-169, 1993.

1 Health Promotion and Prevention of Injury and Disease

The Victorian Active Script Programme: Promising Signs for General Practitioners, Population Health, and the Promotion of Physical Activity
Sims J, Huang N, Pietsch J, et al (Univ of Melbourne, Victoria, Australia; VicFit, Melbourne, Australia; Whitehorse Council, Box Hill, Australia)
Br J Sports Med 38:19-25, 2004   1–1

Introduction.—The Active Script Program (ASP) was established in 1999 to increase the number of general practitioners (GPs) in Victoria, Australia, who give appropriate, consistent, and effective advice regarding physical activity to their patients. A capacity building strategy within Divisions of General Practice was used to augment GP participation. Program objectives were to educate and support GPs in advising sedentary patients and to develop tools and resources to aide GPs. The success and cost of the ASP among GPs in Victoria, Australia, were evaluated.

Methods.—A systems approach was used to promote the ASP strategy in Victorian general practice. Economic analyses were included in the program's evaluation. The primary outcome measures were changes in GP knowledge and behavior and the program's cost-effectiveness, based on modeled estimates of numbers of patients advised and adopting physical activity and gaining the associated health benefits.

Results.—GP awareness and provision of physical activity advice increased because of ASP. Weight control was the most frequent reason for GPs to prescribe physical activity (Table 2). The program's reach was modest, based on actual GP involvement, but the cost-effectiveness was Aus$138 per patient to become adequately active to gain health benefits and Aus$3647 per disability-adjusted life-year saved.

Conclusion.—The ASP increased the ability of the Divisions of General Practice to support GPs in promoting physical activity. These data provide a strong economic argument for governments to invest in such programs, but caution is warranted concerning the maintenance of patients' physical activ-

TABLE 2.—Characteristics of Scripts Written by Phase I General Practitioners (GPs) (n = 628 scripts)

	Male	Female			Missing data
Sex of patients receiving scripts	52.5% (n = 330)	33.3% (n = 209)			14.2% (n = 89)
	Low	Nearly there	Active		Missing data
Activity level* as assessed by GP	41.4% (n = 260)	32.3% (n = −203)	22.1% (n = 139)		4.1% (n = 26)
	Walking only	Walking and other	Other only		
Advice prescribed	85.7% (n = 538)	24.2% (n = 152)	14.3% (n = 90)		
	Review date specified	Referred to activity provider in local area			
Follow up	12.4% (n = 78)	5.5% (n = 34)			

	Weight control	Hypertension	Hyperchol	Arthritis	Diabetes	Past history of heart disease
Benefits identified by GP as relevant to patients receiving script	40.9% (n = 257)	33.9% (n = 213)	26.4% (n = 213)	14.8% (n = 93)	14.2% (n = 89)	6.8% (n = 43)

*Low: 1 or 2 bouts of 30 minutes of activity in 7 days; nearly there: 3 or 4 bouts of 30 minutes of moderate activity in 7 days; active: 5 or more bouts of 30 minutes of moderate activity in 7 days.

Abbreviation: Hyperchol, Hypercholesterolemia.

(Courtesy of Sims J, Huang N, Pietsch J, et al: The Victorian Active Script Programme: Promising signs for general practitioners, population health, and the promotion of physical activity. *Br J Sports Med* 38:19-25, 2004. Reprinted with permission from the BMJ Publishing Group.)

ity levels. Refining the program to encourage GPs to use community support more effectively will help guide future development.

▶ How can physicians play an effective role in encouraging physical activity among their patients? This article reports on an ambitious project in which more than 40% of GPs in a selected area of Victoria, Australia, were given training in advising their patients. Self-reported changes in practice were received from about a third of the doctors involved; these individuals claimed to be advising physical activity more frequently and to be providing a more appropriate exercise prescription. A check with a subsample of patients nominated by 5 GPs (perhaps the most enthusiastic of the doctors in the trial?) found that most of the patients contacted recalled receiving written or verbal advice (generally to walk more); in consequence, most had increased their physical activity moderately. Assuming that, as a result of the program, 10% of patients remained active for long enough to improve their health, a somewhat speculative economic analysis suggested that a disability-adjusted life-year could be saved for a cost of $3647. This supports earlier findings that enhanced interventions by GPs and other health professionals can be cost-effective.[1-3]

R. J. Shephard, MD, PhD, DPE

References

1. Hatziandreu EI, Kaplan JP, Weinstein MC, et al: A cost effective analysis of exercise as a health promotion activity. *Am J Public Health* 78:1417-1421, 1988.
2. Munro J, Brazier J, Davey R, et al: Physical activity for the over 65s; Could it be a cost-effective exercise for the NHS? *J Public Health Med* 19:397-402, 1997.
3. Stevens W, Hillsdon M, Thorogood M, et al: Cost effectiveness of a primary care based physical activity intervention in 45-74 year old men and women: A randomized controlled trial. *Br J Sports Med* 32:236-241, 1998.

Estimating Changes in Daily Physical Activity Levels Over Time: Implications for Health Interventions From a Novel Approach

Vogels N, Egger G, Plasqui G, et al (Maastricht Univ, The Netherlands; Deakin Univ, Melbourne, Australia)

Int J Sports Med 25:607-610, 2004   1–2

Background.—The World Health Organization (WHO) has predicted that obesity will be one of the major pandemics of the 21st century. Obesity has a causal link with many different diseases and is estimated to cost between 5% and 12% of the health budgets of many countries. Obesity and overweight are caused by a chronic energy imbalance, which has become more ubiquitous in contemporary life with the widespread use of time-saving and "time-using" technologies. A novel method was used to examine and compare physical activity levels in 4 different groups of men to investigate the effects of "modernity" on activity levels.

Methods.—Four groups of men were evaluated. The first group was composed of historically active (HA) actors in a historical theme park. These men played the part of Australian settlers 150 years ago. The second group was composed of sedentary modern-day office workers (MS), the third

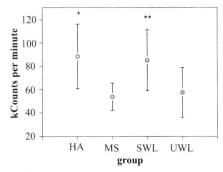

FIGURE 2.—Average weekly Tracmor output (kCounts per minute) and standard deviations for 4 groups of men: men performing activity at level carried out historically (*HA*); modern-day sedentary workers (*MS*); men who have successfully lost weight (*SWL*); and men who have not been successful at losing weight (*UWL*). Statistical significance was determined by Independent-Samples *t*-test between the groups HA and MS (* $P < .05$), and the groups SWL and UWL (** $P < .01$). (Courtesy of Vogels N, Egger G, Plasqui G, Westerterp KR: Estimating changes in daily physical activity levels over time: implications for health interventions from a novel approach. *Int J Sports Med* 25:607-610, 2004. Copyright Georg Thieme Verlag.)

group of men had successfully lost body mass in a modern men's weight-loss program (SWELL), and the fourth group was composed of men who were unsuccessful in losing weight in the same program (UWL).

Results.—The activity of men who were successful in losing weight in a weight-loss program was similar to that of men performing activity at a level carried out historically. Both of these groups were significantly more active than modern-day sedentary workers and men who had not been successful at losing mass (Fig 2). The linear regression between weekly average activity levels and the degree of waist size loss was indicative of a significant positive association.

Conclusions.—A higher activity level appeared to facilitate the maintenance of long-term mass loss, and this level is likely to approximate activity levels in the past. An increase in physical activity is necessary for the successful prevention and treatment of obesity, because long-term loss of body mass or maintenance is unlikely to occur in persons who are as sedentary as the bulk of the population today.

▶ The authors of this report adopted an ingenious method of trying to assess the secular trend to a decrease in the energy cost of daily activities over the past 150 years by comparing the metabolism of workers in a "pioneer village" with values for the current generation of sedentary office workers. There are several limitations to this approach. At least in Canadian pioneer villages, the "pioneers" spend quite a lot of time talking to visitors rather than pursuing their nominal tasks, and they do not depend on constant daily toil in the face of various natural disasters to avoid starvation. Against this, the present-day "pioneers" are probably less familiar with some of the energy-saving tricks that the real pioneers likely learned. Nevertheless, the present generation of "pioneers" do show almost twice the accelerometer counts that are recorded in the office workers. Perhaps more interestingly, among subjects who are engaged in a "weight-loss" program, activity counts were much larger in those who showed a decrease in body mass than among those who did not. This emphasizes the important role of physical activity in achieving both weight loss and replacement of fat by muscle.

R. J. Shephard, MD, PhD, DPE

A Randomised Controlled Trial of Three Pragmatic Approaches to Initiate Increased Physical Activity in Sedentary Patients With Risk Factors for Cardiovascular Disease
Little P, Dorward M, Gralton S, et al (Univ of Southampton, England; Highcliffe Surgery, Christchurch, England; Nightingale Surgery, Romsey, England; et al)
Br J Gen Pract 54:189-195, 2004   1–3

Introduction.—Physical activity is an important modifiable risk factor for cardiovascular disease. It is not clear what combination of feasible approaches, with the use of existing resources in primary care, are the best for initiating increased physical activity. Three approaches for initiating physi-

TABLE 4.—Changes in Main Outcome Measures at 1 Month From Baseline According to Intensity of Intervention

	Control +/-Booklet	P-Value	GP +/-Booklet	P-Value	Nurse +/-Booklet	P-Value	GP/Nurse +/-Booklet	P-Value	Test for Trend
Distance walked (m)	7.1	0.18	9.0	0.32	14.6	0.06	28.5	<0.002	Z = 1.93 P = 0.05
(95% CI)	(-3.5 to 17.7)		(-9.0 to 27.0)		(-0.6 to 30.0)		(11.1 to 45.8)		
Godin score	8.2	0.01	6.8	0.14	13.7	<0.001	14.4	<0.001	Z = 2.42 P = 0.02
(95% CI)	(2.1 to 14.3)		(-2.4 to 16.0)		(6.6 to 20.7)		(7.8 to 21.0)		

Note: Rationale for ordered intensity categories: the nurse intervention (20 minutes) is the most intensive single intervention (Box 1), followed by general practitioner (GP) prescription (a 5- to 10-minute appointment). *P* values in the table are based on the paired *t* test (ie, the difference from baseline). The test for trend assesses a trend in the differences with greater intensity of intervention using nonparametric test for trend in STATA.

(Courtesy of Little P, Dorward M, Gralton S, et al: A randomized controlled trial of three pragmatic approaches to initiate increased physical activity in sedentary patients with risk factors for cardiovascular disease. *Br J Gen Pract* 54:189-195, 2004.)

cal activity were evaluated in a randomized controlled ($2 \times 2 \times 2$) factorial investigation in 4 general practices.

Methods.—A total of 151 sedentary patients with substantiated risk factors for cardiovascular disease were randomly assigned to 8 groups defined by 3 factors: prescription by general practitioners for brisk exercise not necessitating a leisure facility (ie, walking) 30 min/d, 5 d/wk; counseling by practice nurses, based on psychological theory to modify intentions and perceived control of behavior, and using behavioral implementation techniques (ie, contracting, "rehearsal"); use of the Health Education Authority booklet "Getting Active, Feeling Fit."

Results.—Effects were modest with single interventions. A trend was observed from the least intensive interventions (control ± booklet) to the more intensive interventions (prescription and counseling combined ± booklet) for increased physical activity and fitness (test for trend, $P = .02$ and $P = .05$, respectively). Significant increases in both physical activity and fitness were observed from baseline only with the most intense intervention (prescription and counseling combined) (Godin score, 14.4; 95% CI, 7.8-21, which was equivalent to three 15-minute sessions of brisk exercise and a 6-minute walking distance, 28.5 m, respectively, 95% CI, 11.1-45.8) (Table 4). Counseling made a difference only among participants with lower intentions at baseline.

Conclusion.—Feasible interventions with the use of available staff that combine exercise prescription and counseling explicitly based on psychological theory may initiate substantial increases in physical activity.

▶ This survey used the very simple Godin questionnaire[1] to provide an objective assessment of changes in patient behavior as a result of various initiatives designed to increase physical activity. As is usually the case, the sample evaluated was somewhat biased (151 recruited of 444 invitations). The benefit seemed to come mainly from the combination of a nurse using current psychological techniques of motivation plus a booklet; a physician plus a booklet was less effective, and the combination of a nurse plus a doctor plus a booklet was not much better than the nurse plus a booklet. The Godin questionnaire results suggested that the end result was the equivalent of adding three 15-minute sessions of walking per week, which is certainly an improvement for those who were initially sedentary, although it is well below the currently recommended minimum levels of physical activity for health.[2] At a marginal cost of some £20, the intervention was judged to be quite cost-effective.

R. J. Shephard, MD, PhD, DPE

References

1. Godin G, Shephard RJ: A simple method to assess exercise behavior in the community. *Can J Appl Sport Sci* 10:141-146, 1985.
2. Shephard RJ: Whistler 2001: A Health Canada/CDC conference on "Communicating Physical Activity and Health Message: Science Into Practice." *Am J Prev Med* 23:221-225, 2002.

Promoting Walking and Cycling as an Alternative to Using Cars: Systematic Review
Ogilvie D, Egan M, Hamilton V, et al (Univ of Glasgow, Scotland; Univ of Strathclyde, Glasgow, Scotland)
BMJ 329:763-766, 2004   1–4

Introduction.—Increasing physical activity in the population may be the "best buy" for improving public health. The tendency has been to promote physical activity as leisure and through individual behavior changes. The best available evidence on the effects of population level interventions was systematically reviewed for the purpose of determining the best way to promote a shift from the use of cars to walking and cycling.

Methods.—Electronic databases and websites, bibliographies, reference lists, and archives for published and unpublished documents were systematically reviewed to identify experimental or observational trials with a prospective or controlled retrospective design that assessed any intervention applied to an urban population or area by measurement of outcomes within the local population.

Results.—A total of 22 trials met inclusion criteria. Some evidence suggested that targeted behavioral change programs could change behavior within motivated subgroups and resulted in a shift of about 5% of all trips at a population level. Single trials of commuter subsidies and a new railway station also demonstrated positive effects. The balance of the best available evidence concerning publicity campaigns, engineering measures, and other interventions indicates that they have not been effective (Table). Participants in trials of active commuting experienced short-term improvements in particular measures of health and fitness; no evidence was identified concerning the effects on health of any effective intervention at population levels.

Conclusion.—The best available evidence shows that, thus far, the use of targeted behavioral change programs are the most effective way to promote a modal shift; the social distribution of the programs' effects is not known, which makes it clear that other types of interventions need to be examined.

▶ In North American society, physical fitness has commonly been seen as a personal rather than a societal responsibility. However, it has recently been suggested that constraints of urban design contribute to the current sedentary lifestyle and that personal fitness could be enhanced if measures were taken to encourage people to walk or cycle to work.[1,2] The article by Ogilvie and associates is a meta-analysis of both published and unpublished reports that have explored attempts to change population behavior in this respect. In general, any changes induced by municipal initiatives such as extending cycle paths, providing fare subsidies, or building a new railway station have been disappointingly small. Moreover, any increases in active commuting have not been sustained for more than a few months. One issue that needs to be explored further is why the baseline level of active commuting is as much as an order greater in some communities than in others.

R. J. Shephard, MD, PhD, DPE

TABLE.—Summary of Evidence of Effectiveness of Interventions to Promote Modal Shift

Study	Validity Score	Nature of Comparison	Evidence for Shift From Cars Towards Walking and Cycling*			
			Significant Positive Effect	Positive Effect of Uncertain Significance	Inconclusive or No Effect	Negative Effect of Uncertain Significance
Targeted behaviour change programmes						
Glasgow[w1 w2]	9	Controlled	Yes	—	—	—
Perth, Australia (TravelSmart)[w3-9]	7	Controlled	Yes	—	—	—
Frome (TravelSmart pilot)[w10]	9	Controlled	—	Yes	—	—
Gloucester (TravelSmart pilot)[w11]	9	Controlled	—	Yes	—	—
Århus[w12-14]	7	Uncontrolled	—	Yes	—	—
Adelaide[w15-18]	4	Uncontrolled	—	—	Yes	—
Publicity campaigns and agents of change						
Camden-Islington[w19]	8	Controlled	—	—	Yes	—
Maidstone[w20]	7	Controlled	—	—	Yes	—
Phoenix[w21]	5	Uncontrolled	—	Yes	—	—
Eugene[w22]	4	Uncontrolled	—	—	Yes	—
Engineering measures						
Delft[w23-30]	7	Controlled	—	Yes	—	—
Detmold-Rosenheim[w31-33]	6	Uncontrolled	—	—	—	Yes
Stockton[w34]	5	Uncontrolled	—	—	—	Yes
England (20 mph (30 km/h) zones)[w35]	5	Uncontrolled	—	—	Yes	—
Boston[w38-40]	4	Uncontrolled	—	Yes	—	—
England (bypasses)[w36 w37]	3	Uncontrolled	—	—	—	Yes
Financial incentives						
California (cashing out)[w41 w42]	8	Controlled	Yes	—	—	—
Trondheim[w43 w44]	7	Uncontrolled	—	—	—	Yes
Providing alternative services						
San Francisco[w45-47]	7	Controlled	—	—	Yes	—
Voorhout[w48]	7	Uncontrolled	Yes	—	—	—
California (telecommuting)[w49]	4	Controlled	—	—	—	Yes

Note: References to primary studies included in the review (w1-w51) can be found on bmj.com.
*No studies had significant negative effects.
(Courtesy of Ogilvie D, Egan M, Hamilton V, et al: Promoting walking and cycling as an alternative to using cars: Systematic review. *BMJ* 329:763-766, 2004. Reprinted with permission from the BMJ Publishing Group.)

References

1. Carnall D: Cycling and health promotion. *BMJ* 320:888, 2000.
2. Roberts I: Congestion charging and the walking classes. *BMJ* 326:345-346, 2003.

Factors of the Physical Environment Associated With Walking and Bicycling
Wendel-Vos GCW, Schuit AJ, De Niet R, et al (Natl Inst for Public Health and the Environment, Bilthoven, The Netherlands; Maastricht Univ, The Netherlands)
Med Sci Sports Exerc 36:725-730, 2004   1–5

Introduction.—Physical activity is an important modifiable risk factor for various chronic diseases. Physical environments have the capability to obstruct or facilitate physical activity. Factors in the physical environment that may influence walking and bicycling during leisure time and for commuting purposes were evaluated.

Methods.—Demographic factors and time spent walking and bicycling were evaluated via a self-administered questionnaire. GIS databases were used to objectively measure the total square area of green space and recreational space (ie, woods, parks, sport grounds, allotments for vegetable gardens, and grounds for day trips) in a circle surrounding the postal code of a respondent within a radius of 300 and 500 m. Multilevel regression analysis was used to evaluate the association of walking and bicycling with green and recreational space. Adjustments were made for age, gender, and educational level.

Results.—Within the 300-m radius, the square area of sports grounds was correlated with bicycling in general; the square area of parks was linked with bicycling for commuting purposes. It is likely that these results reflect the link between living in the outskirts of town and time spent bicycling.

Conclusion.—Green and recreational space, particularly sports grounds and parks, was correlated with time spent bicycling.

▶ When I was a resident in Toronto, I was impressed by a beautiful network of ravine parks, most of which were rarely used. However, other investigators have been optimistic that a pleasant physical environment would enhance the physical activity of the local population.[1-3] After making a cross-sectional multiple regression analysis, Wendel-Vos and associates suggest that features of the built environment can have a favorable influence on habitual physical activity. In fact, their results show that the hours of walking per week were unrelated to neighboring green space. The impact of such space on cycling was statistically significant ($P < .05$) but little practical or clinical importance; each hectare of sports ground was associated with a 2.4-min/wk increase in cycling. One problem in this analysis is that Maastricht, The Netherlands, is a relatively small town, and those who are near to a sports ground live on the outskirts of the town; this, in itself, may have given them a small incentive to use their bicycles to reach the town or a suburban railway station. Further, the authors were not confident that their analysis eliminated all effects of socio-economic status, which is an important determinant of habitual physical activity. Those of higher socioeconomic status are more likely to live near a park or sports ground.

R. J. Shephard, MD, PhD, DPE

References

1. Ball K, Bauman A, Leslie E, et al: Perceived environmental aesthetics and convenience and company are associated with walking for exercise among Australian adults. *Prev Med* 33:434-440, 2001.
2. Bauman A, Smith B, Stoker L, et al: Geographical influences upon physical activity participation: Evidence of a "coastal effect." *Aust N Z J Public Health* 23:322-324, 1999.
3. Booth S, Sallis JF, Rittenbaugh C, et al: Environmental and societal factors affect food choice and physical activity: Rationale, influences, and leverage points. *Nutr Rev* S231-S239, 2001.

Physical Activity and Television Viewing in Relation to Risk of Undiagnosed Abnormal Glucose Metabolism in Adults
Dunstan DW, on behalf of the AusDiab Steering Committee (Internatl Diabetes Inst, Melbourne, Australia; Deakin Univ, Melbourne, Australia; Univ of Queensland, Brisbane, Australia; et al)
Diabetes Care 27:2603-2609, 2004   1–6

Background.—Many studies have demonstrated a relationship between physical activity and reduction in risk of diabetes and obesity, and other cardiovascular risk factors. The relationship between physical activity, television (TV) viewing time and precursors of type 2 diabetes (impaired fasting glycemia [IFG] and impaired glucose tolerance [IGT]) was evaluated in a large population-based cross-sectional study.

Methods.—The study included 8229 adults who participated in the Australian Diabetes, Obesity and Lifestyle Study (AusDiab) from 1999 to 2000 and who had no known preexisting health conditions. All study participants had a fasting oral glucose tolerance test (OGTT). Obesity was assessed through waist circumference and body mass index (BMI). Demographic information, plus physical activity and TV time during the previous week, were quantified through a questionnaire.

Results.—After adjustment for known confounders and for weekly TV time, the odds ratio (OR) for abnormal glucose metabolism was 0.62 for men and 0.71 for women who engaged in more than 2.5 h/wk of physical activity, compared with the ORs of those who were sedentary. The OR for abnormal glucose metabolism was 1.16 for men and 1.49 for women who watched more than 14 hours of TV per week (Table 3) compared with the ORs of those who were active. TV watching was also associated with an increased risk of newly diagnosed type 2 diabetes in men and women and IGT in women. Physical activity of more than 2.5 h/wk was associated with a re-

TABLE 3.—Adjusted* ORs for the Presence of Abnormal Glucose Metabolism According to Categories of TV

	n		Age-adjusted		Multivariate		Additional Adjustment for Waist Circumference	
	Men	Women	Men	Women	Men	Women	Men	Women
Television viewing								
0-7 h/week	1,106	1,811	1.00	1.00	1.00	1.00	1.00	1.00
7.01-14 h/week	1,257	1,448	0.90 (0.65-1.25)	1.24 (0.91-1.69)	0.89 (0.63-1.25)	1.25 (0.92-1.71)	0.81 (0.60-1.09)	1.21 (0.87-1.69)
>14 h/week	1,338	1,339	1.11 (0.82-1.49)	1.54 (1.13-2.11)	1.16 (0.79-1.70)	1.49 (1.12-1.99)	0.97 (0.68-1.39)	1.34 (0.94-1.92)
P for trend			0.46	0.008	0.41	0.008	0.95	0.10

Note: Data are OR (95% CI)

* Adjusted for age, education, family history of diabetes, cigarette smoking, dietary covariates (total energy, total fat, total saturated fat, total carbohydrates, total sugar, fiber and alcohol), and physical activity time.

(Courtesy of Dunstan DW, on behalf of the AusDiab Steering Committee: Physical activity and television viewing in relation to risk of undiagnosed abnormal glucose metabolism in adults *Diabetes Care* 27:2603-2609, 2004. Copyright 2004, with permission from The American Diabetes Association.)

duced risk of IFG, IGT and new type 2 diabetes diagnoses in both men and women. However, only the association of IGT in women reached significance.

Conclusions.—These findings lend further support to the idea that a sedentary lifestyle is harmful, and physical activity is protective of glucose metabolism. Promotion of physical activity at the expense of sedentary activities, such as TV watching, may be an important public health strategy for the prevention of abnormal glucose metabolism in adults.

▶ A number of previous reports have noted a connection between the time spent watching TV and obesity, particularly in children.[1,2] The present authors argue that physical activity and sedentary behavior are distinct variables, with differing determinants. Nevertheless, it seems obvious that if several hours per day are spent in front of a TV set, this is a period of discretionary leisure that cannot be allocated to other more active pursuits. Indeed, TV watchers are likely to advance "lack of time" as an important reason why they are not more active. In adults, the negative impact of TV watching seems weaker than in children. After adjusting for other relevant variables, including the amount of physical activity taken, a significant increase in the risk of abnormal glucose metabolism is seen only in women who watch TV for 7 to 14 h/wk; in men, even this amount of TV watching is not significantly linked with abnormal glucose metabolism. The presence of an independent effect of TV watching in the women presumably reflects limitations to the physical activity assessment, which ignores physical activities performed around the home.

R. J. Shephard, MD, PhD, DPE

References

1. Anderson RE, Crespo CJ, Bartlett SJ, et al: Relationship of physical activity and television watching with body weight and level of fatness among children: Results from the third National Health and Nutrition Examination Survey. *JAMA* 279:938-942, 1998.
2. Sidney S, Sternfeld B, Haskell WL, et al: Television watching and cardiovascular risk factors in young adults: The CARDIA study. *Ann Epidemiol* 6:154-159, 1996.

Occupational, Commuting, and Leisure-Time Physical Activity in Relation to Total and Cardiovascular Mortality Among Finnish Subjects With Type 2 Diabetes

Hu G, Eriksson J, Barengo NC, et al (Univ of Helsinki; Univ of Kuopio, Finland)
Circulation 110:666-673, 2004   1–7

Background.—It is estimated that the number of persons with diabetes in the world will at least double in the next 25 years. Cardiovascular disease (CVD) is responsible for more than 75% of total mortality among patients with type 2 diabetes. A need exists to control the increasing prevalence of type 2 diabetes to prevent an increase in CVD in the future. Some previous studies have assessed the association between leisure-time physical activity and mortality among patients with diabetes, but the potential effects of occupational and commuting physical activity have not been clarified. Whether occupational, commuting, or leisure-time physical activity is independently associated with a reduced risk of total and CVD mortality was determined among Finnish patients with type 2 diabetes, participating in population-based surveys.

Methods.—The prospective study included 3316 Finnish participants, 25 to 74 years old, with type 2 diabetes. The association of different types of physical activity with mortality was analyzed with Cox proportional-hazard models.

Results.—During a mean follow-up of 18.4 years, 1410 deaths were recorded, of which 903 were due to cardiovascular disease (CVD). The multivariate adjusted hazard ratios associated with light, moderate, and active work were 1.00, 0.86, and 0.60, respectively, for total mortality and 1.00, 0.91, and 0.60, respectively, for CVD mortality. The multivariate-adjusted hazard ratios associated with low, moderate, and high leisure-time physical activity were 1.00, 0.82, and 0.71, respectively, for total mortality and 1.00, 0.83, and 0.67, respectively, for CVD mortality. Active commuting was significantly adversely associated with total and CVD mortality, but these relationships were no longer significant after additional adjustment for occupational and leisure-time physical activity.

Conclusions.—Total and CVD mortality are reduced with moderate or high levels of physical activity in patients with type 2 diabetes. In addition to leisure-time physical activity, occupational and commuting physical activities are also important aspects of a healthy lifestyle among patients with diabetes.

▶ Policy planners are placing a growing emphasis on commuting as a useful method of augmenting daily physical activity, with proposals to establish well-tended walkways that would make self-propelled transportation both esthetically pleasant and safe. The message from this Finnish study is complex—on a univariate analysis, active commuting appears to have a favorable impact on all-cause and cardiac deaths, but this effect is no longer significant with a multivariate analysis that also includes measures of leisure and occupational activity. One problem in disentangling the data is that the sort of person who decides to walk or cycle to work also enjoys an active leisure. It would be difficult to find a group of physically active commuters who were sedentary for the rest of the week just to look specifically at the benefits of active commuting. The other possibility (which could perhaps be applied to the Finnish data) is to replace the simple 3-level classification of commuters with a multilevel classification of the energy expenditures involved in commuting. Even if the immediate health effects are small, active commuting conveys other social benefits; it conserves fossil fuel, reduces urban congestion, and helps to minimize the air pollution that is currently a feature of most large cities.

R. J. Shephard, MD, PhD, DPE

Does Walking 15 Minutes per Day Keep the Obesity Epidemic Away? Simulation of the Efficacy of a Populationwide Campaign

Morabia A, Costanza MC (Geneva Univ)
Am J Public Health 94:437-440, 2004   1–8

Background.—There is an urgent need to design population-wide weight control programs to address the worldwide obesity epidemic. It has been proposed that small increases in physical activity may prevent weight gain in most populations because an extra 420 kJ per day (100 kcal/d) can compensate for observed gain in body mass. However, it is not known how much daily walking is needed to attain that goal. The typical basal metabolic rate of a Western adult is 4.2 kJ/min. The act of walking expends 3.1 times an individual's basal metabolic rate. Thus, an individual with a basal metabolic rate of 4.2 who walks slowly for 15 minutes expends 195 kJ. The total energy expenditure of the adult resident population of Geneva, Switzerland, was measured to simulate the potential effect of campaigns promoting different combinations of duration and intensity of daily walking on the total energy expenditure of that population.

Methods.—A unique monitoring system was used in this study. The residents of Geneva completed validated quantitative physical activity frequency questionnaires from 1997 to 2001. Sedentarism was defined as spending less than 10% of an individual's total energy expenditure in physical activities that required at least a basal metabolic rate of 3.9 METS, which corresponds to moderate walking.

Results.—The estimated (mean) population energy expenditure gain for slow walking would only be about +38 kJ/d if the campaign were 100% successful and only +19 kJ/d if the campaign were 50% successful. It was also found that a 100% or 50% successful campaign to promote slow walking for 30 minutes per day would provide only a modest +105 (or +53) kJ/d gain (Table 2). If the specific goal of a population-wide campaign against obesity is to achieve an energy expenditure of 420 kJ/d through walking, individuals should engage in about 60 minutes of slow walking or about 30 minutes of brisk walking.

Conclusions.—The population-based simulation approach presented in this study can be extended to other activities that can be integrated easily into everyday life by subgroups (such as sports) or by the whole population, such as bicycling instead of driving and climbing stairs instead of taking elevators.

▶ There has been much discussion of recent recommendations concerning the minimum amount of aerobic exercise needed for population health. Most US authorities have suggested that 30 minutes per day of moderate activity is sufficient, whereas Health Canada has cautioned that a minimum of 60 minutes of exercise per day may be required if the intensity is only moderate.[1] Those who are influenced by public health messages seem most likely to begin a walking program; the problem in North America is that most people walk quite slowly. Their additional energy expenditure is correspondingly low. As

TABLE 2.—Population Gains in Energy Expenditure and Reductions in Population Prevalence of Sedentarism for Hypothetical Intervention Campaigns of Varying Degrees of Recommended Walking Intensity and Duration and of Population Compliance: General Adult (35-74 years) Population of Geneva, Switzerland, 1997-2001

Walking Activity	Intensity (× BMR)	Duration, min/d	Maximal Gain, kJ/d*	Compliance by Eligible Adults, %	Population Mean Gain, kJ/d	Sedentarism† Reduction, %
Slow	3.1	15	+195	100	+38	Reduction not possible
				50	+19	(58% sedentary)
		30	+389	100	+105	
				50	+53	
Moderate	3.9	15	+245	100	+150	−4
				50	+76	−2
		30	+490	100	+356	−14
				50	+178	−7
Brisk	4.7	15	+295	100	+255	−10
				50	+127	−5
		30	+590	100	+541	−29
				50	+264	−14
Athletic-brisk	6.0	15	+377	100	+326	−14
				50	+165	−7
		30	+754	100	+690	−40
				50	+336	−19

* Assumes BMR = 4.2 kJ/d.
† Sedentarism is defined as less than 10% of total energy expenditure spent in physical activities with an intensity of 3.9 BMR or more.
Abbreviation: BMR Basal metabolic rate.
(Courtesy of Morabia A, Costanza MC: Does walking 15 minutes per day keep the obesity epidemic away? Simulation of the efficacy of populationwide campaign. *Am J Public Health* 94:437-440, 2004. Copyright 2004, American Public Health Association.)

the article by Morabia and Costanza points out, at least 60 minutes of activity per day are then needed to generate the 420 kJ of added daily energy expenditure[2] that has been proposed to tackle one of the main causes of current morbidity (the obesity epidemic). Notice that the population impact of the recommended energy expenditure is weakened by low compliance rates and, possibly, also by increased food intake and alterations in resting metabolism associated with a negative energy balance.

R. J. Shephard, MD, PhD, DPE

References

1. Shephard RJ: Whistler 2001: A Health Canada/CDC conference on "Communicating physical activity and health messages: Science into practice." *Am J Prev Med* 23:221-225, 2002.
2. Hill JO, Wyatt HR, Reed GW, et al: Obesity and the environment: Where do we go from here? *Science* 299:853-855, 2003.

Physical Activity and Changes in Weight and Waist Circumference in Midlife Women: Findings From the Study of Women's Health Across the Nation
Sternfeld B, Wang H, Quesenberry CP Jr, et al (Kaiser Permanente, Oakland, Calif; Univ of California, Berkeley; Rush Univ, Chicago; et al)
Am J Epidemiol 160:912-922, 2004   1–9

Background.—The extent to which age, menopausal status, or lifestyle factors account for the increased body mass, fat mass, and central adiposity in middle-aged women has not been determined. The Study of Women's

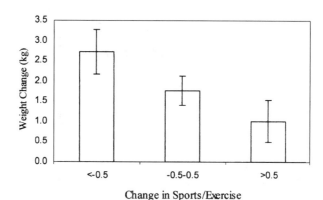

Change in Sports/Exercise

FIGURE 1.—Mean within-woman body mass change between baseline (1996-1997) and year 3 (1999-2000) according to change in the level of sports/exercise (on a scale of 1-5) (Study of Women's Health Across the Nation). Results were adjusted for baseline age, baseline levels of sports/exercise, race/ethnicity, the presence of chronic conditions, and study site. For the F statistic, $P < .0001$; all pairwise comparisons showed a significant difference at $P < .01$. *Bars* indicate 95% confidence interval. (Courtesy of Sternfeld B, Wang H, Quesenberry CP Jr, et al: Physical activity and changes in weight and waist circumference in midlife women: Findings from the Study of Women's Health Across the Nation. *Am J Epidemiol* 160:912-922, 2004. Reprinted by permission of Oxford University Press.)

Health Across the Nation is a multisite, prospective, community-based observational study of menopause in a multiethnic cohort of initially premenopausal or early perimenopausal women. Three-year changes in body mass and waist circumference in the Study of Women's Health Across the Nation cohort were analyzed to determine the contributions of aging, menopause, and physical activity to those changes.

Methods and Findings.—The cohort consisted of 3064 racially diverse women aged 42 to 52 years at baseline. During the 3-year follow-up, mean body mass increased by 2.1 kg or 3%. The mean waist circumference increased by 2.2 cm, or 2.8%. The change in menopausal status did not correlate with body mass gain or increased waist circumference. A 1-unit increase in the reported level of exercise was associated with reductions of 0.32 kg in body mass and 0.10 cm in waist circumference. Inverse relationships were also noted for daily routine physical activity (Fig 1).

Conclusion.—Middle-aged women tend to increase in body mass and waist circumference over time. Maintaining or increasing participation in regular physical activity can prevent or attenuate these increases.

▶ Many women would like to know the secret of avoiding the gain of body mass and accumulation of body fat that are commonly seen around the time of the menopause. A prospective study of women in this age category here finds a significantly smaller body mass gain but no significant difference of waist circumference among individuals who reported engaging in regular sport and/or exercise.

Self-reported activity questionnaires have only a limited reliability, and the true benefit of an active lifestyle may be greater than the rather small differences demonstrated by the present results. Further, no distinction was drawn between lean and adipose mass, and it may be that the active women maintained lean tissue while those who were sedentary accumulated fat.

R. J. Shephard, MD, PhD, DPE

Pairing Personality With Activity: New Tools for Inspiring Active Lifestyles
Gavin J (Concordia Univ, Montreal)
Physician Sportsmed 32(12):17-24, 2004   1–10

Background.—Much publicity has been devoted to promote active lifestyles, yet physical activity levels have not increased. It has been suggested more recently that a match between a physical fitness program and an individual's personality might serve to increase personal motivation and thereby increase participation in an active lifestyle. How these physical activity programs could be matched to an individual's psychosocial characteristics was described.

Identifying Characteristics.—Matching an individual to a fitness program should involve identifying traits common to both the individual and the physical activity. Apparently, 7 personality characteristics should be present

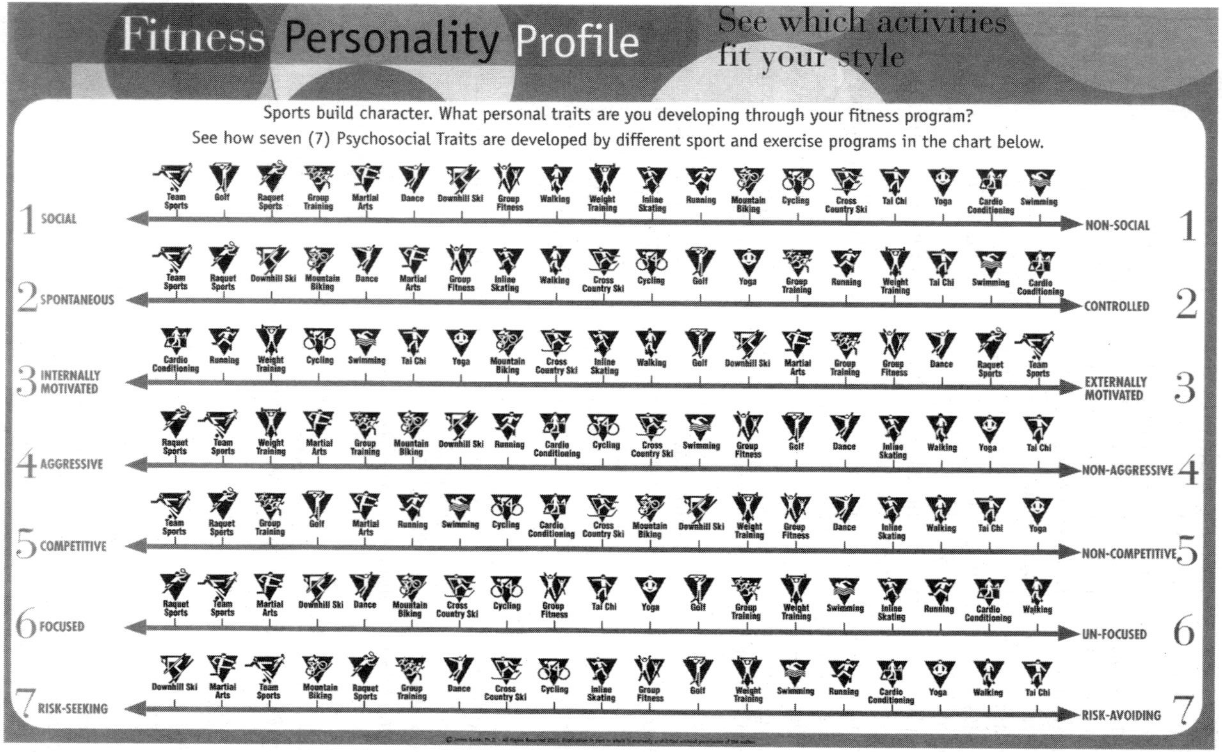

Fitness Personality Profile

See which activities
fit your style

Sports build character. What personal traits are you developing through your fitness program?
See how seven (7) Psychosocial Traits are developed by different sport and exercise programs in the chart below.

1 SOCIAL — NON-SOCIAL 1

2 SPONTANEOUS — CONTROLLED 2

3 INTERNALLY MOTIVATED — EXTERNALLY MOTIVATED 3

4 AGGRESSIVE — NON-AGGRESSIVE 4

5 COMPETITIVE — NON-COMPETITIVE 5

6 FOCUSED — UN-FOCUSED 6

7 RISK-SEEKING — RISK-AVOIDING 7

FIGURE 3.—The psychosocial dimensions can be used to arrange icons representing the demands of 19 popular sports. Patients can select sports they find interesting and see how specific sports fit their personality traits. (Courtesy of Gavin J: Pairing personality with activity: New tools for inspiring active lifestyles *Physician Sportsmed* 32(12):17-24, 2004. Copyright 2004. Reproduced with permission of McGraw-Hill, Inc.)

that are relevant to this activity-based analysis (Fig 3) as follows: (1) sociability, (2) spontaneity, (3) self-motivation, (4) aggressiveness, (5) competitiveness; (6) mental focus, and (7) risk taking. Physical activities can be ranked along these characteristics to allow individuals to match activities to their own preferences.

Conclusions.—Combining personality assessment and physical activity ranking along the 7 characteristics described, individuals can become aware of their personal preferences and the correspondence between these preferences and physical activities. This may increase compliance with advice to increase activity levels and may lead to healthier lifestyles.

▶ I have often suggested that the type of exercise recommended to a patient should be adapted to the individual's personality. Dr James Gavin here develops this thesis at length. A second important issue is how the individual's personality influences the way in which a sport is performed; for example, whether mountain biking is kept to easy trails or extends to very risky routes, and whether running is pursued in a relaxed manner or with a determination to beat previous achievements, despite warning symptoms, such as growing chest pain.

R. J. Shephard, MD, PhD, DPE

Health-Care Costs and Exercise Capacity
Weiss JP, Froelicher VF, Myers JN, et al (Stanford Univ, Palo Alto)
Chest 126:608-613, 2004   1–11

Introduction.—There is general agreement that the health care costs linked with physical inactivity are great and that improvement in fitness may have favorable cost-efficacy. Most of these data were derived from reviews and analytical models, but the effect of measured exercise capacity on health care costs has not been directly examined. The association between exercise capacity and health care costs was evaluated.

Methods.—The Veterans Affairs Health Care System recently executed a Decision Support System that provides data concerning patterns of care, patient outcomes, workload, and costs. Total inpatient and outpatient costs were obtained from existing administrative and clinical data systems, were adjusted for relative value units, and were expressed in relative cost units. Univariate and multivariate analyses were used to assess the 1-year total costs in the year after a standard exercise test. Costs were compared with exercise capacity estimated in metabolic equivalents (METs), other test results, and clinical variables for 881 consecutive patients referred for clinical reasons for treadmill testing between October 1, 1998, and September 30, 2000.

Results.—The mean patient age was 59 years; 95% were men; 74% were white. Eight patients (<1%) died during the 1-year follow-up. Exercise testing revealed an average maximal heart rate of 138 beats/min, 8.2 METs, and a peak Borg scale of 17. Unadjusted analysis showed that costs were incre-

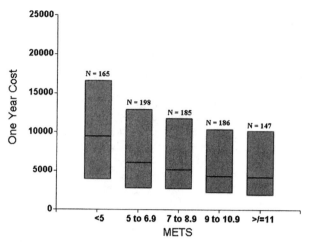

FIGURE 1.—The 1-year cost by exercise test performance given in metabolic equivalents (METs). In unadjusted analysis, costs were incrementally lower by an average of 5.4% per MET increase ($P < .001$). The data shown are the median with 25th and 75th percentiles. (Courtesy of Weiss JP, Froelicher VF, Myers JN, et al: Health-care costs and exercise capacity. *Chest* 126:608-613, 2004.)

mentally lower by an average of 5.4% per MET increase ($P < .001$) (Fig 1). In multivariable analyses adjusted for demographic variables, for treadmill test performance and results, and for clinical history, METs were the most significant predictor of cost ($P < .001$).

Conclusion.—Exercise capacity is a strong predictor of 1-year total health care costs in patients referred for exercise testing for clinical reasons. Exercise capacity is inversely correlated with health care costs.

▶ The likelihood that an increase of physical activity will reduce medical and other social costs has been an important factor motivating governments to encourage increased habitual physical activity on a population basis.[1] One or 2 quasiexperimental studies have looked at the impact of increased physical activity on medical expenditures,[2] but, in general, evidence has been drawn in a less satisfactory manner from cross-sectional comparisons between active and inactive individuals. The study of Weiss and associates has an advantage over some articles, in that careful estimates of accumulated medical costs were available for the individuals under study. A moderately objective assessment of habitual physical activity was also obtained from the individual's treadmill endurance time. However, most of the 881 study participants were referred to the laboratory for possible coronary disease, and this raises the specter that the extent of initial atherosclerotic disease may have influenced both medical costs and the measured physical working capacity.

R. J. Shephard, MD, PhD, DPE

References

1. Katzmarzyck PT, Gledhill N, Shephard RJ: The economic burden of physical inactivity in Canada. *Can Med Assoc J* 163:1435-1440, 2000.

2. Shephard RJ: *Economic Benefits of Enhanced Fitness.* Champaign, Ill, Human Kinetics, 1986.

Effects of Cardiorespiratory Fitness on Healthcare Utilization
Mitchell TL, Gibbons LW, Devers SM, et al (Cooper Clinic, Dallas; Cooper Inst for Aerobics Research, Dallas)
Med Sci Sports Exerc 36:2088-2092, 2004   1–12

Background.—It has been well established that physical activity has beneficial effects on body mass index, hypertension, cholesterol, blood sugar, and some forms of cancer. However, over 50% of American adults do not achieve the level of physical activity recommended by the Centers for Disease Control and Prevention (CDC) and the American College of Sports Medicine, despite the obvious and extremely well-publicized benefits to health and almost daily exhortations regarding the dangers of poor diet and inadequate exercise in the popular media. More than one fourth of adults have reported that they do not engage in any leisure-time physical activity. A number of studies have evaluated the relationship between exercise participation, absenteeism, health care costs, and productivity, often as part of a broader health promotion program. The efficacy of exercise alone has been difficult to assess. One reason for this difficulty is that many studies have examined reported participation versus functional capacity. The relationship between cardiorespiratory fitness and incidence of medical treatments during a 1-year period before each of 2 examinations was investigated.

Methods.—A prospective study was conducted among 6679 healthy male subjects who underwent medical examinations on 2 occasions, including maximal exercise testing. In the second part of the study, a subset of subjects (2974 persons) were evaluated to compare overnight hospital stays between low-fit men who remained low-fit at the second examination and low-fit men who became fit by the second examination.

Results.—In the first part of the study, the division of study subjects by fitness into quartiles (Q1, lowest fitness level; Q4, highest fitness level) showed an inverse relationship between fitness levels and outcome measures. Men in the Q1 fitness group (lowest fitness level) had more office visits and overnight hospital stays than men in the Q4 fitness group (highest fitness level). These differences persisted after adjustment for potential confounding variables, including age, follow-up year, blood pressure, cholesterol, and smoking. In the second part of the study, division of the subjects into fitness tertiles (T1, lowest fitness, to T3, highest fitness level) showed that subjects who improved their fitness by the time of the second examination had a decreased number of overnight hospital stays compared with those who remained unfit at the time of the second examination.

Conclusion.—Men who become fit or maintain fitness are less likely to have physician visits or overnight hospital stays, compared with men who are unfit.

▶ One argument frequently advanced for participation in fitness programs is that they will save health care dollars.[1] However, there is only limited empirical evidence to support this view. The present report has 2 virtues—the sample size was large, and a part of the data was collected prospectively. Thus, one can examine the extent of any benefits from enhancing personal fitness. Health care savings was noted primarily in terms of a decreased frequency of overnight hospital stays. Bed use was almost halved in the group who improved their fitness relative to those who remained unfit. However, because most of the sample subjects were relatively young, the annual savings was relatively small (no more than 0.175 bed-nights per person). There is a need for similar studies on women and on older populations. Details of the fitness program were left to the individual, and it is unclear from the text how large an increase in fitness was needed to achieve the observed cost benefit.

R. J. Shephard, MD, PhD, DPE

Reference

1. Shephard RJ: *The economics of enhanced fitness.* Champaign, Ill, Human Kinetics, 1986.

Do Physical Leisure Time Activities Prevent Fatigue? A 15 Month Prospective Study of Nurses' Aides
Eriksen W, Bruusgaard D (Univ of Oslo, Norway)
Br J Sports Med 38:331-336, 2004   1–13

Background.—Physical leisure time activities may decrease the risk of persistent fatigue. This hypothesis was tested in a prospective cohort study.

Methods.—The cohort consisted of 6234 female Norwegian nurses' aides who were not on leave because of pregnancy or illness. The women completed an initial questionnaire in 1999, and 5341 (85.7%) completed another questionnaire 15 months later. Persistent fatigue was defined as always or usually feeling fatigue in the daytime during the preceding 14 days.

Findings.—Among participants without persistent fatigue at baseline, a decreased risk of persistent fatigue at follow-up was associated with engagement in physical leisure time activities for at least 20 minutes once a week or more during the 3 months before baseline. The odds ratio was 0.70. Adjustments were made for age, affective symptoms, sleeping problems, musculoskeletal pain, long-term health problems, smoking, marital status, tasks of a caring nature during leisure time, and work factors at baseline (Table 3).

Conclusions.—Physical leisure time activity reduces the risk of persistent fatigue. Clinicians should question patients with fatigue about their level of physical activity.

TABLE 3.—Relation Between Physical Leisure Time Activities at Baseline and Prevalence of Persistent Fatigue (Always or Usually Fatigued During Daytime) at the 15-Month Follow-up in Respondents Without Persistent Fatigue at Baseline

Physical Leisure Time Activities at Baseline	N	% (n)	Persistent Fatigue at Follow Up	
			OR (95% CI)	Adj OR (95% CI)
No regular exercise	1080	13.1 (141)	1.00	1.00
Slow walks†	815	11.4 (93)	0.86 (0.65 to 1.13)	0.80 (0.58 to 1.12)§
Brisk walks‡	968	9.7 (94)	0.72 (0.54 to 0.94)**	0.66 (0.48 to 0.91)**
Aerobics or gymnastics‡	269	8.9 (24)	0.65 (0.41 to 1.03)*	0.81 (0.49 to 1.35)¶
Other regular exercise	1315	8.4 (111)	0.61 (0.47 to 0.80)***	0.64 (0.47 to 0.87)***
Any regular exercise	3367	9.6 (322)	0.70 (0.57 to 0.87)***	0.70 (0.55 to 0.89)***

N, Total number of subjects in each category; n, number of cases in each category; %, proportion of cases in each category; OR, crude odds ratio; 95% CI, 95% confidence interval; Adj OR, odds ratio adjusted for age, baseline health characteristics (level of fitness, affective symptoms, sleeping problems, musculoskeletal pain, widespread pain, long term health problems of any kind), daily consumption of cigarettes, former smoking, number of preschool children, engagement with special tasks of a caring nature during leisure time, number of hours worked a week, frequency of night shifts, quantitative work demands, positive challenges in the job, the extent to which the work required physical endurance, the extent to which the culture in the work unit was supportive and encouraging, and personal engagement in the work unit, in logistic regression analysis (N = 3971. Overall rate of correct classification = 90.1%. Hosmer-Lemeshow test: χ^2 = 6.823; df = 8; p = 0.56).
    Area under the ROC curve = 0.95.
    *p<0.10;**p<0.05;***p<0.01; §p = 0.19; ¶p = 0.43.
    †As the only activity.
    ‡As the only activity or in combination with slow walks.
    (Courtesy of Eriksen W, Bruusgaard D: Do physical leisure time activities prevent fatigue? A 15-month prospective study of nurses' aides. *Br J Sports Med* 38: 331-336, 2004. Reprinted with permission from the BMJ Publishing Group.)

▶ It seems logical that when persons are required to engage in a fixed amount of heavy physical work, fatigue is more likely in those who are unfit than in those who have maintained their fitness by an adequate volume of regular physical activity. The present study of nurses' aides appears to bear out this thesis, as previously supported by both cross-sectional studies[1-3] and one longitudinal study[4] (where benefit was seen only in men). One weakness in the current analysis is that the questionnaire did not distinguish between physical and mental or psychological fatigue. Much of the job-related physical work presumably involved the lifting of patients, and it would have been helpful to distinguish muscle-building from aerobic leisure activity. None of the sample were fatigued when baseline data were collected, but some may have been nursing for only a short time. It is thus just conceivable that subsequent work-induced fatigue kept those with symptoms from engaging in leisure-time activity, rather than the reverse. The amount of leisure activity associated with protection against fatigue (20 minutes of brisk walking at least once a week) is only moderate, and it may be that a different answer would have been obtained in workers whose job did not itself involve a substantial amount of walking.

R. J. Shephard, MD, PhD, DPE

References

1. Chen MK: The epidemiology of well-perceived fatigue among adults. *Prev Med* 15:74-81, 1986.
2. Stewart WD, Abbey S, Meana M, et al: What makes women tired? A community sample. *J Women's Health* 7:69-76, 1998.

3. Kristal-Boneh E, Froom P, Harari G, et al: Fatigue among Israeli industrial employees. *J Occup Environ Med* 38:1145-1150, 1996.
4. Bültmann U, Kant U, Kasl SV, et al: Lifestyle factors as risk factors for fatigue and psychological distress in the working population: Results from the Maastricht Cohort Study. *J Occup Environ Med* 44:116-124, 2002.

Associations Between Physical Activity Dose and Health-Related Quality of Life

Brown DW, Brown DR, Heath GW, et al (Ctrs for Disease Control and Prevention, Atlanta, Ga)
Med Sci Sports Exerc 36:890-896, 2004   1–14

Introduction.—The beneficial effects of participation in regular physical activity are widely accepted. However, the association between physical activity and health-related quality of life (HR-QOL) is unclear.

Methods.—Associations between frequency, duration, and intensity of physical activity and HRQOL were evaluated among 175,850 adults with the use of data from the 2001 Behavioral Risk Factor Surveillance System. Logistic regression was used to determine odds ratios (ORs) and 95% CIs, which were adjusted for age, gender, race/ethnicity, education, smoking status, and body mass index.

Results.—The age-standardized prevalence of 14 or more unhealthy (physical or mental) days during the prior 30 days was 28.4% in physically inactive adults, 16.7% among participants with insufficient levels of physical activity, and 14.7% among those who met recommended levels. Overall, participation in no moderate physical activity (OR, 2.02; 95% CI, 1.85-2.21) was linked with an increased likelihood of having 14 or more unhealthy days. For moderate physical activity, participation every day of the week (5-6 d/wk as referent) (OR, 1.35; 95% CI, 1.26-1.46) was linked with an increased likelihood of 14 or more unhealthy days, as was participation in physical activity for less than 20 minutes (OR, 1.43; 95% CI, 1.30-1.58) or 90 minutes or more (OR, 1.22; 95% CI, 1.14-1.31) per day (30-59 min/d as referent). Similar correlations were seen for those who participated in vigorous physical activity.

Conclusion.—Participants who achieved the recommended levels of physical activity were more likely to report fewer unhealthy days than were those who were inactive or insufficiently active. Participation in daily moderate or vigorous physical activity and participation in very short (<20 min/d) or extended (≥90 min/d) periods of physical activity were linked with poorer HRQOL. Further data is needed to determine the relationship between the dose of physical activity and HRQOL.

▶ This article takes data from the massive US behavioral risk factor survey of 2001. It looks at the prevalence of 14 or more unhealthy days in the past month in relation to the respondent's pattern of physical activity. All the information is self-reported, and it necessarily excludes the poorer stratum of society who do not have access to a personal telephone. In general, good health was associated with the adoption of currently recommended minimum patterns of weekly physical activity, although, because of the cross-sectional nature of the data, the analysis could not answer the fundamental question of whether physical activity promotes good health or whether the converse is true. Perhaps more interestingly, an association was shown between poor health and participation in excessive amounts of physical activity (ie, exercise on more than 6 d/wk or for more than 90 minutes per session). Possibly, further surveys of this type might enable us to define more clearly an optimal upper limit for exercise prescriptions.

R. J. Shephard, MD, PhD, DPE

Normative Ethics in Sports Medicine
Bernstein J, Perlis C, Bartolozzi AR (Univ of Pennsylvania, Philadelphia; 3B Orthopaedics, PC, Philadelphia)
Clin Orthop 420:309-318, 2004   1–15

Background.—The medical problems typically addressed in sports medicine are usually far removed from the issues usually associated with medical ethics. However, there are moral challenges in the field of sports medicine, and the unique position of the athlete as patient can make it difficult for the team physician to do the "right" thing.

In most medical encounters, there are 3 basic assumptions: that the physician works exclusively on the patient's behalf; that the patient and physician have the common goal of improving the patient's health; and that the physician-patient relationship is private. However, these 3 assumptions may not apply in sports medicine. This study attempted to better define the ethical norms and ideals in sports medicine.

Methods.—Six case scenarios were selected for this survey, and each case was followed by 3 to 6 statements. Respondents were asked to indicate the extent to which they agreed or disagreed with the given statement on a visual analogue scale. A total of 23 statements were included.

The survey was sent to a convenience sample of academic ethicists in the United States and to all members of the physician groups of the National Football League, National Hockey League, and Ivy League. Respondents were asked to accept the assumptions given in the case scenarios for the purpose of determining their agreement with the statements.

Results.—Of the 50 ethicists contacted, 35 replied, and 4 of these respondents declined to participate (a response rate of 62%). A total of 131 of 253 team physicians responded to the survey (response rate, 52%). Responses were converted from scores ranging from 0 to 100, and a difference greater than 20 points was determined to represent significant disagreement. According to this standard, there was agreement between the physicians and ethicists for 18 of 23 statements.

Conclusion.—Team physicians and ethicists hold many of the same ethical views on common ethical issues in sports medicine. However, the high degree of variance in the responses in both groups suggested that there are still many unresolved areas in the field of ethics in sports medicine.

▶ This is a comparative study and survey of team physicians of the National Football League, National Hockey League, and Ivy League and those of ethicists regarding advertising, conflicting health care goals, confidentiality, innovative treatments, and enabling dangerous behavior of professional athletes, as well as treating children. The views are those of 31 ethicists and 131 team physicians. The wide variance in responses points out the many unresolved ethical areas in sports medicine.

R. C. Cantu, MD, MA

Analysis of Injury Rates and Treatment Patterns for Time-Loss and Non–Time-Loss Injuries Among Collegiate Student-Athletes
Powell JW, Dompier TP (Michigan State Univ, East Lansing)
J Athletic Train 39:56-70, 2004   1–16

Introduction.—In recent years, numerous collegiate programs have had an increase in the participation time of their athletes. This increases greater exposure concerning of chances for injury and places a higher demand for service on the athletic health care team, particularly athletic trainers. There is concern that some athletic programs are not sufficiently staffed to meet the changing medical coverage needs of the student athlete.

The injury rates for time-loss and non–time-loss were compared among selected intercollegiate athletic programs. The number of treatments associated with these injuries were examined in a volunteer cross-sectional cohort investigation of 50 athletic programs representing the 3 National Collegiate Athletic Association divisions, the National Association of Intercollegiate Athletes, and the National Junior College Athletic Association during the 2000 to 2002 academic year.

Methods.—Athletes listed on the team rosters for the participating institutions and representing the sports associated with the institutions' athletic programs were evaluated. The athletic training staff and students documented the injury and treatment data for the participating institutions, including information for time-loss and non–time-loss injuries, daily treatments, and daily athlete-exposures.

Results.—Non–time-loss injury rates were 3.5 (confidence interval [CI], 3.4-3.6) times the time-loss rate for men and 5.1 (CI, 4.9-5.2) times the time–loss rate for women. Non–time-loss injuries necessitated more treatments during the year compared to time-loss injuries. For male athletes, 22% of injuries resulted in loss of participation time; 47% of treatments were associated with these injuries. In female athletes, 16% of injuries and 34% of treatments were linked with time-loss injuries.

Conclusion.—Throughout the sports medicine year, athletic training staff and students spent more time delivering treatments to athletes who did not miss participation time, compared with those who missed time. These numbers reflect the nature of care and management patterns of injuries so that players are able to continue sports competition.

▶ This is a comparison study of collegiate student athletes who lose time with their injuries and those who lose no time with their injuries. This study finds that sports medicine staff spent as much if not more time delivering treatment to athletes who were not missing participation than those who lost participation time. This study is reflective of treatment of student athletes so that they can continue to compete.

R. C. Cantu, MD, MA

Physical Fitness, Injuries, and Team Peformance in Soccer
Arnason A, Sigurdsson SB, Gudmundsson A, et al (Univ of Sport & Physical Education, Oslo, Norway; Univ of Iceland, Reykjavik, Iceland)
Med Sci Sports Exerc 36:278-285, 2004   1–17

Introduction.—During a 90-minute soccer match, an elite player averages traveling between 10 and 11 km. Overall, the mean work rate is about 70% to 75% of maximum oxygen intake and close to the anaerobic threshold. Midfielders travel farther than defenders or attackers. Among defensive players, fullbacks typically cover more distance than centerbacks. There may be a difference in the requirements between different playing positions. It is not known whether this is reflected by differences in fitness. The association between physical fitness and team success in soccer was evaluated, along with differences in physical fitness between different player positions.

Methods.—A total of 306 male soccer players from 17 teams within the 2 highest divisions in Iceland were evaluated. Just before the beginning of the 1999 soccer season, players underwent determinations of height and body mass, body composition, flexibility, leg extension power, jump height, and peak oxygen intake. Injuries and player participation in matches and training were documented throughout the 4-month competitive season. Team average physical fitness was compared with team success (final league standing) by means of a linear regression model. Physical fitness was also compared between players in various playing positions.

Results.—A significant association was seen between team average jump height (countermovement jump and standing jump) and team success ($P = .009$ and $P = .012$, respectively). The same trend was also seen for leg extension power $P = .097$), body composition (percent body fat; $P = .07$), and total number of injury days per team ($P = .09$).

Goalkeepers had different fitness characteristics than outfield players. They tended to be taller and heavier, more flexible in hip extension and knee flexion, and had higher leg extension power and a lower peak oxygen intake. Only minor differences were seen between defenders, midfield players, and attackers. The association between team average performance on various tests and team success were usually weak.

Conclusion.—It is recommended that coaches and medical support teams focus more attention on jump and power training, preventive measures, and adequate rehabilitation of prior injuries to increase team success.

▶ This study looked at position-specific as well as overall physical fitness in soccer. It stressed specific preventive and rehabilitative measures and correlated those with team success in soccer.

R. C. Cantu, MD, MA

A Congested Football Calendar and the Wellbeing of Players: Correlation Between Match Exposure of European Footballers Before the World Cup 2002 and Their Injuries and Performances During That World Cup
Ekstrand J, Waldén M, Hägglund M (Linköping Univ, Sweden)
Br J Sports Med 38:493-497, 2004   1–18

Background.—The overall risk of injury for professional soccer players has been reported to be about 1000 times higher than that of a high-risk industrial worker. Many of these injuries can be prevented if appropriate prophylactic measures are taken. However, the mechanisms behind football injuries are complex, and many factors are involved. The way in which the season is planned has an important influence on injuries. One study of training and matches at amateur levels found that a high training/match quotient with many training sessions in relation to the number of matches played provided greater success with fewer injuries. However, this relationship has not been studied at the professional level. In this study, the exposure of soccer players in European teams to match play in the months leading up to World Cup 2002 was correlated with their injuries and performances during that World Cup.

Methods.—The team physicians of 11 of the best soccer teams in Europe were asked to prospectively record players' exposure and injuries during the 2001-2002 season. A total of 65 players participated in the World Cup in Korea and Japan in June 2002. The teams reported injuries sustained by these players during the World Cup, and the players' performance was evaluated by 3 international experts.

Results.—The number of matches for each team during the season varied from 40 to 76, depending on the countries involved. The mean number of matches per player was 36. Top players played more matches, particularly during the final period of the season. Players who took part in the World Cup played more matches during the season than those who did not (46 vs 33 matches). The World Cup players did not show any increased risk of injury during the season. About 29% incurred injuries during the World Cup, and 32% of these players performed below their normal standard. The underperforming players had played more matches during the 10 weeks before the World Cup than did those who performed above expectations (12.5 vs 9 matches).

Conclusions.—Significant variation exists in the number of matches played per season in European professional soccer leagues. Top-level players are expected to play many matches, especially in the final period of the season. A period in which many matches are played can increase the risk of injury and poor performance in the following period.

▶ This was a comparison study of the performance of European footballers before the World Cup of 2002 and during World Cup play. The study showed that the number of matches played varies considerably per season and that top-level players are obligated to play many matches, especially during the final part of the season. This increase in matches played at the end of the season can result in fatigue, poor performance during play, and an increased risk of injury to the players.

R. C. Cantu, MD, MA

The Risk of Death in Running Road Races: Does Race Length Matter?
Frere JA, Maharam LG, Van Camp SP (San Diego State Univ, Calif; New York Road Runners; Alvarado Med Group, San Diego, Calif)
Physician Sportsmed 32(4):33-40, 2004   1–19

Introduction.—The risk of death for marathon participants and for high school and collegiate athletes has been quantified. Data concerning the risk of death in running shorter road races are limited. The incidence and causes of exercise-associated death in running road races were evaluated to help identify runners at risk.

Methods.—The number of finishers and the number of deaths between 1996 through 2000 were evaluated in 62 of the largest races (according to the USA Track and Field in 1999) from 10-km, 12-km, 15-km, and half-marathon distances. Differences in the risk of death among these races were compared.

Results.—Thirty-eight (61%) of the officials from the 62 races returned questionnaires. Five deaths occurred during the 5-year evaluation period among 1,636,720 finishers. All fatalities were men (age range, 38-84 years). Four deaths were during 10-km races, and 1 occurred in a half-marathon race. All 3 of the deaths for which additional data were available were attributed to coronary artery disease. The overall incidence of death in running road races was about 3.1 per 1 million finishers. This risk and that for 10-km races are significantly lower than is the risk reported for marathons from combined data from other sources.

Conclusion.—The risk of death from running road races is significantly lower than is the risk for running marathons. This data may help physicians and their patients determine the appropriateness of participating in a road race and may help race directors and medical doctors determine emergency medical needs.

▶ These authors compared the risk of death from running marathons with the risk of death from running shorter road races and found that running a shorter road race carried a significantly lower risk than did running a marathon.

R. C. Cantu, MD, MA

Injury Patterns in Big Ten Conference Football
Albright JP, Powell JW, Martindale A, et al (Univ of Iowa, Iowa City; Michigan State Univ, East Lansing; Univ of Illinois, Urbana-Champaign; et al)
Am J Sports Med 32:1394-1404, 2004   1–20

Background.—The safety of participants in sports was evaluated by the National Collegiate Athletic Association (NCAA) in 1997, which led to a review of existing fall and spring football practice data in the Big Ten Injury Surveillance System (B10-ISS). An increased risk of injuries was found in the spring and was termed the *spring risk factor.* Injury rates and the type of practice session in which the injuries occurred were determined, a comparison was made of the types of injuries, and why the risk of injuries during the spring is increased was assessed. Based on findings, new NCAA regulations were formulated to level the seasonal injury patterns. Whether this outcome was obtained was investigated.

Methods.—In the phase 1 analysis, review of the B10-ISS covering the spring of 1992 through the fall of 1997 was undertaken and included all reportable injuries. On the basis of these findings, the NCAA updated their regulations with the goal of reducing injury rates for the spring to levels equal to or lower than those for fall practices. In phase 2, which covered the spring of 1998 through the fall of 2000, a prospective evaluation was done not only to document the same injuries found in the phase 1 analysis but also to update individual player position descriptions and string and exposures for these categories in the spring and fall practices. The previous fall and spring practice categories had been scrimmages, full contact, and limited contact, but the rule changes had introduced the new spring practice designations as full pads with and without tackling, helmets only, spring game, and other scrimmages.

Results.—The phase 1 analysis identified 3950 fall injuries and 1007 spring injuries over the period covered. The fall practice– and spring practice–related injury rates were 10.6 and 19.8 per 1000 athlete exposures, respectively. The injury rate for spring football conditions was nearly 2-fold higher than that for the fall football conditions. The greatest risk of injury was found during scrimmages in both the fall and the spring, and a higher risk was also noted for contact practices over both seasons. However, it was found that reducing the number of contact sessions had less effect than reducing the number of limited-contact sessions. It was believed that a greater effect in reducing the high injury rate associated with the spring season would be achieved by increasing the number of full-contact practices in full protective gear.

In the phase 2 analysis, 1502 injuries occurred in the fall and 648 in the spring, so the fall average per team per year rate was 46 and the spring average per team per year rate was 20. When the overall injury rate per 1000 athlete exposures was determined, the spring rate was 3 times higher than the fall rate: an estimated 40 injuries per team in 3 years were attributable to spring practice. Scrimmages produced the highest injury rates in both the fall and the spring, and the second highest risk of injury in the spring occurred with full pads without tackling. Skill position players run a higher risk than linemen or linebacker–tight end positions in the spring. The highest risk of injury was among nonplayers in both seasons. Each of the anatomical regions had a significant increase in the number of soft tissue and bony injuries, and the greatest incidence involved the forearm–wrist–hand area.

Conclusions.—The NCAA spring football rule changes did not equalize the risk of injuries between the fall and the spring sessions. The analysis permitted the identification of the complexity of the process and will inform further investigations into sports injuries.

▶ This study focused on the 1998 NCAA's rule change decreasing the number of scrimmages and contact practices allowed during the spring season and compared injuries before this rule change to those after the rule change. The authors concluded that the 1998 rule change resulted in a greater increase in spring practice injury rates.

R. C. Cantu, MD, MA

Incidence of Injury in Junior and Senior Rugby League Players
Gabbett TJ (Queensland Academy of Sport, Sunnybank, Australia)
Sports Med 34:849-859, 2004   1–21

Background.—Rugby league players at all playing levels frequently incur musculoskeletal injuries in this collision sport. A rugby game consists of 2 30- to 40-minute halves (depending on level of play) separated by a 10-minute rest. High-intensity and low-intensity activity periods alternate throughout the game, requiring players to excel in speed, agility, muscle strength and power, and aerobic power. The incidence, type, site, and cause of training and match injuries were explored in a review of the extent of the injury problem in rugby leagues at all competitive levels.

Methods.—Comparisons were made between studies defining injuries as pain or disability incurred during a match or training session and injury causing a player to miss later matches. Injury exposure was defined as the number of hours players are exposed to injury. Injury incidence was expressed as number per 1000 player-position game hours.

Results.—Injury rates usually increase at higher playing levels. The overall incidence of injury is 160.6 per 1000 player-position game hours for amateur rugby players and up to 346 injuries per 1000 player-position game hours for professionals. The rates for semiprofessional players are even higher at 824.7 per 1000 player-position game hours, reflecting the high fitness/moderate skill levels at this competitive level compared with the low fitness/low skill levels of amateurs and high fitness/high skill levels of professionals. Injury rates of prepubertal, peripubertal, and postpubertal rugby players increase progressively at higher playing levels. Professional rugby league players' incidence of injury is 34 to 52.3 injuries per 1000 player-position game hours, with 15.6% to 30.0% being major injuries. Long-term job limitations, medical costs, and loss of income can accompany these injuries. Between 4% and 6% of retired professional rugby players still incur losses caused by injuries while playing.

Most recent studies find head and neck injuries are the most common, seen in 25.3% of amateur and 28.8% (head) and 33.3% (neck) of professional injuries. Semiprofessional players are more often injured in the thigh and calf, with only 10.0% incurring head and neck injuries. Junior rugby players (aged 6-17 years) more often have fractures, but senior rugby players have more hematomas and strains. Players are more likely to miss matches because of severe joint injuries. Tackling is the activity most often causing injury, responsible for 46.3% to 91.0% of injuries. The tackled player usually is the one injured. Forwards receive tackling injuries at a higher rate than backs. Fatigue is a factor in amateur rugby injuries but not at other levels. Injury rates climb as the season progresses, except among junior players.

The injury rates for training are much lower at all playing levels, and few cause missed matches. The thigh and calf are the most common sites of training-related injuries, which are usually muscular strains caused by overuse and overexertion. Forwards are more often involved than backs. Training injuries tend to occur in the latter stages of training and the early stages of the rugby season, except among professional rugby players.

Prevention and Conclusions.—Prevention strategies to minimize tackling injuries are needed, including teaching defensive skills, correct tackling technique, correct falling technique, and ways to minimize the absorption of impact forces in tackles. Injuries related to fatigue may be reduced by training players in skills and decision-making abilities under fatigue conditions during matches. Reduced training loads could also reduce training injury rates for the preseason preparation period. Further studies are needed to assess risk factors for injury in junior and senior players, injuries related to specific player positions, and the effect injuries have on performance.

▶ This author looked at not only the incidence of injury in junior and senior rugby players but also the type of injuries. It is a well-known fact that the incidence of rugby league injuries increases as the playing level increases. The author discusses this as well as those types of injuries seen most often in junior and senior players.

R. C. Cantu, MD, MA

Soccer Injuries: A Review on Incidence and Prevention
Junge A, Dvorak J (FIFA Med Assessment and Research Centre, Zurich, Switzerland)
Sports Med 34:929-938, 2004   1–22

Background.—Soccer injuries have been investigated previously, but few data have focused on preventive efforts and the effectiveness of such interventions. The incidence and prevention of soccer injuries were reviewed.

Methods.—A review of the current literature on the exposure-related incidence of soccer injuries, covering both male and female players at various levels of play, the characteristics and causes of injury, and areas targeted for preventive efforts was performed.

Results.—Most studies focused on male adult players at the professional level. Players in the professional league in the United States and the national division league of Iceland have the highest incidences of injury; the lowest levels are noted for Dutch and Danish low-level players. Match injuries occur 4 to 6 times more often than training injuries. Male elite soccer players sustain an average of 1 performance-limiting injury annually. Female soccer players have a lower injury incidence than men, but some types of injury are more prevalent among female athletes. The incidence of injury increases with age in young players, with those aged 17 to 18 years having an incidence similar to that of adult players. The areas affected most often are the ankle, knee joints, and thigh and calf muscles. Sprains, strains, and contusions are reported most often. Trauma is the principal cause of injury. Between 9% and 34% of injuries result from overuse. Player contact is an important cause of injury, with 12% to 28% resulting from foul play, although international tournaments have a higher incidence attributable to such tactics. Noncontact injury accounts for 26% to 59% of injuries and usually occurs during running and turning. Reinjury occurs often, accounting for 20% to 25% of all injuries.

Prevention efforts have focused on reducing all injuries or injuries to the knee and ankle areas. Specific preventive activities include doing warm-up exercises that emphasis stretching, regularly performing cool-downs, permitting adequate rehabilitation and sufficient recovery time from injury, having proprioceptive training, wearing protective equipment, maintaining good playing field conditions, and adhering to the rules. In 1 study, players following a prevention regimen reduced injuries by 75%. Female high-school players (14-19 years old) in a preseason conditioning program that combined sport-specific cardiovascular conditioning, plyometric work, sport-cord drills, strength training, and flexibility had a 14% injury incidence compared with a 34% injury incidence for an untrained group. Education and supervision interventions reduced injuries in male youth players by 21%. Mild injuries, overuse injuries, and training injuries were reduced most, with low-level teams benefiting more than those at a high skill level. Knee injuries have been significantly reduced by proprioceptive and neuromuscular training approaches. A reduction in ankle sprains occurred when orthosis use and coordination training programs were implemented.

Conclusions.—Multimodal training programs appear to reduce soccer injuries. Specific injuries such as knee injuries and recurrent ankle sprains have responded to proprioceptive and neuromuscular training. Further well-designed studies are needed to identify the effects of preventive interventions. In addition, more data are needed concerning differences between male and female soccer players regarding the incidence and types of injuries as well as preventive efforts that have proved successful.

▶ These authors looked at injury data available on male and female soccer players. Although there are data available on injuries to male soccer players, there are limited data on female injuries. This article discusses prevention programs for male and female soccer players.

R. C. Cantu, MD, MA

A One Season Prospective Cohort Study of Volleyball Injuries
Verhagen EALM, Van der Beek AJ, Bouter LM, et al (Inst for Research in Extramural Medicine and TNO Vumc, Amsterdam; Norwegian Univ of Sport and Physical Education, Oslo; VU Univ, Amsterdam)
Br J Sports Med 38:477-481, 2004   1–23

Introduction.—Few prospective reports on volleyball injuries and their prevention have been performed, despite the popularity of the sport and the large number of players. The overall incidence of acute and overuse volleyball injuries was evaluated. Factors associated with ankle sprains were analyzed.

Methods.—A total of 486 players from the second and third Dutch national volleyball divisions were prospectively followed up during a whole season in a cohort investigation. Measurements were taken at 3 time points during the season (baseline, follow-up 1, and follow-up 2). The player questionnaire addressed demographics (only at baseline), sports participation, use of preventive measures, and prior injuries. Volleyball exposure during physical training and matches was documented for each player by the coach by means of a weekly exposure form. In the event of injury, the coach provided the injured player with an injury registration form, which was completed within 1 week after injury onset.

Results.—A total of 100 injuries were reported. The overall injury incidence was 2.6 per 1000 hours; the incidence of acute injuries was 2.0 per 1000 hours. Most of the injuries were ankle sprains. Thirty-one of the 41 players (75%) with an ankle sprain reported a prior ankle sprain. There were 25 overuse injuries. The overall incidence of overuse injuries was 0.6 per 1000 hours, with the back and shoulder being the most common sites.

Conclusion.—Ankle sprain is responsible for 41% of all volleyball-associated injuries. Prior injury appears to be an important risk factor for an ankle sprain. Injury prevention programs for volleyball players should concentrate on ankle sprains, particularly for players with prior injury.

▶ This is a limited study of 1 season of 486 volleyball players from the Dutch national volleyball divisions and the overall acute injuries and overuse injuries associated with the sport. The article focuses on ankle sprains, which represent 41% of injuries seen in these athletes.

R.C. Cantu, MD, MA

A Numerical Model for Risk of Ball-Impact Injury to Baseball Pitchers
Nicholls RL, Miller K, Elliott BC (Univ of Western Australia, Crawley, Perth)
Med Sci Sports Exerc 37:30-38, 2005   1–24

Introduction.—Baseball and softball cause more injuries necessitating medical attention than any other sport in the United States. Of 88 fatalities documented between 1973 and 1995, 76% were caused by impact from the batted, pitched, or thrown ball. A decrease in the incidence and severity of such impact injuries necessitates understanding of the biomechanical mechanisms underlying trauma and rigorous quantification of equipment performance to establish risk of such injury occurring. Metal baseball bats produce higher ball exit velocity than wood bats; this increases the risk of impact injuries to infield players. A model of bat-ball impact based on experimental data for bat kinematics and ball time-dependent behavior was used to assess the maximum risk of a pitcher being struck by a baseball from bat type.

Methods.—Three-dimensional bat kinematics at the instant of impact were measured by high-speed videography in 17 high-performance batters. A linear viscoelastic constitutive model was created for stiffer and softer types of baseballs. The risk of impact injury was ascertained by using available movement time data from adult pitchers. Data showed that 0.400 seconds is needed to evade a batted ball.

Results.—The highest ball exit velocity (61.5 m/s) was achieved with the metal bat and the stiffer ball model, equating to 0.282 seconds of available movement time. For 5 impacts along the long axis of each bat, the best case scenario involved the use of the wood bat and the softer ball (46.0 m/s, 0.377 seconds).

Conclusion.—The performance difference between the metal and wood bats was attributed to the preimpact linear velocity of the bat impact point and to differences in orientation on the horizontal plane. Reducing the swing moment of the baseball bat, along with the shear and relaxation moduli of the baseball, increased the available movement time.

▶ These authors looked at batted-ball injuries in baseball relative to metal and wooden bats and the baseballs themselves. Their research suggests ways that ball exit velocity may be reduced and thus make metal bats safer. Much more work is needed in this area. These authors feel that prevention of such injuries is more efficacious than treatment of these injuries on the field after they occur.

R. C. Cantu, MD, MA

Acute Hand and Wrist Injuries in Experienced Rock Climbers
Logan AJ, Makwana N, Mason G, et al (Wrexham Maelor Hosp, Wales)
Br J Sports Med 38:545-548, 2004   1–25

Background.—As the sport of rock climbing is increasing in popularity, so are associated injuries, particularly to the hand and wrist. The incidence of acute wrist and hand injuries for the membership of The Climbers' Club of Great Britain was assessed.

Study Design.—A questionnaire was sent to the membership of The Climbers' Club, asking about rock climbing history and associated acute injury to wrist and hand. A total climbing intensity score was calculated for each respondent, representing lifetime exposure to rock climbing. This score was then related to incidence of injury.

Findings.—Complete questionnaires were returned by 545 (50%) of the members. The majority of responders were men whose average age was 50 years. There were 155 climbers with 235 wrist and hand injuries. Finger tendon injuries were the most common, followed by abrasions or laceration or both and fractures. Climbing intensity scores were significantly higher for those with hand and wrist injuries.

Conclusions.—Increasing lifetime climbing intensity was associated with increased injury among the climbers. The most common type of climbing-associated injury was to the finger tendons or pulleys.

▶ These authors studied 545 members of The Climbers' Club of Great Britain looking historically at common injuries in this particular sport. They found that injuries to the wrist and hand are the most common injuries in rock climbers. These results were correlated with the increase in climbing intensity over the climbers' career.

R. C. Cantu, MD, MA

Evaluation of Physiological Standard Pressures of the Forearm Flexor Muscles During Sport Specific Ergometry in Sport Climbers
Schoeffl V, Klee S, Strecker W (Klinikum Bamberg, Germany; Humboldt Univ Berlin)
Br J Sports Med 38:422-425, 2004   1–26

Introduction.—Chronic exertional compartment syndrome (CECS) is well described in sports medicine. The most frequently affected is the tibialis anterior muscle compartment in runners and walkers. Few cases of CECS of the forearm flexor muscles have been reported. Standard pressure levels inside the deep flexor compartment of the forearms during a sport-specific test (climbing ergometry) were evaluated.

Methods.—Ten healthy high-level climbers were prospectively enrolled. All participants underwent climbing-specific ergometry using a rotating climbing wall (step test, total climbing time 9 to 15 minutes). Pressure was determined by means of a slit catheter positioned in the deep flexor compartment of the forearm. Pressure, blood lactate, and heart rate were documented every 3 minutes and during recovery.

Results.—Physical exhaustion of the forearms defined the end point of the climbing ergometry in all participants. Blood lactate increased with physical stress, achieving a mean of 3.48 mmol/L. Compartment pressure was associated with physical stress. It exceeded 30 mm Hg in only 3 participants. A critical pressure of over 40 mm Hg was not seen. After the test, the pressure diminished to normal levels within 3 minutes in 7 participants. The 3 participants with higher pressure levels (more than 30 mm Hg) needed a longer time to recover.

Conclusion.—An algorithm was created to ascertain further clinical and therapeutic consequences of climbing ergometry. Basic pressure below 15 mm Hg and stress pressure below 30 mm Hg, as well as pressures during the 15-minute recovery period below 15 mm Hg, are physiologic. Pressures of 15 to 30 mm Hg during recovery are indicative of high risk of CECS. Pressures above 30 mm Hg affirm CECS.

▶ CECS in forearms of sport climbers is the subject of this article.

R. C. Cantu, MD, MA

A Prospective Study of Kitesurfing Injuries
Nickel C, Zernial O, Musahl V, et al (Klinikum Elmshorn, Germany; Univ Hosp Schleswig Holstein, Kiel, Germany; Univ of Pittsburgh, Pa; et al)
Am J Sports Med 32:921-927, 2004   1–27

Background.—In kitesurfing, the athlete uses a small board and transfers the energy of the wind into speed by means of a large maneuverable kite. Even in light surf conditions, the athlete can perform high jumps. The kites used are generally between 9 and 16 m², and the boards range from 120 to 200 cm in length. Boards may be directional, which means they are like small windsurfing boards with a nose and a tail, or bidirectional, which means they are shorter than directional boards and have fins at both ends. Kitesurfers move downwind and upwind at about 48 to 64 km/h. Injuries in a kitesurfing population over an entire season were prospectively evaluated for common injury patterns and potential areas where preventive measures could be used.

Methods.—Over the course of 6 months, or 1 season, data were collected via questionnaire from 235 kitesurfers, who ranged in age from 14 to 48 years (mean, 27.2 years). The average experience was 2.8 years, and most participants (225) were men.

Results.—One hundred twenty-four injuries were reported over the 17,728 kitesurfing hours. In 25 athletes, multiple injuries occurred. The overall injury rate was 7.0 injuries per 1000 hours of kitesurfing. During competition, the injury rate was 16.6 injuries per 1000 hours, and during practice, the rate was 6.8 injuries per 1000 hours. The risk of injury was 2.5 times higher during competition than during training. Most injuries were contusions, followed by abrasions, lacerations, joint sprains, and fractures. The foot and ankle were injured more than any other body part, followed by the head, knee, and thorax. Most of the injuries fell into the mild category (77%); however, 19% were considered medium, and 3% were considered severe. One female athlete (age, 25 years) died. Fifty-four percent of the injuries occurred on the water more than 50 m from the beach, 26% were on the water less than 50 m from the beach, and 20% occurred on the beach. Contusions generally occurred when the athlete was pulled against an obstacle. Overestimation of expertise was reported by 30 athletes, and misinterpretation of weather conditions was reported by 19. Technical mistakes were reported by 55 kitesurfers. Most injuries occurred when the wind speed was 11 to 18 knots at flat-water conditions. Twenty-one percent of kitesurfers used protective devices, including a helmet (7%) and a quick-release system (18%). The injury rates tended to be lower among athletes who used the quick-release system, and none of the athletes who used helmets sustained head injuries.

Conclusions.—Based on the injury rates from these data, kitesurfing can be classified as a high-risk sport. Prevention strategies could lower the injury rate. Protective equipment such as a quick-release system and helmets, athlete awareness of the distance to the beach, and regulations that specify areas for use by kitesurfers on the beach and over the water could potentially improve the safety of the sport.

▶ This is a study of 235 kitesurfers over a 6-month period (1 season) and the types of injuries associated with this sport. The findings of 1 death and 11 severe injuries during this period have caused this sport to be ranked as high risk.

R. C. Cantu, MD, MA

Snowmobile Trauma: 10 Years' Experience at Manitoba's Tertiary Trauma Centre
Stewart RL, Black GB (Univ of Manitoba, Winnipeg, Canada)
J Can Chiroprac Assoc 47:90-94, 2004   1–28

Background.—As snowmobiling has increased in popularity, so have snowmobile-related injuries and deaths. Factors associated with injury include alcohol use, excessive speed, and suboptimal lighting. The Winnipeg, Manitoba, Health Science Center's experience with snowmobile injuries was reviewed retrospectively to identify risk factors.

Study Design.—A chart review was performed of all snowmobile-related injuries from 1988 through 1997.

Findings.—Data from the charts identified 480 snowmobile-related injuries in 260 men and 34 women. Of these patients, 27.6% died. Collisions accounted for 72% of the injuries. More than 30% of injuries were sustained on roadways (as opposed to snowmobile trials). Of the injured patients, excessive speed was a risk factor in 54%, suboptimal lighting in 86%, and alcohol in 70%. More than half of all injuries were musculoskeletal.

Conclusions.—Recreational snowmobile use remains a significant cause of serious injury. These injuries are associated with potentially preventable human factors. In addition to the previously reported risk factors of alcohol consumption, poor lighting, and excessive speed, an additional factor was identified related to snowmobiling injuries—snowmobiling on roads. Trail monitoring would not prevent these injuries, which do not occur on designated snowmobiling trails.

▶ These authors studied whether the previously determined risk factors associated with snowmobile use continue, and they identified previously unknown risk factors associated with the use of snowmobiles. They concluded that snowmobile injuries are primarily caused by human error and that efforts must focus on prevention of injuries and on the drivers who have the ultimate control of the snowmobile.

R. C. Cantu, MD, MA

Effectiveness of Helmets in Skiers and Snowboarders: Case-Control and Case Crossover Study
Hagel BE, Pless IB, Goulet C, et al (Univ of Alberta, Edmonton, Canada)
BMJ 330:281-283, 2005   1–29

Objective.—To determine the effect of helmets on the risk of head and neck injuries in skiers and snowboarders.

Design.—Matched case-control and case crossover study.

Setting.—19 ski areas in Quebec, Canada, November 2001 to April 2002.

Participants.—1082 skiers and snowboarders (cases) with head and neck injuries reported by the ski patrol and 3295 skiers and snowboarders (controls) with non-head or non-neck injuries matched to cases at each hill.

Main Outcome Measures.—Estimates of matched odds ratios for the effect of helmet use on the risk of any head or neck injury and for people requiring evacuation by ambulance.

Results.—The adjusted odds ratio for helmet use in participants with any head injury was 0.71 (95% confidence interval 0.55 to 0.92), indicating a 29% reduction in the risk of head injury. For participants who required evacuation by ambulance for head injuries, the adjusted odds ratio for helmet use was 0.44 (0.24 to 0.81). Similar results occurred with the case crossover design (odds ratio 0.43, 0.09 to 1.83). The adjusted odds ratio for helmet use for participants with any neck injury was 0.62 (0.33 to 1.19) and for participants who required evacuation by ambulance for neck injuries it was 1.29 (0.41 to 4.04).

Conclusions.—Helmets protect skiers and snowboarders against head injuries. We cannot rule out the possibility of an increased risk of neck injury with helmet use, but the estimates on which this assumption is based are imprecise.

▶ Injury epidemiology is a growing field. In studies examining the role of equipment, some authors simply count the number of people who were injured and determine what percentage participated in a particular prevention strategy. For example, only about 25% of injured persons wore helmets in this study. To know whether helmets are truly protective, we have to compare the injury rates in helmeted snowboarders and nonhelmeted snowboarders. Traditional methodology would use a case-control approach for a rare event such as head injury. In a case-control study, the controls should resemble the cases as much as possible, except for the probability of being exposed to the intervention of interest. However, the choice of controls is difficult as helmeted snowboarders may be more aggressive than nonhelmeted snowboarders. A more novel approach is the case cross-over design. In this design, subjects are compared to themselves at 2 different times to determine whether the odds of wearing a helmet are decreased when an injury occurs compared to the odds when an injury does not occur. Because the cases and controls are the same subjects, one expects increased similarities between cases and controls compared to a traditional case-control approach (note that in this study, subjects may snowboard differently when they are not wearing their helmet). In this particular study, the point estimate is similar with the 2 methods (confidence intervals are wider with the case cross-over design because the number of subjects was restricted for this analysis), which may be partly due to the researchers adjusting for the most important covariates in the case-control study. Researchers in the field of injury epidemiology should consider the case cross-over design as a potential model when examining rare injuries.

I. Shrier, MD, PhD

Effect of Trail Design and Grooming on the Incidence of Injuries at Alpine Ski Areas
Bergstrøm KA, Ekeland A (Orthopaedic Surgery and Sports Medicine, Voss, Norway; Martina Hansens Hosp, Bærum, Norway)
Br J Sports Med 38:264-268, 2004   1–30

Introduction.—The effect of trail design and grooming on the incidence of injuries at alpine ski areas has not been delineated, although there are recommendations that better slope preparation would reduce injury risk. The effect of trail design and grooming on the incidence of ski injuries, injury rate, and the mean injury severity score (ISS) was examined in the Hafjell and Voss alpine ski areas in Norway.

Methods.—A total of 1410 skiing injuries were documented between December 1990 and the 1996 season for both ski areas. In Hafjell, 183 injuries were plotted on an area map during the first 2 ski seasons and 214 were plotted during the same period in Voss. During the last 3 seasons in Hafjell, 835 ski injuries were linked to 6712 snow-grooming hours and 6,829,084 lift journeys.

Results.—The mean injury rate was 2.2 injuries/1000 skier days. The mean ISS was 3.1. Accumulations of injuries at 3 sites (black spots) were documented on the Hafjell area map and represented 40% of all injuries in the alpine area ($P < .05$). Seven injury accumulation sites were documented at the alpine area map of Voss and represented 22% of total injuries ($P < .05$).

Grooming of the slopes was rated as poor for the 49% of injuries that occurred at the sites of injury concentration. This differed significantly (27%) from injuries that occurred at random in Hafjell. Corresponding rates for Voss were 50% and 25%, respectively. Grooming hours appeared to be inversely proportional to the number of injuries at both sites ($R = -0.99$; $P < .02$). The mean ISS diminished significantly in Hafjell during the evaluation period ($P < .001$).

Conclusion.—Inappropriate trail design and slope grooming appear to result in an accumulation of injuries at certain sites. Modification in construction and maintenance of the trails may decrease the number of injuries and the mean ISS.

▶ These authors sought to determine the effects of trail design and identify conditions of slopes and correlate those with injury rates.

R. C. Cantu, MD, MA

The Effect of Pre-season Dance Training on Physical Indices and Back Pain in Elite Cross-Country Skiers: A Prospective Controlled Intervention Study

Alricsson M, Werner S (Karolinska Institutionen for Kururgisk Vetenskap, Stockholm)

Br J Sports Med 38:148-153, 2004   1–31

Introduction.—Cross-country skiing is a monotonous sport that frequently causes muscle tightness, which can result in injuries or impaired sports performance. Good range of motion and joint mobility are important for acquiring good technique and developing speed. There is some evidence that dance training provides these fitness components for cross-country skiers. A long-term dance training period combined with ski training is not possible. The effect of preseason dance training on back pain, joint mobility, muscle flexibility, and speed and agility for elite cross-country skiers was evaluated.

Methods.—Twenty-six skiers (mean age, 19 years) participated in either an intervention group that gave 12 weeks of dance training or a control group that did not dance. The 2 groups had a similar preseason physical training program. Joint mobility and muscle flexibility of the spine, hip, and ankle were assessed. Two sports-related functional tests (slalom and hurdle) were also given. All measurements and tests were performed before and after the dancing period.

Results.—Four (of 6) participants who initially reported ski-associated back pain did not report back pain after dance training. Three with back pain from the control group continued to report back pain. At baseline, the intervention group had a slightly impaired range of motion in the spine compared to controls.

After dance training, there was a better relationship between kyphosis of the thoracic spine and lordosis of the lumbar spine, along with a 7.1° increase in hip flexion with the knee extended ($P = .02$). In control subjects, hip extension dropped by 0.08 m on average ($P = .01$). No positive effects of dance training on sports-associated functional tests were seen.

Conclusion.—Preseason dance training improved the range of hip motion and joint mobility and flexibility of the spine. These improvements may explain the decrease in ski-associated back pain in the intervention group.

▶ In 26 elite cross-country skiers who used preseason dance training as a means of improving hip range of motion and joint mobility, as well as flexibility of the spine, there was a reduction in low back pain.

R. C. Cantu, MD, MA

Knee Pain and Bicycling: Fitting Concepts for Clinicians

Asplund C, St Pierre P (Dewitt Army Community Hosp, Fort Belvoir, Va; Uniformed Services Univ of Health Sciences, Bethesda, Md)
Physician Sportsmed 32(4):23-30, 2004   1–32

Background.—The number of cycling-related injuries has increased along with the increased interest in cycling as a low-impact form of exercise. These injuries are related to overuse, an improper bicycle fit or equipment, poor technique, or inappropriate training patterns. Because of the repetitive nature of cycling, any malalignment can lead to dysfunction, impaired performance, and pain.

Considerations.—The fit of the bicycle, the training distance and intensity, and anatomical factors (eg, leg-length discrepancy, muscle imbalance, and inflexibility) must be considered in assessing knee pain and cycling-related overuse injuries. Cycling consists of repeating 2-phase pedal cycles in which the power phase begins with the pedal in the 12 o'clock position and ends in the 6 o'clock position and the recovery phase begins in the 6 o'clock position and ends in the 12 o'clock position. In these phases, the knee can undergo repetitive stresses that produce an injury, particularly when the muscles are inflexible or weak. An inappropriate saddle height or improperly aligned shoe cleats can also transmit abnormal forces to the knee repetitively and can produce an injury.

Evaluation.—The assessment of cyclists with anterior knee pain must include the fit of the bicycle because the saddle may be too low, too far forward, or both, which can create excessive stresses for the knee. Exaggerated tibial rotation caused by cleats that are excessively rotated internally or externally places more stress on the knee. For cyclists with medial knee pain, the culprit may be an improper saddle height, the saddle position being too far forward or aft, or an improper cleat position. Poor flexibility of the legs and training errors can also produce medial knee pain, as can anatomical abnormalities or inflammatory conditions such as pes anserine bursitis or mediopatellar plica syndrome. Lateral knee pain is most often the result of anatomical factors and an improper bike fit. Iliotibial band syndrome may be caused by a tight iliotibial band that repeatedly rubs over the lateral condyle with flexion and extension. Having tight, inflexible leg muscles can add to the problem. Although posterior knee pain is rare, it can be caused by biceps tendinosis or medial hamstring tendinosis. When the saddle is too high or too far back, the biceps tendon can be stressed, which increases the stress on the posterior knee.

Treatment and Prevention.—The management of an overuse injury includes protection, rest, ice, compression, elevation, medication, and modalities to control inflammation and permit healing of the tissues. Once healing and rehabilitation have been accomplished, the cyclist requires further training to achieve the above-normal endurance and power needed to excel in the sport. Adjustments to the bike fit, saddle position, and cleat rotation are needed to avoid further problems. Anatomical problems may require customized orthoses. A slow return to training is important, and the focus should be on doing a condensed version of normal training with the use of lower resistance and higher cadence. A rule of thumb is that each week of cycling-specific training missed requires 1 to 2 weeks of training to return to previous form. A preparticipation physical examination can forestall problems. The athlete can benefit from developing a sensible training plan. If a history of overuse injuries exists, early-season stretching and strengthening programs can be useful. A stretching routine before and after riding for all riders can promote continuous pain-free riding.

▶ These authors studied overuse injuries in cycling and identified factors that clinicians need to consider when evaluating cyclists and returning them to cycling after their injuries. The authors recommend that clinicians take into consideration not only the cyclist's biomechanical factors and training issues but also have an understanding of bicycle fitting and how that contributes to injuries.

R. C. Cantu, MD, MA

Mountain Bike Injuries and Clipless Pedals: A Review of Three Cases
Patel ND (Cardiff, Wales)
Br J Sports Med 38:340-341, 2004   1–33

Background.—The injuries associated with off-road mountain biking are generally skin abrasions and contusions from falling off the bike. However,

3 cases were reported in which the cycle itself was the cause of significant soft tissue injuries.

> *Case Reports.*—The 3 men ranged in age from 23 to 42 years, and their injuries occurred within 10 months of each other. In each case, the rider lost control of the cycle at moderate to high speed and came off to the side rather than over the handlebars. All had major soft tissue injuries to their right lower legs but no other injuries. In 2, ragged lacerations extended over the medial border of the tibia. One had delayed primary closure, and 1 required split-skin grafting. The third rider had an injury that extended more proximally and that included damage to the middle third of the patellar tendon. Primary closure was achieved, but the knee joint was thoroughly irrigated to prevent joint contamination. All riders received antibiotics and were able to return to cycling within 3 months of their injuries.

Mechanisms.—All 3 cyclists used a clipless pedal system, in which it is necessary to twist the foot to release the foot from the pedal. In each of the cases, the cyclist struggled to release the foot quickly when he lost control. To maintain balance, the cyclist forcibly placed his foot on the ground; however, the right leg did not have time to clear the cycle, and it became caught on the exposed teeth of the chain ring. The resulting injuries can be simple abrasions or the serious soft tissue injuries described in these cases.

Conclusions.—The safe and effective use of clipless pedals may require better information to be supplied to the rider, correct adjustment of the pedals to facilitate quick release, or the addition of a chain ring guard. In the cases described, serious soft tissue injuries were caused by the inability to extract the foot from the clipless pedal in time for the right leg to clear the chain ring.

▶ This article affords a comprehensive discussion of mountain biking injuries from the use of clipless pedals; thus, it serves as a useful reference source on this topic.

R. C. Cantu, MD, MA

Tree Stand Falls: A Persistent Cause of Sports Injury

Metz M, Kross M, Abt P, et al (Univ of Rochester, NY; Washington County Hosp, Hagertown, Md; Univ of Miami, Fla)
South Med J 97:715-719, 2004   1–34

Objective.—Tree stand falls are a well-known cause of hunting-related injury. Spine and brain injuries associated with these falls result in a significant incidence of permanent disability. Prior studies indicate that hunting tree stand injuries are largely preventable with the proper use of safety belts; however, compliance with safety belt use is variable. The purposes of this study were to determine 1) current compliance with safety belt use, 2) alterations in the spectrum of injury, and 3) causes of the falls.

Methods.—From January 1996 to October 2001, 51 tree stand-related injuries referred to either of two regional trauma centers or their region's medical examiner's office were reviewed. Data had been recorded in each hospital's trauma registry, and the registries were searched for falls. Medical records were reviewed for additional data retrospectively, with an emphasis on determining the use of safety belts, and mechanisms contributing to the fall.

Results.—Fifty-one cases of tree stand-associated injuries were identified. These injuries all occurred in men, with a mean age of 42.6 years (range, 22-69 years). Alcohol use was present in 10% of patients and in two of the three deaths. The mean Injury Severity Score was 18.1 (range, 2-75). The most common injuries were spinal fractures (51% of series) and extremity fractures (41% of series). Closed head injuries were identified in 24% and lung injuries were identified in 22% of patients. Abdominal visceral injuries were present in 8% and genitourinary injuries were present in 4%. Three patients died. In addition to injury from the fall, a significant number (six patients [12%]) had additional morbidity from exposure. Only two patients reported the use of a safety belt (4% of series). There were no cases of gunshot wounds in this review, either self-inflicted or hunter-related. The chief reasons reported for these falls were errors in placement that resulted in structural failure of the stand, or errors made while climbing into or out of the stand (50% of falls).

Conclusion.—Devastating spine and brain injuries continue to occur after falls from tree stands during recreational hunting when safety belts are not used. Our results suggest a continuing need for the education of hunters concerning safe tree stand hunting practices, including proper methods of stand placement, assessment of tree branch strength, avoidance of fatigue and alcohol, anticipation of firearm recoil, and proper methods of stand entrance and exit. Trauma prevention programs directed toward heightened public awareness of these injuries during hunting season are still needed.

▶ Standing high in trees as a vantage point is apparently useful in big game hunting in the United States. Such positions, often 10 to 15 feet above the forest floor, provide a wide field of view and minimize the hunter's scent on the ground. One can also purchase commercially made stands that strap or bolt onto a convenient tree and can be optionally fitted with a safety strap in case the rig collapses or the hunter slips. This study reports 51 injuries to hunters falling from these devices. Spinal injuries were the most common result, with limb fractures a close second. Closed head injury was the third most common injury. A significant number of injuries occurred related to alcohol consumption. Intriguingly, 3 of 51 hunters fell asleep and then fell out of the stand, and 2 of 51 were knocked out of the stand by the rifle recoil. Clearly, an education campaign would be of benefit to minimize risky behavior (eg, alcohol use) or to ensure safe methods of accessing these stands. One disturbing complication of the safety strap device was asphyxiation—when the strap prevented the fall, it slipped up around one hunter's neck, resulting in strangulation.

P. McCrory, MBBS, PhD

Exercises to Prevent Lower Limb Injuries in Youth Sports: Cluster Randomised Controlled Trial
Olsen O-E, Myklebust G, Engebretsen L, et al (Norwegian Univ of Sport and Physical Education, Oslo, Norway)
BMJ 330:449-452, 2005   1–35

Objective.—To investigate the effect of a structured warm-up programme designed to reduce the incidence of knee and ankle injuries in young people participating in sports.

Design.—Cluster randomised controlled trial with clubs as the unit of randomisation.

Setting.—120 team handball clubs from central and eastern Norway (61 clubs in the intervention group, 59 in the control group) followed for one league season (eight months).

Participants.—1837 players aged 15-17 years; 958 players (808 female and 150 male) in the intervention group; 879 players (778 female and 101 male) in the control group.

Intervention.—A structured warm-up programme to improve running, cutting, and landing technique as well as neuromuscular control, balance, and strength.

Main Outcome Measure.—The rate of acute injuries to the knee or ankle.

Results.—During the season, 129 acute knee or ankle injuries occurred, 81 injuries in the control group (0.9 (SE 0.09) injuries per 1000 player hours; 0.3 (SE 0.17) in training v 5.3 (SE 0.06) during matches) and 48 injuries in the intervention group (0.5 (SE 0.11) injuries per 1000 player hours; 0.2 (SE 0.18) in training v 2.5 (SE 0.06) during matches) (Table 2). Fewer injured players were in the intervention group than in the control group (46 (4.8%) v (76 (8.6%); relative risk intervention group v control group 0.53, 95% confidence interval 0.35 to 0.81).

Conclusion.—A structured programme of warm-up exercises can prevent knee and ankle injuries in young people playing sports. Preventive training should therefore be introduced as an integral part of youth sports programmes.

▶ This is a critical study designed to prospectively test the usefulness of a structured warm-up program on the incidence of knee and ankle injuries in young athletes. Given that preparticipation stretching has not been found to be a useful injury countermeasure,[1] the efficacy of warm-up as a strategy has been questioned. In this study, 1837 Norwegian adolescents playing handball were followed up over the course of a competitive season. Clubs were randomly assigned to perform either a 20-minute structured warm-up (designed to improve running, cutting, and landing technique as well as balance and

TABLE 2.—Number of Acute Injuries, Acute Knee or Ankle Injuries, and Incidence of Injuries During Matches and Training

	Intervention Group (n=958)		Control Group (n=879)		Rate Ratio(95% CI)*	P Value (z Test)
	Injuries	Incidence	Injuries	Incidence		
No of acute injuries:	85	0.9 (0.08)	156	1.8 (0.06)	0.51 (0.39 to 0.66)	<0.0001
Match	53	4.7 (0.06)	111	10.3 (0.04)	0.46 (0.33 to 0.64)	<0.0001
Training	32	0.4 (0.14)	45	0.6 (0.12)	0.66 (0.42 to 1.04)	0.07
No of acute knee or ankle injuries:	48	0.5 (0.11)	81	0.9 (0.09)	0.55 (0.39 to 0.79)	0.001
Match	28	2.5 (0.06)	57	5.3 (0.06)	0.47 (0.30 to 0.74)	0.001
Training	20	0.2 (0.18)	24	0.3 (0.17)	0.78 (0.43 to 1.41)	0.41

Note: Incidence is reported as the number of injuries per 1000 player hours, with standard errors.
*Rate ratio obtained from Poisson model.
Abbreviation: CI, Confidence interval.
(Courtesy of Olsen O-E, Myklebust G, Engebretsen L, et al: Exercises to prevent lower limb injuries in youth sports: Cluster randomised controlled trial. *BMJ* 330:449-452, 2005, with permission from the BMJ Publishing Group.)

strength) or their usual training strategy. The striking finding was that the structured warm-up group had a 50% reduction in knee and ankle injuries, and this was most marked in game play situations. This supports the premise that warm-up should be a routine part of preparticipation training.

P. McCrory, MBBS, PhD

Reference

1. Shrier I: Stretching before exercise does not reduce the risk of local muscle injury: A critical review of the clinical and basic science literature. *Clin J Sports Med* 9:221-227, 1999.

Sport-Induced Lipoma

Copcu E (Adnan Menderes Univ, Aydin, Turkey)
Int J Sports Med 25:182-185, 2004   1–36

Background.—Lipoma of the subcutaneous fat is a common human neoplasm. Trauma may be a significant factor in lipoma etiology. The cases of 2 athletes who had fast-growing lipomas in the right scapular area were discussed.

Case 1.—Woman, 21, professional table-tennis player, had a large right subcutaneous mass in the scapular area. She had no history of lipoma, no blunt trauma to the back and no functional impairment. The tumor was very fast growing. Physical examination revealed a 12 × 10 cm soft-tissue mass with a smooth surface located between the bone and the skin. It had poor mobility but did not adhere to the skin. Systemic and laboratory tests were normal. US confirmed a diagnosis of lipoma. At surgery, histologic analysis also confirmed the diagnosis. No postsurgical complications occurred. Lipoma did not recur within 6 months of follow-up.

Case 2.—Woman, 24, professional volleyball player, had a subcutaneous mass in her right-scapular area. She had no history of lipoma and no other signs or symptoms. She noticed the mass 6 months before admission and went to the clinic because of its fast growth. Systemic and laboratory tests were normal. Physical examination indicated a 15 × 12 cm soft-tissue mass in her right-scapular area. Like Case 1, the tumor was mobile and did not adhere to the skin. US and a subsequent histologic analysis at surgery confirmed the diagnosis of lipoma. No postsurgical complications occurred, and no recurrence was detected within 6 months of follow-up.

Conclusions.—These reports describe fast-growing lipomas that occurred in athletes. Lipomas may be triggered by chronic microtrauma of the subcutaneous fat tissue combined with exercise-induced hormones. Treatment was by complete surgical removal.

▶ These are case study reports of 2 athletes with a fast-growing lipoma on their scapular area. One athlete was a professional volleyball player, and the other was a table-tennis player. The article discusses reasons for the formation of these lipomas and also discusses their treatment.

R. C. Cantu, MD, MA

2 Injuries to the Head, Neck, and Spine

Mechanisms of Head Injuries in Elite Football
Andersen TE, Árnason Á, Engebretsen L, et al (Norwegian Univ, Oslo, Norway)
Br J Sports Med 38:690-696, 2004   2–1

Objectives.—The aim of this study was to describe, using video analysis, the mechanisms of head injuries and of incidents with a high risk of head injury in elite football.

Methods.—Videotapes and injury information were collected prospectively for 313 of the 409 matches played in the Norwegian (2000 season) and Icelandic (1999 and 2000 season) professional leagues. Video recordings of incidents where a player appeared to be hit in the head and the match was consequently interrupted by the referee were analysed and cross referenced with reports of acute time loss injuries from the team medical staff.

Results.—The video analysis revealed 192 incidents (18.8 per 1000 player hours). Of the 297 acute injuries reported, 17 (6%) were head injuries, which corresponds to an incidence of 1.7 per 1000 player hours (concussion incidence 0.5 per 1000 player hours). The most common playing action was a heading duel with 112 cases (58%). The body part that hit the injured player's head was the elbow/arm/hand in 79 cases (41%), the head in 62 cases

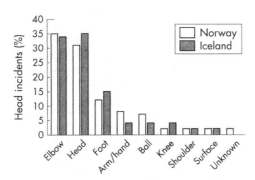

FIGURE 2.—The opponent body part hitting the head of the exposed player in Norway (n = 124 incidents, *white bars*) and in Iceland (n = 68 incidents, *gray bars*). (Courtesy of Andersen TE, Árnason Á, Engebretsen L, et al: Mechanisms of head injuries in elite football. *Br J Sports Med* 38:690-696, 2004, with permission from the BMJ Publishing Group.)

(32%), and the foot in 25 cases (13%) (Fig 2). In 67 of the elbow/arm/hand impacts, the upper arm of the player causing the incident was at or above shoulder level, and the arm use was considered to be active in 61 incidents (77%) and intentional in 16 incidents (20%).

Conclusions.—This study suggests that video analysis provides detailed information about the mechanisms for head injuries in football. The most frequent injury mechanism was elbow to head contact, followed by head to head contact in heading duels. In the majority of the elbow to head incidents, the elbow was used actively at or above shoulder level, and stricter rule enforcement or even changes in the laws of the game concerning elbow use should perhaps be considered, in order to reduce the risk of head injury.

▶ This is an excellent study prospectively examining the mechanisms of head injury in soccer. The authors collected TV videotape of 313 matches played in Norway and Iceland over a 2-year period in the elite professional leagues. From these, 192 head injury incidents (19 per 1000 player hours) were noted when a head contact occurred and the referee had to stop the match while the player was treated or removed from the field. Of these incidents, a total of 17 head injuries were noted including 5 concussions (concussion incidence, 0.5 per 1000 player hours). Of the 192 head contacts, 43% were upper limb to head contact and 32% were head to head contact. In the majority of cases, no free kick was awarded to the injured player. It was proposed by the authors that rule enforcement and penalizing arm-head contact may be an effective injury prevention strategy.

P. McCrory, MBBS, PhD

The Management of Facial Injuries in Rugby Union
Hayton MJ, Stevenson HI, Jones CD, et al (Musculo-Skeletal Science, Crosby, England; Arrows Park Hosp, Liverpool, England)
Br J Sports Med 38:314-317, 2004   2–2

Introduction.—Guidelines have yet to be defined within the rugby union concerning the management of facial lacerations, which account for one third of total injuries. A number of facial injuries treated at rugby union have been treated in an inadequate fashion with poor wound cleaning, inappropriate suture material, and advice concerning suture removal. These issues, along with the use of sterile suture equipment, were addressed in a questionnaire.

Methods.—A postal questionnaire was sent to the medical officers of 64 rugby union clubs at the end of the 2001/2002 season. Questions were open-ended to permit free self-explanation of current practice.

Results.—The response rate was 57% (39/68 questionnaires). Respondents providing medical assistance came from a variety of backgrounds; most were general practitioners. Some practitioners were paid, but most had honorary posts. Most rugby clubs had dedicated medical rooms. Most respondents suture facial wounds at the club, use local anesthetic, use gloves, irrigate the wounds with sterile saline or water, use monofilament sutures on facial skin (not mucosal areas) or steristrips, do not use glue on the face, allow immediate return to play, and advise suture removal before game/training if ready for removal rather than after the game.

When used, sterile suture packs were usually sterilized by the practitioner or the hospital. About the same proportion of respondents did and did not use a dry dressing and did and did not use ointment. The suture size used varied; most used either 6/0 or 5/0 suture material. Nearly all respondents had been shown suture techniques; 25 would and 14 would not consider attending a short techniques class. Twenty clubs paid for equipment and 19 did not pay.

Recommendations/Conclusion.—A dedicated medical room should be available, physicians should always use gloves and local anesthetic, and sterile suture packs and instruments should be provided. Small monofilament sutures are recommended. Complex facial lacerations require special management. Rugby players should be encouraged to wear protective gear. Some physicians may benefit from a suture techniques course.

▶ These authors present guidelines to be used for caring for facial injuries in rugby union players including wound cleansing, use of sterile equipment, appropriate suture materials, and suture removal.

R. C. Cantu, MD, MA

Sports Related Maxillofacial Injuries: The First Maxillofacial Trauma Database in Switzerland
Exadaktylos AK, Eggensperger NM, Eggli S, et al (Univ Hosp Bern, Switzerland)
Br J Sports Med 38:750-753, 2004   2–3

Background.—With the increase in the amount of medical data handled by emergency units, advances in computerisation have become necessary. New computer technology should have a major influence on accident analysis and prevention and the quality of research in the future.

Objectives.—To investigate the occurrence of sports related maxillofacial injuries using a newly installed relational database. To establish the first sports trauma database in Switzerland.

Methods.—The Qualicare databank was used to prospectively review 57 248 case histories of patients treated in the Department of Emergency Medicine between January 2000 and December 2002. Pre-defined key words were used to collect data on sports related maxillofacial injuries.

Results.—A total of 750 patients with maxillofacial injuries were identified. Ninety (12%) were sports related maxillofacial fractures. Most (27%) were sustained during skiing and snowboarding, 22% during team sports such as soccer or ice hockey, and 21% were from cycling accidents. Sixty eight per cent of the cyclists, 50% of the ice hockey players and soccer players, and 48% of the skiers and snowboarders had isolated fractures of the midface. Fractures of the mandible were noted predominantly in contact sports.

Conclusions.—Computerisation of trauma and emergency units and the introduction of customised software can significantly reduce the workload of researchers and doctors. The effective use of new computer technology should have a considerable influence on research and the quality of future prospective and retrospective studies.

▶ Although the title of this study reads as though maxillofacial injuries are the main focus, in fact it really describes the implementation of a computerized software strategy to assist clinicians in the emergency department and researchers to develop injury surveillance techniques as well as injury countermeasures. This software combines a medical recordkeeping facility with a relational database capacity to search for meaningful injury data. In the example given, the software enabled the rapid understanding of incidence, risk factors, and disposition of maxillofacial injuries, a fairly rare sporting injury that has not been well studied previously.

P. McCrory, MBBS, PhD

Statistical Procedures for Determining the Extent of Cognitive Change Following Concussion
Collie A, Maruff P, Makdissi M, et al (Univ of Melbourne, Parkville, Victoria, Australia; CogState Ltd, Carlton South, Victoria, Australia; La Trobe Univ, Bundoora, Victoria, Australia)
Br J Sports Med 38:273-278, 2004   2–4

Background.—An estimated 300,000 sports-related concussions are reported annually in the United States. However, this figure may underestimate the incidence of concussions because of nonreporting or lack of awareness of concussive symptoms. Other studies have also suggested that the incidence of concussions in junior and community-based sports may also be higher than in previous estimates. Considerable attention has been given to methodological problems associated with the assessment of cognitive functioning before and after a concussion, but there has been much less investigation of the statistical techniques used to guide decisions about the presence or absence of cognitive impairment after a concussion.

Overview.—Neuropsychological (NP) testing is often used to aid in determining whether the cognitive functioning of a concussed athlete has declined. The NP test score after a concussion is compared with the baseline test score. In many cases, clinicians simply subtract one from the other and make a clinical decision about the significance or nonsignificance of the resulting difference score. However, these techniques do not account for the many factors that may affect interpretation of serially acquired cognitive test scores. A number of alternative approaches used in other areas of medicine for differentiating "true" changes from those caused by these confounding factors are presented, along with a case example to demonstrate the effect that the statistical approach may have on clinical decision making.

Conclusions.—The use of appropriate techniques for the determination of both the clinical and statistical significance of a change in the NP test score after a concussion is advocated. Among these techniques are reliable change calculations and regression methods, which are designed to minimize sources of measurement error. The use of inappropriate techniques in determining the extent of a cognitive change after a concussion may lead to erroneous clinical decisions that could endanger an athlete's health.

▶ This article discusses NP testing to determine the extent of cognitive changes after a concussion. Because of the many confounding factors involved, it is inadequate to simply compare baseline test scores to scores after a concussion. The article discusses alternative approaches to determine true cognitive changes after a concussion and the effect on clinical decision making.

R. C. Cantu, MD, MA

A Prospective Controlled Study of Cognitive Function During an Amateur Boxing Tournament
Moriarity J, Collie A, Olson D, et al (Univ of Notre Dame, Ind; CogState Ltd, Melbourne, Australia; Univ of Melbourne, Australia; et al)
Neurology 62:1497-1502, 2004   2–5

Background.—It is well known that chronic neurocognitive sequelae may accompany participation in the sport of boxing. Among these sequelae are the clinical effects of chronic traumatic encephalopathy (the "punch drunk" syndrome), neuropathologic injury, and cognitive impairment. There has been speculation that many of these neurologic and cognitive phenomena may reflect a genetic risk rather than exposure to head impact.

Few studies have reported acute postbout cognitive effects in amateur boxers, and none have documented the effects of repeated boxing bouts within a short time frame. Whether participation in a 7-day amateur boxing tournament is associated with acute deterioration in cognitive test performance was investigated.

Methods.—A prospective study was conducted of 82 collegiate amateur boxers participating in a 7-day single elimination tournament and a group of 30 matched nonboxing control participants. None of the participants had a history of recent concussion or past history of brain injury. For the boxers, cognitive assessment using a computerized test battery was performed before the tournament and within 2 hours of completing each bout.

The subjects completed tests of simple and choice reaction time, working memory tasks, and learning. Analysis of variance was used to compare the serial performance of control participants with that of the boxers after 1, 2, and 3 bouts.

Results.—The 82 boxers participated in 159 fights. Cognitive testing was performed after 142 of these bouts. The serial performance of boxers participating in 3 bouts was equivalent to that of boxers participating in 2 bouts and 1 bout and to nonboxing control participants in the areas of simple reaction time, choice reaction time, and working memory tasks. There was an observable improvement in the learning task for boxers participating in 3 bouts. Boxers whose bout was stopped by the referee demonstrated significant slowing in simple and choice reaction time.

Conclusion.—With the exception of boxers whose bouts were stopped by the referee, amateur boxers who participated in multiple bouts during a 7-day tournament showed no evidence of cognitive dysfunction immediately after the bout.

▶ Eighty-two amateur boxers participating in a 7-day amateur boxing tournament were studied and no deterioration in cognitive function in the postbout period was seen.

R. C. Cantu, MD, MA

Ocular Complications of Boxing
Bianco M, Vaiano AS, Colella F, et al (Catholic Univ, Rome)
Br J Sports Med 39:70-74, 2005   2–6

Objectives.—To investigate the prevalence of ocular injuries in a large population of boxers over a period of 16 years, in particular, the most severe lesions that may be vision threatening.

Methods.—Clinical records of the medical archive of the Italian Boxing Federation were analysed. A total of 1032 boxers were examined from February 1982 to October 1998. A complete ophthalmological history was available for 956, who formed the study population (a total of 10 697 examinations). The following data were collected: age when started boxing; duration of competitive boxing career (from the date of the first bout); weight category; a thorough ocular history. The following investigations were carried out: measurement of visual acuity and visual fields, anterior segment inspection, applanation tonometry, gonioscopy, and examination of ocular fundus. Eighty age matched healthy subjects, who had never boxed, formed the control group.

Results.—Of the 956 boxers examined, 428 were amateur (44.8%) and 528 professional (55.2%). The median age at first examination was 23.1 (4.3) years (range 15-36). The prevalence of conjunctival, corneal, lenticular, vitreal, ocular papilla, and retinal alterations in the study population was 40.9% compared with 3.1% in the control group ($p \leq 0.0001$). The prevalence of serious ocular findings (angle, lens, macula, and peripheral retina alterations) was 5.6% in boxers and 3.1% in controls (NS).

Conclusions.—Boxing does not result in a higher prevalence of severe ocular lesions than in the general population. However, the prevalence of milder lesions (in particular with regard to the conjunctiva and cornea) is noteworthy, justifying the need for adequate ophthalmological surveillance.

▶ One of the underrecognized medical problems in boxing is the presence of ophthalmologic injury.[1-3] In this study, more than 1000 Italian amateur (45%) and professional (55%) boxers were assessed over a 16-year period during their ring careers, and 40.9% were found to have demonstrable ocular pathology. In a group of matched controls, the incidence of ocular abnormalities was 3.1% ($P < .0001$). With regard to serious eye injuries (those threatening vision), the incidence was 5.6% in boxers and 3.1% in controls (not statistically significant). This study demonstrates the usefulness of a formal ophthalmologic assessment as a routine part of the assessment of boxers, both at the commencement of and serially throughout their careers.

P. McCrory, MBBS, PhD

References

1. Unterharnscheidt F: A neurologist's reflections on boxing. V. Concluding remarks. *Rev Neurol* 23:1027-1032, 1995.
2. Whiteson A: Ocular injuries from boxing. *BMJ* 304:574, 1992.
3. Giovinazzo VJ, Yannuzzi LA, Sorenson JA, et al: The ocular complications of boxing. *Ophthalmology* 94:587-596, 1987.

Summary and Agreement Statement of the 2nd International Conference on Concussion in Sport, Prague 2004
McCrory P, Johnston K, Meeuwisse W, et al (Univ of Melbourne, Australia; McGill Univ, Montreal; Univ of Calgary, Alta, Canada; et al)
Br J Sports Med 39:196-204, 2005   2–7

Background.—The consensus recommendations of the 1st International Symposium on Concussion in Sport are updated in this report. This report, known as the Prague agreement statement, is intended to expand on the principles outlined in the original consensus recommendations.

Overview.—The 1st International Symposium on Concussion in Sport was held in Vienna, Austria, in 2001. The original goals of the symposium were to provide recommendations for improving the safety and health of athletes who had a concussion in a variety of sports, including ice hockey and soccer. The current document is reflective of the expanded representation at the second meeting of trauma surgeons, sports psychologists, and other interested disciplines. The recommendations from the Vienna meeting that injury grading scales for concussion be abandoned in favor of combined measures of recovery to determine injury severity and to individualize recommendations regarding a return to play. A new classification of concussion in sport is presented, including simple versus complex concussion. In simple concussion, the athlete's injury progressively resolves without complication in 7 to 10 days. In complex concussion, the athlete experiences persistent symptoms, specific sequelae, prolonged loss of consciousness, or prolonged cognitive impairment after injury. The importance of a preparticipation physical examination, including a concussion history, is stressed. To aid the diagnosis, a sport concussion assessment tool (SCAT) was developed as a standardized tool for patient education, as well as physician assessment of sports concussion. Management of concussion, including protocol for the return of the athlete to participation and the roles of pharmacologic treatment and sports psychology, are discussed. At present, there is no clinical evidence that the currently available protective equipment will prevent concussion. However, protective equipment in certain sports may prevent other forms of head injury, which may be an important issue for those sports. Risk compensation is an important concept in the consideration of the use of protective equipment.

Conclusion.—A revised and updated version of the consensus recommendations of the International Symposium on Concussion in Sport is presented. These revised recommendations from the second meeting in Prague were intended to expand on recommendations developed at the first Vienna symposium.

▶ This article is a summary statement from the recent international consensus meeting on sports-related concussion that was held in Prague in November 2004 sponsored by the International Ice Hockey Federation, FIFA (Fédération International de Football Association), and the International Olympic Commission. It is a revision and update of the document produced after the 1st International Conference on Concussion in Sport held in Vienna in 2001.[1] The article discusses the definition, severity grading, symptoms, and management of concussion. For the first time, pediatric concussive injury is discussed and the document also provides a sideline assessment card that summarizes the previous work in this area. The article is also notable for a speculative new categorization of concussion subtype based on clinical presentation. The article represents an international consensus based on conference discussions by most, if not all, the major clinicians and researchers in this field.

P. McCrory, MBBS, PhD

Reference

1. Aubry M, Cantu R, Dvorak J, et al: Summary and agreement statement of the first International Conference on Concussion in Sport, Vienna 2001. *Br J Sports Med* 36:6-10, 2002.

Concussion in Professional Football: Injuries Involving 7 or More Days Out—Part 5

Pellman EJ, Viano DC, Casson IR, et al (ProHEALTH Care Associates LLP, Lake Success, NY; ProBiomechanics LLC, Bloomfield Hills, Mich; New York Univ; et al)
Neurosurgery 55:1100-1119, 2004   2–8

Introduction.—Most athletes who receive a concussion (mild traumatic brain injury [MTBI]) have a relatively quick recovery and return to play in a short period. The small group of National Football League (NFL) players who do not return to play for 7 or more days after MTBI were compared during a 6-year period with the majority of NFL players who do return to play within 7 days to help determine the demographic and clinical differences between the 2 groups that could explain the extended period of missed playing. This information may provide prognostic factors and aid physicians in the early evaluation, grading, and management of MTBI in professional athletes.

Methods.—The 7-day dividing line between players does not reflect an arbitrary distinction. Because NFL teams play games only once weekly, all participants missed at least 1 game, which is considered a significant loss of playing time because the season has only 16 games. Between 1996 and 2001, the reporting of concussion was performed by NFL teams by a special standardized reporting form completed by team physicians. Signs and symptoms were grouped according to general symptoms, somatic complaints, cranial nerve effects, cognitive problems, memory problems, and unconsciousness. Medical action and management of MTBI were documented. A total of 887 MTBIs were reported in practices and games during the 6-year evaluation period.

Results.—Seventy-two concussions (8.1%) involved more than 7 days away from play. The highest incidence was among quarterbacks (14.8%), the return unit on special teams (11.8%), and secondary players (10.8%). Quarterbacks had the highest odds ratio (OR) of more than 7 days out with MTBI (OR, 2.10; $P = .049$); running backs had the lowest relative risk (OR, 0.13; $P = .021$). The highest fraction of more than 7 days out involved passing plays (36.1%) and kickoffs (22.2%). Several signs and symptoms occurred at a higher frequency on initial examination in players out for more than 7 days; the average number per player was 4.46 with more than 7 days out compared with 2.58 among those who played within 7 days ($t = 6.02$; degrees of frequency, 77.1). The signs and symptoms with the highest incidence among those in the group out more than 7 days were disorientation to time, retrograde amnesia, fatigue, and the general category of cognitive problems (all, $P = .001$). Loss of consciousness for more than 1 minute was a predictor of more than 7 days out ($P = .001$); this occurred in 7.9% of cases. Among players with more than 7 days out, 72.2% were removed from the game and 12.5% were hospitalized. These rates were significantly higher than those for players with fewer than 7 days out ($P < .0001$). Management for approximately 90% of players was rest, regardless of the number of days out; those with more than 7 days out were more likely to receive drug or medical therapies.

Conclusion.—Quarterbacks and secondary players were the most vulnerable for more than 7 days out with MTBI among professional football players. Although 8.6% of MTBIs involved more than 7 days out, only 1.6% involved a prolonged postconcussion syndrome. These players recovered from symptoms and had a consistent return to NFL play.

▶ This article discusses concussion in NFL players and deals with those football players held out 7 or more days after a concussion. As with the other clinical articles in this series, the limitations section is 6 paragraphs and nearly a page in length and bears careful reading and reflection.

R. C. Cantu, MD, MA

Can We Manage Sport Related Concussion in Children the Same as in Adults?

McCrory P, Collie A, Anderson V, et al (Univ of Melbourne, Parkville, Victoria, Australia; CogState Ltd, Carlton South, Victoria, Australia; Royal Children's Hosp, Parkville, Victoria, Australia; et al)
Br J Sports Med 38:516-519, 2004   2–9

Background.—The consensus guidelines for the management of sport-related concussion in adults have been widely implemented. However, there are no guidelines for the management of sport-related concussion in children. The presence of important anatomic, physiologic, and behavioral differences between adults and children suggest that the guidelines for adults will need modification or revision to facilitate management of sport-related concussion in children.

Overview.—The estimated incidence of traumatic brain injury (TBI) in children age 15 years and under is 180 per 100,000 children per year, of which about 85% are classified as mild injuries. In the United States, it is estimated that over 1 million children per year sustain a TBI, accounting for over 250,000 pediatric hospital admissions and more than 10% of all visits to emergency departments. The most common cognitive sequelae of concussion in children are the same as those for adults, including reduced speed of information processing, poor attention, and impaired executive function. However, these processes are crucial to educational and social achievement in children, which magnifies the detrimental effects of concussion on this age group (Fig 1). In addition, brain tolerance to biomechanical force differs between adults and children. A 2 to 3-fold greater force of impact is required to produce clinical symptoms in children compared with adults. Thus, if a child manifests clinical symptoms after head trauma, it is a reasonable assumption that the child has sustained a much greater impact force compared with an adult with the same postconcussive symptoms. Further complicating the picture is the fact that the brain is cognitively maturing during childhood, which makes assessment of the cognitive effects of concussion more difficult in chil-

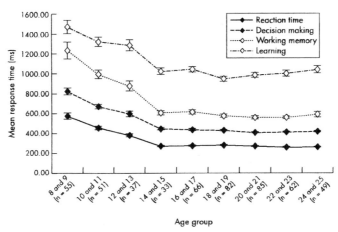

FIGURE 1.—Mean (and standard error) response speed on four cognitive tasks in nine different age bands, from 8 to 25 years of age. (Courtesy of McCrory P, Collie A, Anderson V, et al: Can we manage sport related concussion in children the same as in adults? *Br J Sports Med* 38:516-519, 2004. Reprinted with permission from the BMJ Publishing Group.)

dren. In terms of the risk factors for sequelae and poor recovery after concussion in children, there is circumstantial evidence that a prior history of brain injury is a risk factor for subsequent concussive injury in children. Other risk factors are the fact that the child's brain is less mature and that premorbid cognitive, attention, and behavioral impairments may be present.

Conclusions.—At present there are no evidence-based guidelines for the treatment of sport-related concussion in children and adolescence. It has been suggested that concussive symptoms take longer to resolve in children than in adults, so it is critical that they not resume sport participation until all of their physical symptoms are fully resolved. There is a need for increased awareness of the issues presented in this report among those involved in the management of sport-related concussion in children so that the sequelae and poor recovery that can be associated with these injuries can be avoided.

▶ The management of sport-related concussion in adults has evolved significantly in the past decade; however, similar pediatric injury has received little or no interest. Concussive injury is relatively common in children and adolescents and there are particular concerns in these age groups given that far more of the task of daily life is acquiring knowledge and learning new skills and even a temporary disruption of cognitive function may lead to substantial consequences in terms of academic progress, social competence, and self-esteem. This article summarizes the literature in regard to this topic and provides new information regarding cognitive maturation throughout this period. In broad terms, the generic adult concussion guidelines of no play or training (or school) until symptom free, both at rest and exercise is appropriate in this age group. It becomes more problematic when considering cognitive testing in the same manner as used in adult concussion given the rapidly changing cognitive maturation that may confound accurate assessment. This article is the first in the sports medicine literature raising this important topic and many of the questions posed require further study.

P. McCrory, MBBS, PhD

Decreased Neck Muscle Strength Is Highly Associated With Pain in Cervical Dystonia Patients Treated With Botulinum Toxin Injections

Häkkinen A, Ylinen J, Rinta-Keturi M, et al (Central Hosp, Jyväskylä, Finland; Univ of Jyväskylä, Finland; Rheumatism Found Hosp, Heinola (Kautiainen), Finland)
Arch Phys Med Rehabil 85:1684-1688, 2004   2–10

Objectives.—To compare the isometric neck muscle strength of cervical dystonia patients treated with botulinum toxin injections with that of healthy control subjects and to evaluate the association between neck strength, neck pain, and disability in these patients.

Design.—Clinical cross-sectional study.

Setting.—Outpatient rehabilitation and neurology clinics in a Finnish hospital.

Participants.—Twenty-three patients with cervical dystonia with botulinum toxin-treated neck muscles and 23 healthy control subjects.

Interventions.—Not applicable.

Main Outcome Measures.—Isometric neck strength was measured by a special neck strength measurement system (Fig 1). Disability was measured

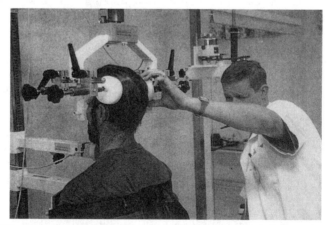

FIGURE 1.—Positioning of the subjects during the strength measurements in the isometric neck strength testing machine. The chest and waist were held with broad straps to eliminate contribution of the trunk musculature. (Reprinted from Häkkinen A, Ylinen J, Rinta-Keturi M, et al: Decreased neck muscle strength is highly associated with pain in cervical dystonia patients treated with botulinum toxin injections. *Arch Phys Med Rehabil* 85:1684-1688, 2004. Copyright 2004 with permission from The American Congress of Rehabilitation Medicine and the American Academy of Physical Medicine and Rehabilitation.)

by the Neck Disability Index, and pain and symptoms of cervical dystonia by a visual analog scale.

Results.—Isometric neck strength in all directions measured was significantly lower (25%-44%) in the cervical dystonia patients than in the healthy controls. Neck pain levels reported during the strength tests (*r* range, −.36 to −.70) and neck pain experienced during the preceding week (*r* range, −.52 to −.63) were inversely associated with isometric strength results. The difference between sides in rotation strength was 35% in the patient group (*P* < .001), whereas no significant difference between sides was found in the healthy controls. Fifty-one percent of the patients reported moderate or severe disability. Pain, stiffness, and incorrect position of the head were the most prominent symptoms.

Conclusions.—Cervical dystonia patients with botulinum toxin-treated neck muscles showed significantly lower maximal neck strength than healthy controls. The patients also had a statistically significant difference between sides in neck rotation strength. Thus, strength measures may be useful to detect disturbance in the function of the neck muscles.

▶ Cervical dystonia is characterized by tonic and intermittent spasms of the neck muscles that typically cause an involuntary deviation of the head from center position. It is often treated with botulinum toxin (BTX) to reduce pain and muscle spasm. It was reported that isometric neck strength was significantly less in all directions in cervical dystonia patients treated with BTX injections compared with that of healthy controls. In addition, there was a large variation in maximal strength and a higher difference between sides in rotation strength. It was suggested that neck muscle strength should be monitored on a regular basis to determine the extent of function losses in this patient group.

M. J. L. Alexander, PhD

Experience With Cervical Stenosis and Temporary Paralysis in Athletes
Bailes JE (West Virginia Univ, Morgantown)
J Neurosurg: Spine 2:11-16, 2005   2–11

Object.—Transient spinal cord injury (TSCI) in athletes presents one of the most challenging clinical scenarios. Management difficulties in and subsequent return-to-play decisions are especially important in those with cervical canal stenosis.

Methods.—Ten athletes (nine male and one female patients) were evaluated for TSCI. The diagnostic survey included physical and neurological examinations, plain radiographs with flexion-extension dynamic studies, computerized tomography, and magnetic resonance (MR) imaging. Clinical courses were followed and, in those who returned to contact sports activities, subsequent experience was noted. Symptoms consisted of paralysis, weakness, or numbness in all four extremities, their duration ranging from 15 minutes to 48 hours. Radiography revealed no evidence of fracture/dislocation or ligamentous instability. Spinal stenosis of 8 to 13 mm in length at three or more levels was evident in all cases. Four patients returned to competition without recurrent TSCI (mean follow-up duration 40 months); six individuals retired. The occurrence of TSCI is not uncommon in athletes involved in contact sports. The diagnostic workup focuses on excluding fracture/dislocation, cord contusion, ligamentous infolding or instability, herniated nucleus pulposus, syrinx, or other surgically correctable lesions. There appear to be two groups of athletes who sustain TSCI: those who experience TSCI yet in whom radiographic studies are normal, and those with cervical stenosis, the most difficult management group.

Conclusions.—It does not appear that a single episode of TSCI in an athlete with spinal stenosis will substantially increase the risk of subsequent catastrophic spinal cord injury in those in whom MR imaging demonstrates preservation of cerebrospinal fluid signal.

▶ Transient cervical spinal cord injury is a rare but dramatic phenomenon, with an estimated incidence of 0.7 cases per 1000 athletes in US football.[1] Although occasionally seen, no epidemiologic studies exist for other sports. Athletes may present with motor or sensory symptoms that can last up to several days. Athletes who experience this condition fall into 2 radiologically defined groups: those with cervical canal stenosis and those with a normal spinal canal. Such differentiation is best made with MRI rather than CT or plain radiography. There are surprisingly few prospective studies to guide clinical management of this condition. Torg et al[2] reported that 35 of 63 patients (56%) with canal stenosis defined on *plain radiography* had recurrent episodes of transient cord injury after return to sports, and none sustained a permanent spinal cord injury. In another study, Torg et al[3] noted that in a survey of 117 athletes with permanent spinal cord injuries, none had reported a prior history of transient cord motor symptoms; however, 1 athlete had reported transient limb paresthesias. In this study, 6 of 10 athletes with canal stenosis reported recurrent episodes with continued sports participation. At the present time, there are only anecdotal guidelines (class 3 evidence) upon which to guide clinical recommendations. It is clear, however, that catastrophic spinal cord injury is not typically associated with prior episodes of transient cord injury and that cervical canal stenosis alone does not predict a high risk of future catastrophic spinal injury.

P. McCrory, MBBS, PhD

References

1. Cantu RC: Cervical spine injuries in the athlete. *Semin Neurol* 20:173-178, 2000.
2. Torg JS, Corcoran TA, Thibault LE, et al: Cervical cord neurapraxia: Classification, pathomechanics, morbidity and management guidelines. *J Neurosurg* 87:843-850, 1997.
3. Torg JS, Pavlov H, Genuario SE, et al: Neurapraxia of the cervical spinal cord with transient quadriplegia. *J Bone Joint Surg Am* 68:1354-1370, 1986.

Cervical Spinal Cord Injury in Sumo Wrestling: A Case Report

Nakagawa Y, Minami K, Arai T, et al (Kyoto Univ, Japan; Nippon Med School, Chiba, Japan; Kishiwada City Hosp, Osaka, Japan; et al)

Am J Sports Med 32:1054-1058, 2004   2–12

Introduction.—The increase in participation in sumo wrestling has resulted in a higher incidence in injuries. In sumo, dislocations of the spine and spinal cord are unusual. Reported was a case of dislocation of the lower cervical spine and cervical spinal cord injury in a collegiate sumo wrestler.

Case Report.—Man, 19, was a collegiate sumo wrestler who had been practicing sumo for 10 days. He was 166 cm tall and weighed 78 kg. During an intercollegiate sumo championship in October 1999, he competed with a 120-kg opponent during his third match of the day. The opponent pushed him and he escaped by going around the *dohyo* (sumo ring). They both stopped in the center of the dohyo and the patient got under his opponent in a position in which the back of his head was situated on the abdomen of his opponent. His opponent forced him to step outside the dohyo by fixing the back of his head. The patient fell down near the corner of the dohyo, which forced hyperflexion of his cervical spine.

Examination by a physician on the dohyo revealed that the patient was conscious, respiration was good, and mobility of his upper extremities was normal. His lower extremities were paralyzed. He had sensory loss below T4, and it was assumed he had motor loss below T2. He was immediately transported to the emergency department where he was given a high-dose steroid. Radiologic examination of the cervical spine revealed that the spinous process of T1 was displaced inferiorly (anteroposterior view). Dislocation of the seventh cervical spinal body was suspected and MRI was performed.

The patient had an anterior dislocation of C7 on T1 and a cervical spinal cord injury at the same level. Manual repositioning of the cervical spine with skull traction without anesthesia was not successful, and surgical repositioning and posterior fixation were subsequently performed. Postoperatively, his sensory loss was slightly improved below T7. Paralysis of his lower extremities did not improve.

On November 5, 1999, an anterior cervical body fusion was performed to stabilize the spine. After 1 year of rehabilitation, the patient was able to attend the university by using a wheelchair and drive a car modified for his handicap. There was no motor or sensory improvement at 1 year after the injury.

Conclusion.—It is recommended that measures be taken to improve the education of sumo wrestlers concerning preventive techniques to reduce the likelihood of cervical spinal cord injury.

▶ This is a case study of a 19-year-old collegiate sumo wrestler who suffered hyperextension of his cervical spine and subsequent C7-T1 dislocation with spinal cord injury. The authors discuss the mechanics of this rare injury in sumo wrestling and its prevention.

R. C. Cantu, MD, MA

Pseudarthrosis of the First Rib in the Overhead Athlete
Mithöfer K, Giza E (Hosp for Special Surgery, New York; Harvard Med School, Cambridge, Mass)
Br J Sports Med 38:221-222, 2004   2–13

Introduction.—Fractures of the first rib are rare in athletes and are different from traumatic first rib fracture associated with a high energy thoracic trauma. These fractures are induced by stress and precipitated via chronic muscular forces acting on the first rib. They usually heal with conservative treatment. Described was a fracture of the first rib in a tennis player in whom a symptomatic pseudarthrosis developed due to persistent overhead activities.

Case Report.—Man, 21, right dominant competitive tennis player, was seen for a persistent low-grade right shoulder pain of several months duration. He reported a popping sensation during preseason serving practice that had occurred 6 months previously. The patient had been practicing 5 times weekly, up to twice a day. He was treated conservatively at that time for a rotator cuff impingement.

The patient improved initially, yet continued to experience activity-associated right shoulder and neck pain, especially with overhead activities. The pain progressively interfered with his ability to compete. He had an unremarkable medical history with no prior shoulder or neck symptoms. Results of cervical spine and neurovascular examinations of his right upper extremity were normal. The shoulder range of motion was painful, especially with resisted forward flexion and abduction.

Impingement signs and cross arm adduction testing results were positive, and he had point tenderness in the right supraclavicular fossa. Radiographs revealed hypertrophic pseudarthosis of the right first rib. The patient avoided overhead activity for 2 weeks, then progressed to a supervised, sport-specific exercise program below the pain threshold for 4 weeks. At 6 weeks, he gradually advanced to overhead activity.

He was able to return to competitive tennis at 2 months. At 12-month follow-up, he remained free of pain and had no limitations with any overhead activities, despite radiographic persistence of the pseudarthosis.

Conclusion.—It appears that healing of the first rib fracture is not needed before return to athletic activity. The athlete may gradually return to the sport-specific activities at below symptom threshold level, thereby effectively preventing long periods of inactivity and prolonged absence from competition.

▶ A 21-year-old tennis player with low-grade shoulder pain with an initial diagnosis of rotator cuff impingement was found to have a first rib fracture/pseudarthrosis. The need to consider this rare condition in the overhead athletes with chronic shoulder pain is stressed.

R. C. Cantu, MD, MA

Acute Traumatic First-Rib Fracture in the Contact Athlete: A Case Report
Colosimo AJ, Byrne E, Heidt RS Jr, et al (Univ of Cincinnati, Ohio; Wellington Orthopaedic and Sports Medicine, Cincinnati, Ohio)
Am J Sports Med 32:1310-1312, 2004   2–14

Background.—Rarely is the first rib fractured during contact sports; the 2 cases reported here both occurred in football players. A traumatic first-rib fracture was sustained by a football player in a collision.

Case Report.—Adolescent male, 17 years, was playing high school varsity football and sustained a direct contact blow to his right shoulder and neck area when he collided with another player. He had immediate discomfort in the area but continued to play the last 2 quarters of the game. The next day, he noted a popping sensation and pain in his right shoulder and neck area. A physical examination revealed decreased cervical range of motion in extension, flexion, and left-side bending because of pain. The right shoulder was pain free and moved through a full range of motion. Tenderness was noted in the area of Erb's point and over the right distal sternocleidomastoid and scalene muscles, but no abnormal results were found on neurologic, vascular, or cardiovascular evaluations. An isolated, nondisplaced, right middle-third first-rib fracture was found fortuitously on routine cervical radiographs. He was given nonsteroidal anti-inflammatory drugs and physical therapy, including therapeutic modalities, massage, and stretching to reduce the pain and to increase cervical mobility. Full cervical motion was regained in 6 days, but the patient still had mild neck pain. At 12 weeks, he had full cervical and shoulder range of motion and normal strength but described soreness in the right first rib area with overhead activities and right arm paresthesias with heavy overhead weight lifting. A persistent fracture line was found on his 12-week radiograph and CT scan with 3-dimensional reconstruction. He was then limited to activities that did not provoke right arm symptoms. At 9 months, he had no complaints, and radiographs confirmed significant callus formation at the fracture line. He completed the football season with no further injuries.

Conclusions.—Contact athletes who have neck or shoulder pain should be evaluated for a possible isolated first-rib fracture if no other injuries are apparent. This athlete was able to return to sports once the first-rib fracture had sufficiently healed and after he no longer had pain or tenderness over the affected area.

▶ This is a case study of a 17-year-old high school varsity football linebacker who sustained a direct blow to his right shoulder and neck area when he collided with another player. A first-rib fracture is rare. The authors recommend that contact sport athletes who present with complaints of neck or shoulder pain should have the differential diagnosis of a first-rib fracture considered in their evaluation if no other cause is found.

R. C. Cantu, MD, MA

Collegiate Football Players Display More Active Cervical Spine Mobility Than High School Football Players
Nyland J, Johnson D (Univ of Louisville, Ky; Univ of Kentucky, Lexington)
J Athletic Train 39:146-150, 2004   2–15

Background.—Age has been established as a contributing factor to reductions in the active mobility of joints, including the cervical spine. The most dramatic reduction in active mobility in the cervical spine occura between 30 and 39 years and 40 and 49 years of age. The progression of cervical spine degeneration is accelerated by a history of excessive or repetitive loading caused by sports or occupation. Decreased range of motion in the cervical spine increases the difficulty in moving out of the way of the path of the torso during impact loading, which increases the risk of neck injury, an effect that is particularly germane to football players.

Adequate cervical spine mobility is crucial to neuromuscular readiness. Neck injuries are an unavoidable aspect of the sport, but effective preparticipation cervical spine screening may facilitate the detection of players who are at risk for sustaining a neck injury.

The active cervical spine range of motion and resting cervical spine alignment (sagittal plane) of collegiate and high school football players were compared by means of the Cervical Range of Motion (CROM) measurement system. Normative values for these populations were also identified.

Methods.—A convenience sample was collected of 189 unimpaired collegiate (70) and high school (119) football players. The subjects were measured for active cervical spine range of motion using the CROM system and the manufacturer's recommended measurement techniques. A 2 × 7 factorial design for main effects was used to evaluate the influence of level of play (college vs high school) on the cervical spine range of motion of the players. All data were collected during preparticipation physical examinations.

Results.—College football players had increased active cervical spine range of motion for flexion, extension, left cervical rotation, and left lateral flexion (overall mean increase = 4.3 ± 2°) compared with high school players. The collegiate players also assumed a more flexed resting sagittal-plane cervical spine posture.

Conclusion.—Collegiate players generally demonstrate greater active cervical spine range of motion than high school players, as well as increased resting sagittal plane cervical spine flexion alignment, compared with high school players, which is supportive of the influence of activity level and sport requirement. The CROM system can provide a portable, valid, and reliable method of measuring aggregate active cervical spine range of motion. This system will allow the early identification of athletes with impaired or excessive cervical spine mobility and facilitate proactive injury prevention.

▶ Active cervical spine range of motion in flexion, extension, and lateral cervical rotation was found to be greater in 189 collegiate football players as compared with 119 high school football players. The authors caution that further study is warranted using radiographic or MRI techniques.

R. C. Cantu, MD, MA

Flexion-Distraction Injury of the Thoracolumbar Spine During Squat Exercise With the Smith Machine
Gallo RA, Reitman RD, Altman DT, et al (Allegheny Gen Hosp, Pittsburgh, Pa; Texas Ctr for Joint Replacement, Plano; Drexel Univ, Philadelphia; et al)
Am J Sports Med 32:1962-1967, 2004   2–16

Introduction.—Flexion-distraction injuries of the lumbar spine are usually associated with lap belt–restrained passengers involved in motor vehicle collisions. Reported are 2 weightlifters with flexion-distraction injuries sustained while performing squatting exercises with probable improper technique and use of the Smith machine. The Smith machine is an apparatus that allows only vertical displacement of the barbell; it consists of a barbell linked to a vertical tract by cylinder bearings. To secure the barbell on the Smith machine, the barbell has to be rotated clockwise and secured on a set of pegs.

Case 1.—Man, 24, (190 lb, 5 feet 10 inches tall) was performing 405-lb squatting exercises during first-time use of a Smith machine. He failed on repetition 6 and the barbell crashed down the machine and he was pinned under the weight. He was wearing a lifting belt and was not using a spotter. Several bystanders removed the barbell. He reported severe mid to low back pain. He was not able to move his lower extremities. He had bilateral, diffuse lower extremity weakness; diminished light-touch sensation in patchy distribution; and bilaterally absent patellar and Achilles tendon jerk reflexes and clonus. Radiographs showed widening of the T12 to L1 interspinous distance, bilateral facet joint subluxation, mild kyphosis, and a left T12 transverse process fracture. CT verified intact vertebral bodies and bilateral facet dislocation. He was taken to the operating room and underwent decompression, reduction, and fusion of the thoracolumbar spine. The posterior elements were obliterated from the level of T12 to L2. The facet joints were dislocated bilaterally at T12 to L1. The facet joints were reduced and the spine was stabilized with segmental compression instrumentation from T11 to L2, pedicle screws at L1, and autologous iliac crest bone grafting posterolaterally. His neurologic function improved postoperatively. At 2-year follow-up, he had good strength against manual resistance in all lower extremity muscle groups. He returned to his previous job as a hospital transporter. He continued to have difficulty with urinary control. Radiographs showed maturation of the posterolateral arthrodesis without progression of kyphosis.

Case 2.—Man, 32, (140 lb, 5 feet 8 inches tall) was performing 350-lb squats during first-time use of the Smith machine. He was wearing a weight belt and did not have a spotter. When he was improperly securing the machine, the mechanism released and he was trapped underneath the barbell. The weight was removed by other weightlifters. He reported severe mid to low back pain. He denied weakness of the lower extremities In the emergency department, he had focal interspinous tenderness, complete motor strength of the lower extremities, normal sensory function in the lumber dermatomal distributions, and good rectal tone and normal perianal sensation. Radiographs and CT scans showed a superior T11 vertebral body compression fracture, 10° kyphosis, and bilateral transpedicular fracture. He underwent nonemergency surgery for stabilization of his thoracolumbar spine, reduction of fractures, and spinal fusion from T10 to T12. At 1-year follow-up, he reported no significant back pain and returned to weightlifting.

Conclusion.—These 2 cases of flexion-distraction injuries in weightlifters underscores the importance of proper knowledge of equipment before lifting heavy loads to ensure the safety of the lifter.

▶ This is a case study of 2 weightlifters who sustained flexion-distraction injury of the thoracolumbar spine while performing squats on the Smith machine. Lack of instructional technique played a part in these injuries. The authors state that this type of injury underscores the need for proper knowledge of weightlifting techniques.

R. C. Cantu, MD, MA

Hyperconcavity of the Lumber Vertebral Endplates in the Elite Football Lineman

Moorman CT III, Johnson DC, Pavlov H, et al (Duke Univ, Durham, North Carolina; Hosp for Special Surgery, New York)
Am J Sports Med 32:1434-1439, 2004   2–17

Background.—Spondylolysis, spondylolisthesis, herniated nucleus pulposus, and varying degrees of lumbosacral strain are among the recognized lumbar spine problems identified in elite football linemen. The activity of these players exposes them to high loads on their spinal columns during practice and games and requires intense single-event loads even during off-season training. Hyperconcavity of the vertebral endplates with expansion of the disk space (HEPS) has been noted in a high percentage of pre–National Football League (NFL) linemen. The incidence and clinical significance of this finding in elite football linemen were investigated.

Methods.—Data were collected during 1992-1993 at the NFL scouting combine in Indianapolis and included 266 elite football linemen. The lumbosacral spine was assessed, each athlete's history was documented, and each athlete underwent a physical examination and had lateral radiographs taken. All vertebral endplate defects of involved vertebrae were measured and compared with those of 110 patients serving as an age-matched control group.

Results.—Eighty-eight (33%) of the pre-NFL linemen and 9 (8%) of the control patients had HEPS, which was a statistically significant difference between the 2 groups. HEPS was present in 4 times as many linemen as patients. Sixty-six (75%) of the linemen with HEPS played on offense, and 22 (25%) played on defense. Players who had HEPS had a lower incidence of lumbosacral spine symptoms than did those without HEPS. Fourteen players with HEPS reported back symptoms, but most were minor complaints that could be handled without taking time off playing. Nonoperative management was effective in 13 of the 14 cases, but 1 player required a laminotomy with a diskectomy for a herniated nucleus pulposus. Ballooning of the disk was associated with HEPS and usually included all 5 lumbosacral disk spaces in both players and patients. Twenty-seven percent of patients with HEPS had endplate sclerosis that affected more than 2 vertebral levels.

Conclusions.—The percentage of elite football linemen with HEPS was about 4 times that found in age-matched control subjects. Players who have HEPS seem to be less likely to have lumbosacral spine symptoms. Generally, when HEPS is present, all 5 lumbosacral disk spaces are involved. It is likely that this condition is an adaptive change that occurs with time in response to the repetitive high loading and axial stress that football linemen experience.

▶ These authors studied 266 elite football linemen from the NFL and found that HEPS is about 4 times more common in these players than in age-matched nonelite football linemen. The reasoning for this outcome is that it is a response to the repetitive loading and axial stress experienced in football line play over time.

R. C. Cantu, MD, MA

Differences in Back Extensor Strength Between Smokers and Nonsmokers With and Without Low Back Pain

Al-Obaidi SM, Anthony J, Al-Shuwai N, et al (Kuwait Univ; Kuwait Dalhousie Physiotherapy and Rehabilitation Centre; Univ of British Columbia, Canada)

J Orthop Sports Phys Ther 34:254-260, 2004   2–18

Study Design.—Cross-sectional study comparing isometric lumbar extensor strength (ILES) in individuals who smoke and nonsmokers with and without low back pain (LBP).

Objectives.—To examine the differences in ILES between individuals who smoke and nonsmokers with and without LBP.

Background.—Given the evidence for general muscle weakness in individuals who smoke and in individuals with LBP, we were interested in examining the interrelationships between back strength, in particular ILES, and LBP in individuals who smoke and nonsmokers.

Methods and Measures.—The study involved 76 men (age range, 30-50 years) in 4 groups, namely, nonsmokers with LBP (NS-LBP), a control group of nonsmokers without LBP (NS-C), smokers with LBP (S-LBP), and a control group of smokers without LBP (S-C). ILES was measured at 7 angles of lumbar flexion, specifically 72°, 60°, 48°, 36°, 24°, 12°, and 0° (Figure). ANOVA and Scheffe post hoc comparison tests were used to analyze the data.

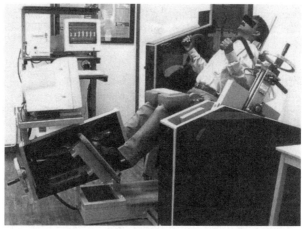

FIGURE.—Setup for testing isometric lumbar extensor strength on the MedX machine at the 7 spinal angles. Setup shows a typical setup, in this case for testing a subject at 0° spinal flexion. (Reprinted from Al-Obaidi SM, Anthony J, Al-Shuwai N, et al: Differences in back extensor strength between smokers and nonsmokers with and without low back pain. *J Orthop Sports Phys Ther* 34:254-260, 2004, with permission of the Orthopaedic and Sports Sections of the American Physical Therapy Association.)

Results.—Nonsmokers with LBP had less muscle strength than those without LBP ($P < .01$). However, the strength of smokers with and without LBP was comparable ($P < .05$). Both groups of individuals who did not smoke were stronger than the 2 groups comprised of smokers.

Conclusions.—Individuals who smoke were weaker than those who did not smoke, but no difference in strength was noted between smokers with and without LBP. Although smoking appears to be an important cofactor in the etiology of LBP, the degree to which smoking is a primary, secondary, or a component of a combined etiology warrants further study.

▶ It has previously been suggested that smoking is a risk factor for LBP, although the reason for the relationship is unclear. It may be that smokers are less active than nonsmokers so they tend to have weaker back muscles because of their lower activity levels. This study reiterated the weaker strength levels of smokers compared to nonsmokers, who were significantly weaker on 7 isometric tests of back strength. However, within the smoking group, those with and without LBP had comparable strength levels. It was suggested that smoking history be included as part of the assessment of subjects with and without LBP.

M. J. L. Alexander, PhD

A Controlled Randomized Study of the Effect of Training With Orthoses on the Incidence of Weight Bearing Induced Back Pain Among Infantry Recruits
Milgrom C, Finestone A, Lubovsky O, et al (Hadassah Univ, Jerusalem; Central Orthopaedic Clinic, Zerifin, Israel)
Spine 30:272-275, 2005   2–19

Study Design.—Randomized controlled trial.

Objectives.—To determine if the use of custom shoe orthoses can lessen the incidence of weight bearing–induced back pain.

Summary of Background Data.—The scientific basis for the use of orthoses to prevent back pain is based principally on studies that show that shoe orthoses can attenuate the shock wave generated at heel strike. The repetitive impulsive loading that occurs because of this shock wave can cause wear of the mechanical structures of the back. Previous randomized studies showed mixed results in preventing back pain, were not blinded, and used orthoses for only short periods of time.

Methods.—A total of 404 eligible new infantry recruits without a history of prior back pain were randomly assigned to received either custom soft, semirigid biomechanical, or simple shoe inserts without supportive or shock absorbing qualities. Recruits were reviewed biweekly by an orthopaedist for back signs and symptoms during the course of 14 weeks of basic training.

Results.—The overall incidence of back pain was 14%. By intention-to treat and per-protocol analyses, there was no statistically significant difference between the incidence of either subjective or objective back pain among the 3 treatment groups. Significantly more recruits who received soft custom orthoses finished training in their assigned orthoses (67.5%) than those who received semirigid biomechanical orthoses (45.5%) or simple shoe inserts (48.6%), $P = 0.001$.

Conclusions.—The results of this study do not support the use of orthoses, either custom soft or semirigid biomechanical, as prophylactic treatment for weight bearing–induced back pain. Custom soft orthoses had a higher utilization rate than the semirigid biomechanical or simple shoe inserts. The pretraining physical fitness and sports participation of recruits were not related to the incidence of weight bearing–induced back pain.

▶ Back pain is a common symptom in all age groups, and one of the risk factors for this is intermittent impulsive skeletal loading. Previous prospective studies have produced conflicting results as to whether foot orthoses can modify such back pain by attenuating the shock wave at heel strike during normal gait. This well-designed randomized controlled trial of more than 400 military recruits during basic training compared the effects of soft and semirigid orthoses with simple shoe inserts (without any shock-absorbing or supportive function). The incidence of back pain in this population was approximately 14%, and there was no statistically significant difference between the groups in regard to this symptom. The usefulness of expensive orthoses in conditions other than biomechanical lower limb overuse injuries remains questionable.

P. McCrory, MBBS, PhD

Can a Patient Educational Book Change Behavior and Reduce Pain in Chronic Low Back Pain Patients?

Udermann BE, Spratt KF, Donelson RG, et al (Univ of Wisconsin, La Crosse; Univ of Iowa, Iowa City; Dartmouth-Hitchcock Med Ctr, Lebanon, NH; et al)
Spine J 4:425-435, 2004   2–20

Background Context.—This study was prompted by 1) the almost universal use of patient education as an initial or at least an ancillary step in the treatment of patients presenting with low back pain, 2) the relative dearth of studies evaluating the effectiveness of patient education and 3) the complete lack of support in the few existing studies for the efficacy of education in improving patients' long-term health status.

Purpose.—A feasibility study to evaluate the efficacy of an individualized biomechanical treatment educational booklet to effect improvement in health status.

Study Design.—A prospective, longitudinal cohort study.

Patient Sample.—Sixty-two subjects (35 female, 27 male), average age 42.4 years, reported a mean duration of back pain before inclusion of 10.4 years. However, because of attrition, only 48 subjects had complete data across the 18-month follow-up period.

Outcome Measures.—Outcome measures included pain status, number of back pain episodes, subject compliance with self-care behaviors, knowledge and opinion of booklet content.

Methods.—Volunteers with chronic low back pain were provided a copy of an individualized biomechanical treatment educational book and told they would undergo a written survey of its content 1 week after reading the book. Subjects' health status at 9 and 18 months was evaluated using a structured telephone interview.

Results.—One week after the 62 subjects, with an average of 10.4 years of symptoms and extensive use of the medical system, finished reading the index book, 51.62% reported noticeable improvement in their pain, their content comprehension was good and opinions about the text were generally positive (Fig 2). At 9-month follow-up, there was statistically significant and clinically relevant improvement in reported pain magnitude ($P < .03$), number of episodes ($P < .0001$) and perceived benefit ($P < .04$). At 18-month follow-up, these gains held or demonstrated even further improvement.

Conclusion.—This study's results suggest that the *Treat Your Own Back* book may have considerable efficacy in helping readers decrease their own low back pain and reduce the frequency of, or even eliminate, their recurrent episodes. These findings also justify conducting a randomized controlled clinical trial to assess this book's efficacy in improving health status in subjects with low back pain with the study design including internal controls to

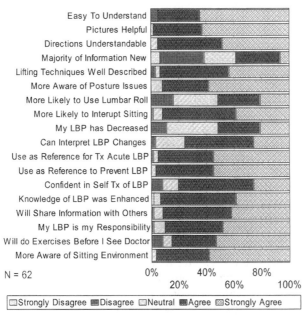

FIGURE 2.—Subjects' perceptions and attitudes regarding the content, style, and philosophy of the *Treat Your Own Back* text. *Abbreviations: LBP,* Low back pain; *Tx,*treatment. (Reprinted by permission of the publisher from Udermann BE, Spratt KF, Donelson RG, et al: Can a patient educational book change behavior and reduce pain in chronic low back pain patients? *Spine J*4:425-435, 2004. Copyright 2004 by Elsevier Science Inc.)

minimize bias issues and a wider range of outcomes, including measures of pain, function, disability, patient satisfaction, utilization of health care services and psychosocial measures.

▶ Although there is a large amount of printed material available for patients with low back pain, little research has been conducted to examine the effectiveness of patient education on recovery. In this pilot study, the subjects were given a book of individualized biomechanical treatment for low back pain which they were asked to study and follow closely. There was 94% compliance with the exercises in the book after 9 months, and 90% compliance after 18 months. This high compliance rate was due to the positive effects on their back pain that occurred because of their following the exercises in the book. The study suggests that there is strong evidence that a randomized controlled trial should be performed to determine the books' efficacy in improving health status in subjects with LBP.

M. J. L. Alexander, PhD

Low Back Pain in Professional Golfers: The Role of Associated Hip and Low Back Range-of-Motion Deficits
Vad VB, Bhat AL, Basrai D, et al (Hosp for Special Surgery, New York; Cornell Univ, New York; Association of Tennis Professionals Circuit, Ponte Verda Beach, Fla; et al)
Am J Sports Med 32:494-497, 2004   2–21

Background.—Low back pain is the most common musculoskeletal complaint experienced by both amateur and professional golfers. The modern golf swing is the primary suspect as the major source of injury for golfers, likely caused by the twisting motion of the lumbar spine at the top of the backswing, with subsequent derotation and hyperextension through the downswing and follow-through. Amateur golfers tend to have poor swing mechanics, and it has been shown that a greater torque develops in the lumbar spine compared with professional golfers.

However, there has been limited investigation of the prevalence of low back pain among professional golfers, and there is limited research on the cause of such injuries. The hypothesis that there is a positive correlation between decreased hip rotation and lumbar range of motion with a prior history of low back pain in professional golfers was investigated.

Methods.—This cross-sectional study was conducted among 42 consecutive professional male golfers. The golfers were categorized as having a history of low back pain of greater than 2 weeks duration that had affected quality of play within the previous year (group 1) or having no such history (group 2). All of the golfers underwent measurements of hip and lumbar range of motion, FABERE's distance, and finger-to-floor distance. Differences in measurements were analyzed by the Wilcoxon signed rank test.

Results.—Previous experience of low back pain was reported by 33% of golfers. A statistically significant correlation was observed between a history of low back pain with decreased lead hip internal rotation, FABERE's distance, and lumbar extension. There was no statistically significant difference noted in nonlead hip range of motion or finger-to-floor distance with a history of low back pain.

Conclusion.—A correlation was observed in golfers between a history of low back pain and range-of-motion deficits in the lead hip rotation and lumbar extension.

▶ This is a look at the biomechanical mechanism associated with the known prevalence of low back pain in golfers. Forty-two consecutive professional male golfers were studied. The results concluded that range-of-motion deficits in lead hip rotation and lumbar spine extension correlated with a history of low back pain in professional golfers.

R. C. Cantu, MD, MA

Trunk Muscle Strength and Disability Level of Low Back Pain in Collegiate Wrestlers
Iwai K, Nakazato K, Irie K, et al (Nippon Sport Science Univ, Tokyo)
Med Sci Sports Exerc 36:1296-1300, 2004   2–22

Background.—Low back pain (LBP) is a common complaint of active athletes. In some cases, radiologic abnormalities (RAs) have been identified as a possible cause of LBP, but no consensus exists on this point. Low strength of the trunk muscles has also been hypothesized to cause chronic LBP. Improvement of low trunk muscle strength could then be an effective treatment for chronic LBP. The relationship between isokinetic trunk muscle strength and the functional disability level associated with chronic LBP was investigated in wrestlers with and without RAs.

Methods.—Fifty-three collegiate wrestlers took part in the investigation. Their trunk extensor and flexor muscle strength was determined at angular velocities of 60°, 90°, and 120° per second. The trunk muscle strength was determined by measurement of peak torque, work, average torque, and average power. Two questionnaires were completed to determine the degree of disability of LBP in the research subjects. Thirty-five wrestlers were assigned to the RA group, and 18 were assigned to the non-RA group based on the results of radiographs and MRI. The trunk muscle strength and disability levels of LBP in each group were determined and compared.

Results.—The variables involved in chronic LBP were comparable between the 2 groups. Trunk muscle strength variables did not differ significantly between the groups, except for the extensor strength of work at 120°/s. The non-RA group had a high correlation between the extensor muscle strength variables and LBP, but a low or nonexistent correlation was found for the RA group. Fourteen wrestlers in the RA group and 8 in the non-RA group had LBP. No significant correlation was found between the trunk flexor variables and the disability level of LBP.

Conclusions.—Only the non-RA group showed high correlation coefficients and significant differences between the isokinetic trunk extensor strength and disability level of chronic LBP. Thus, the relatively low strength of trunk extensors may contribute to nonspecific chronic LBP in collegiate wrestlers.

▶ This is a study of 53 collegiate wrestlers with chronic LBP. The authors found that low strength of the trunk extensors is one of the factors associated with nonspecific chronic LBP in wrestlers without neurologic abnormalities or RAs.

R. C. Cantu, MD, MA

Young Athletes With Low Back Pain: Skeletal Scintigraphy of Conditions Other Than Pars Interarticularis Stress
Connolly LP, Drubach LA, Connolly SA, et al (Children's Hosp, Boston)
Clin Nucl Med 29:689-693, 2004   2–23

Purpose.—Skeletal scintigraphy is an important method for showing evidence of stress injuries affecting the partes interarticulares of young athletes with low back pain. Other etiologies of low back pain may also cause uptake abnormalities in these patients. How often do the results of skeletal scintigraphy support diagnoses other than stress injuries to the partes interarticulares and what are these diagnoses?

Materials and Methods.—We retrospectively reviewed the records of 209 young patients (149 females, 60 males; age range: 8-21 years, mean: 15.7 years) with low back pain and no previously treated vertebral condition who were consecutively referred from a sports medicine clinic to skeletal scintigraphy.

Results.—Sites of high uptake supportive of diagnoses other than pars interarticularis stress were shown in 36 (17%) of the 209 patients. Other diagnoses supported by skeletal scintigraphy included stress at the articulation between a transitional vertebra and the sacrum, injuries to the vertebral body ring apophysis, sacral fracture, spinous process injury, and sacroiliac joint stress.

Conclusion.—Skeletal scintigraphy shows uptake abnormalities supportive of diagnoses other than pars interarticularis stress in a significant number of young patients with low back pain. The uptake abnormalities shown are usually stress-related in this select population.

▶ The authors reviewed records of young athletes who were referred for skeletal scintigraphy for low back pain. Although this technique is typically used to indicate stress injuries affecting the pars interarticularis, in 17% of the cases there was increased uptake at other sites. The authors conclude that these uptake abnormalities are often stress related and that young athletes may have stress injuries to other structures of the vertebrae. This may represent an important diagnostic tool for stress injuries in young athletes.

D. E. Feldman, PhD, PT

Failure of Operative Treatment in a Fast Bowler With Bilateral Spondylolysis
Ranawat VS, Heywood-Waddington MB (Broomfield Hosp, London)
Br J Sports Med 38:225-226, 2004   2–24

Introduction.—Modern day fast bowling places enormous strain on the spine. Stress fractures of the lumber region occur frequently. Surgery is considered for these athletes if conservative treatment fails. Good results are obtained by means of a direct screw repair of the spondylolytic defect. A case of failed surgical intervention with an alternative technique was described.

Case Report.—Man, 19, a fast bowler, experienced bilateral L5 spondylolysis after an acute episode during a cricket competition. He was not able to resume bowling after 3 months of conservative treatment involving wearing a corset and rest. He underwent fusion of L3/L4/L5/S1, which involved posterior stabilization of the lumbar spine using Meurig-Williams plates secured on either side of the midline by screw fixation through the respective spinous processes. The patient's recovery and rehabilitation were uneventful.

He returned during the next season at full fitness and without pain. Early in the season, the man noticed swelling in the lumbar region that increased as the exertion of bowling increased. Radiographs identified a break in the lowermost screw; it was removed as was considered to be the cause of the swelling. His postoperative recovery was quick and he returned to full fitness again.

The patient noticed reappearance of lumbar swelling, yet did not curtail performance because he was selected to play at the international level. Repeat radiographs revealed that more screws were broken and that the metalwork was loose. A large, fluctuant inflammatory swelling about 25 cm in diameter was observed that necessitated regular drainage over the 5 days of his debut test match. Microbiological evaluation detected no evidence of infection. Over 1 L of fluid was aspirated. He completed the remainder of the season and the swelling persisted.

At season end, the man underwent surgery to remove the remaining metalwork. The spondylolytic defects were stable and no further intervention was performed. He returned to bowling the following season and played successfully for 8 years at both the international and national levels without back symptoms. He retired due to a knee injury.

Conclusion.—Posterior spinal stabilization was a poor surgical option for this elite cricket player.

▶ A 19-year-old fast bowler with spondylolysis refractory to conservative treatment serves to discuss the conservative and, when refractory, surgical treatment of this condition in fast bowlers. Localized screw fixation of the spondylolytic defect with bone grafting is the preferred surgical technique of these authors.

R. C. Cantu, MD, MA

Internal Coxa Saltans (Snapping Hip) as a Result of Overtraining: A Report of 3 Cases in Professional Athletes With a Review of Causes and the Role of Ultrasound in Early Diagnosis and Management
Wahl C, Warren RF, Adler RS, et al (Yale Univ, New Haven, Conn; Hosp for Special Surgery, New York; New York Football Giants Inc, East Rutherford, NJ)
Am J Sports Med 32:1302-1309, 2004   2–25

Background.—No single cause is accepted for internal coxa saltans, or snapping hip. Symptoms usually begin insidiously, with a dull deep catch or clunk in the groin during hip flexion and extension. Changing hip position can relieve symptoms, and with progression, the patient may be able to voluntarily reproduce the symptoms. Athletes at highest risk for internal coxa saltans make frequent hip movements at high flexion angles and internal and external rotation. Three athletes were evaluated shortly after progressive internal iliopsoas tendon snapping developed.

Case 1.—Man, 26, was a 4-year veteran National Football League (NFL) offensive lineman. A snapping had developed insidiously and painlessly over several months; pain eventually developed over the course of a month. It was minimally responsive to treatment with rofecoxib, indomethacin, and stretching. On physical examination, a palpable anterior snap occurred as the hip was brought from hyperflexion, abduction, external rotation (FAbER) to extension, adduction, and internal rotation (EAdIR). A break from drills for 2 to 3 weeks brought relief, but the painful snapping returned with a return to practice. An MRI scan showed increased signal intensity around the musculotendinous junction of the iliopsoas tendon at the femoral head level on T2-weighted imaging and mild diffuse hyperintensity of the iliacus muscle belly. US was used to guide injections and monitor therapy, which included peritendinous and intrabursal steroids and rest. His symptoms gradually resolved over 26 months, and he was able to resume playing professionally.

Case 2.—Man, 25, was a 2-year veteran NFL offensive lineman who experienced an acute onset of pain and tenderness in the anterior inferior iliac spine area after repetitive practice drills similar to those in Case 1. Therapy improved the pain, but a catching or vibration with flexion and extension moves developed, and palpable snapping occurred with the FAbER to EAdIR test. An MRI was obtained to differentiate labral tearing from coxa saltans, then a dynamic US revealed a palpable and visible translation of the iliopsoas tendon corresponding to the snap the patient described when he actively loaded his iliopsoas. He was given US-guided injections of steroids and local anesthetics, which promptly relieved his discomfort and permitted him to return to play.

Case 3.—Woman, 25, was a professional soccer player who had a painless loud snap of her hip when doing hyperflexion and rotation maneuvers at an entrance examination. She also reported infrequent intermittent snapping at the hip sometimes accompanied by "locking." She developed anterior groin pain, and described her hip as being "stuck" with no way to unlock it when a new regimen of intensive high step–jump maneuvers was introduced. MRI showed asymmetrical, chronic thickening of the affected iliopsoas tendon, and static and dynamic US found relative hypertrophy of the iliopsoas tendon. Her treatment consisted of rest, intensive cryotherapy, oral nonsteroidal anti-inflammatory drugs, and stretching; she was allowed to gradually return to training, except for the high-step maneuvers. After 29 months, she returned to full participation at an elite level, having infrequent snapping with hyperflexion but no other symptoms.

Conclusions.—Internal coxa saltans was manifest in various ways and responded to various treatments. The condition arose in each case from repetitive activities that included high-flexion hip drills. Imaging methods were chosen based on findings, and dynamic US provided a way to monitor ongoing progress as well as guide injections.

▶ This is a case study of 3 professional athletes—2 NFL players and 1 soccer player—who presented with snapping of the hip. Differing factors were seen in each case, and the diagnosis and treatment were individualized to each case.

R. C. Cantu, MD, MA

Clinical Examination of Athletes With Groin Pain: An Intraobserver and Interobserver Reliability Study
Hölmich P, Hölmich LR, Bjerg AM (Amager Univ, Copenhagen)
Br J Sports Med 38:446-451, 2004   2–26

Introduction.—Groin pain is a diagnostically and therapeutically challenging injury in sports medicine. The literature offers no consensus on definitions of diagnostic criteria for groin pain among athletes. The intraobserver and interobserver variation in the results of standardized clinical examination techniques for groin pain in athletes were calculated.

Methods.—Two physicians and 2 physiotherapists evaluated 18 athletes, 9 with sport-associated groin pain and 9 without groin pain. All examiners were educated in the examination techniques used to assess the athletes. All examiners were blinded to the symptoms and identity of participants. All research subjects were evaluated twice by each examiner in random order.

Examinations involved evaluation of adductor muscle–associated pain and strength; iliopsoas muscle–associated pain, strength, and flexibility; abdominal muscle–associated pain and strength; and pain at the symphysis joint. Kappa statistics and percentage of agreement were used to assess the data.

Results.—Overall, the values and the percentage of agreement were in accordance and demonstrated good reliability of the examinations. The values for the intraobserver agreement were higher than 0.60 in 11 of 14 tests; for interobserver agreement, the values were above 0.60 in 8 of 10 tests. The only test that did not have acceptable interobserver reliability was the strength test for the iliopsoas muscle.

Conclusion.—All except 1 of the tests were reproducible and subject only to limited intraobserver and interobserver variation.

▶ This study of 18 athletes with sports-related groin pain and 9 with no groin pain stresses which clinical examination techniques used to evaluate these athletes are most reliable.

R. C. Cantu, MD, MA

Delayed Onset of Transversus Abdominus in Long-Standing Groin Pain
Cowan SM, Schache AG, Brukner P, et al (Univ of Melbourne, Australia; Royal Children's Hosp, Parkville, Victoria, Australia; Univ of Queensland, Australia: et al)
Med Sci Sports Exerc 36:2040-2045, 2004   2–27

Introduction.—Groin pain in athletes is often difficult to resolve. Given the potential stabilizing role for the transversely oriented abdominal muscles at the anterior pelvic ring, optimal control of these muscles may be a significant consideration in the context of longstanding groin pain. Motor control of the abdominal muscles was examined in Australian football players with and without longstanding groin pain.

Methods.—Ten players with longstanding groin pain and 12 asymptomatic control subjects were evaluated. All participants were elite or subelite Australian football players. Fine-wire and surface electromyography electrodes were used to document the activity of the selected abdominal and leg muscles during a visual choice reaction-time task (active straight-leg raising).

Results.—The transversus abdominus contracted in a feed-forward fashion during an active straight-leg raise (ASLR) in asymptomatic control subjects. When participants with longstanding groin pain completed the ASLR task, the onset of transversus abdominus was delayed ($P < .05$) compared with control subjects. No significant between-group differences were found in the onset of activity of internal oblique, external oblique, and rectus abdominus (all $P < .05$).

Conclusion.—The finding of delayed onset of transversus abdominus in persons with longstanding groin pain supports a relation between longstanding groin pain and transversus abdominus activation.

▶ These authors studied Australian football players. They found a longstanding complaint of groin pain had a delayed onset of transversus abdominus muscle contraction.

R. C. Cantu, MD, MA

Footballer's Hip: A Report of Six Cases
Saw T, Villar R (BUPA Cambridge Lea Hosp, Cambridge, England)
J Bone Joint Surg Br 86-B:655-658, 2004   2–28

Introduction.—A significant proportion of individuals seen with labral pathology caused by trauma are athletes. Arthroscopy has led to a greater understanding of the nature of labral tears and has contributed to their management. A consecutive series of 6 professional footballers seen for intractable hip pain attributed on arthroscopy to an anterior acetabular tear with adjacent chondral damage were evaluated.

Findings.—Detailed medical and athletic histories were obtained from all 6 patients to identify the nature of the labral injury and its impact on their professional athletic careers. Rehabilitation after arthroscopy and date of return to full fitness were also documented. Provocation testing and arthroscopic findings were reviewed.

Two of the 6 footballers injured their dominant side, the leg with which they would normally kick the ball. Two players had defensive positions, 2 were midfielders, and 2 were attackers. All players had an identical injury to the anterior acetabular labrum, along with articular chondral defects adjacent to the labral tear visible at arthroscopy.

All unstable tissues underwent resection back to a stable margin. The most significant chondral damage was observed in a player who needed further surgery to stabilize the chondral flap. No operative or postoperative complications were observed. All patients had symptomatic improvement postoperatively. Five of the 6 footballers were able to return to football at the same level.

Conclusion.—The long-term outcome of hips with anterior acetabular tear remains of concern. Progression to further degeneration is likely due to the early signs of damage observed. Players with more severe chondral defects may progress to osteoarthritis over time.

▶ This is a study of 6 professional football players who had intractable hip pain secondary to an anterior acetabular labral tear with adjacent chondral damage. The study suggests that football players who present with hip or groin pain should have the differential diagnosis of acetabular labral pathology considered by the clinician.

R. C. Cantu, MD, MA

Laparoscopic Repair of Groin Pain in Athletes

Genitsaris M, Goulimaris I, Sikas N, et al (Interbalkan European Med Ctr, Thessaloniki, Greece)
Am J Sports Med 32:1238-1242, 2004   2–29

Background.—Treatment of groin pain can be difficult for professional athletes. Deficiency of the external inguinal ring is a diagnosis of exclusion. Initial treatment is conservative. For those who do not respond to conservative management, bilateral inguinal myorrhaphy is a common surgical treatment. The results of bilateral laparoscopic repair for the treatment of persistent groin pain in 131 professional athletes were presented.

Study Design.—The study group included 131 male professional athletes who were treated for persistent groin pain with bilateral laparoscopic transabdominal preperitoneal (TAPP) mesh implantation in the posterior wall of the inguinal canal from October 1993 to October 2002. A retrospective review of the prospectively collected data was done.

Findings.—A deficiency of the posterior inguinal wall was detected in all patients during laparoscopy. All 131 patients left the hospital within 24 hours, discontinued oral analgesics within 72 hours, and were back to full athletic activities within 3 weeks. Thigh pain was a problem in 3%. There was 1 recurrence during an average of 5 years of follow-up.

Conclusions.—Laparoscopic repair is safe and effective for the treatment of groin pain caused by deficiency of the posterior inguinal wall. The advantages of a laparoscopic approach include less postoperative pain, faster recovery and return to full activities, and excellent long-term results.

▶ These authors studied 131 athletes with groin pain unrelieved with 2 to 8 months of conservative treatment. They found that on laparoscopic study, there was a deficiency of the posterior wall of the inguinal canal of these athletes. Surgical repair was an efficient method of treatment with fast recovery and excellent long-term results.

R. C. Cantu, MD, MA

3 Injuries of the Shoulders and Arms

Rupture of the Pectoralis Major Muscle
Äärimaa V, Rantanen J, Heikkilä J, et al (Turku Univ, Finland; Mehiläinen Hosp, Turku, Finland)
Am J Sports Med 32:1256-1262, 2004   3–1

Background.—Total rupture of the pectoralis major muscle is a rare injury, with fewer than 200 cases reported in the literature. The treatment of this more serious injury to the pectoralis major muscle is controversial. Surgical treatment by anatomic repair is generally advised, but meticulous surgical technique and thorough rehabilitation are needed to obtain the original function and strength of the upper limb. Presented is the largest single series of patients treated with anatomic repair of pectoralis major muscle rupture.

Methods.—A case series of 33 operatively treated pectoralis major ruptures was reviewed in conjunction with a meta-analysis of the previously published cases in the English literature. A statistical analysis was conducted of the difference in outcome between groups of acute operation, delayed operation, and conservative treatment in both the case series and the meta-analysis.

Results.—Findings in the case series and analysis of the cases in the literature showed that early operative treatment is associated with better outcome than delayed treatment. The delayed surgical repair was associated with a better outcome than was conservative treatment.

Conclusion.—Early surgical treatment by anatomic repair will provide the most favorable outcomes in the treatment of total and near-total ruptures of the pectoralis major muscle.

▶ These authors did a retrospective study of 33 operatively treated pectoralis major muscle tears and concluded that early operative intervention gave the best outcome in the treatment of this rare occurrence.

R. C. Cantu, MD, MA

Shoulder MR Arthrography: Which Patients Group Benefits Most?

Magee T, Williams D, Mani N (Neuroskeletal Imaging, Merritt Island, Fla; Univ of Miami, Fla)
AJR 183:969-974, 2004   3–2

Background.—Injuries to the shoulder are common in athletes who participate in throwing sports. Performance of MR arthrography on all patients undergoing MR imaging of the shoulder has been suggested to increase the accuracy of diagnosis. However, MR arthrography of all patients undergoing shoulder MRI may be difficult because of scheduling constraints and patient reluctance to undergo an invasive test. The diagnostic accuracy of conventional MRI was compared with that of MR arthrography of the shoulder in the assessment of high-performance athletes (professional baseball players). The findings in these patients were compared with conventional MRI and MR arthrographic findings in an age-matched control group of amateur athletes.

Methods.—A retrospective review was conducted of conventional MRI and MR arthrographic examinations of the shoulder performed in 20 consecutive professional baseball players with shoulder pain. The interpretations of 2 musculoskeletal radiologists in consensus were compared with retrospective consensus interpretations of conventional MRI and MR arthrographic examinations of the shoulder in a control group of 50 consecutive amateur athletes with shoulder pain.

Results.—Findings in the 20 professional athletes included 2 full-thickness and 6 partial-thickness undersurface supraspinatus tendon tears detected but MR arthrography but not seen on conventional MRI as well as 6 superior labral anteroposterior (SLAP) tears, 2 anterior labral tears, and 1 posterior labral tear. Three patients had both SLAP tears and full- or partial-thickness supraspinatus tendon tears. Of the 14 patients with findings on MR arthrography not seen on MRI, 11 had arthrographic correlation; in all these patients, the arthroscopic findings confirmed the findings on MR arthrography. Findings in the 50 amateur athletes included 5 patients with additional findings on MR arthrography not seen on conventional MRI, including 2 anterior labral tears, 2 partial-thickness supraspinatus tendon tears, and 2 SLAP tears. One patient had both a partial-thickness supraspinatus tendon tear and a SLAP tear seen on MR arthrography. The 5 patients with additional findings on MR arthrography were also evaluated with arthroscopy. Arthroscopic findings confirmed the findings on MR arthrography in all 5 patients.

Conclusions.—MR arthrography was found to be significantly more sensitive for the detection of partial-thickness supraspinatus tears and labral tears than conventional MRI. MR arthrography showed injuries beyond those visualized on conventional MRI in 14 of 20 high-performance athletes in this study. These athletes may be representative of a subgroup of patients for whom MR arthrography can provide significantly more diagnostic information than conventional MRI.

▶ These authors studied 20 professional baseball players with shoulder pain and compared MRI studies with MR arthrography and determined that MR arthrography was more sensitive for detection of partial-thickness supraspinatus tears and labral tears than was conventional MRI.

R. C. Cantu, MD, MA

Shoulder Pathoanatomy in Marathon Kayakers
Hagemann G, Rijke AM, Mars M (Univ of Natal, Durban, South Africa; Univ of Virginia, Charlottesville)
Br J Sports Med 38:413-417, 2004   3–3

Introduction.—An understanding of shoulder injuries in kayakers begins with an appreciation of the kinesiologic, biomechanical, and physiologic demands of the sport. The rotator cuff muscles supply the forces to generate movement in the shoulder and are intimately involved in stabilizing and controlling the humeral head in the glenoid during the kayak stroke. The effectiveness of the cuff depends on its force of action, which is associated with its size, type, and speed of contraction, along with its moment arm or leverage and to its angle of pull. The prevalence of soft and hard tissue abnormalities and their interrelationships in the shoulders of marathon kayakers were evaluated. The pathoanatomical factors that predispose these athletes to injury were assessed.

Methods.—Fifty-two kayakers who had participated in kayaking events for 7 or more years and had completed at least 1 endurance race per year with a minimum of 7 races (an endurance race is longer than 120 km) completed questionnaires and underwent physical examination for range of motion, pain, and stability by means of a standard set of 10 clinical tests. MRI was performed in 3 planes and assessed for evidence of injury or other abnormality. The association between clinical symptoms and MRI findings was examined with respect to age, number of years of kayaking, and number of marathon races completed.

Results.—Thirty kayakers were asymptomatic at the time of scanning. Of these, 22 showed symptoms of pain or instability. The MRI revealed acromioclavicular hypertrophy, acromial or clavicular spur, supraspinatus tendinitis, and partial tear of the supraspinatus as the most common abnormalities. Age, number of years of kayaking, and number of races completed were not significantly associated with symptoms or with the presence of an abnormality on MRI scan. Of all the pathoanatomical findings reported to predispose to rotator cuff injury, only acromial and clavicular spurs correlated highly with supraspinatus muscle pathology.

Conclusion.—Rotator cuff injuries are responsible for a large proportion of injuries observed in marathon kayakers. This is about twice the number reported for sprint kayakers. These injuries are due to secondary impingement factors related to overuse, possibly specific to kayakers, and not due to bony restrictions around the shoulder joint. Acromioclavicular hypertrophy is often seen in marathon kayakers. It may be due to portaging or prior injury.

▶ Not surprising in a study of 52 long distance kayakers, and of the injuries seen in this sport, rotator cuff injuries were the majority owing, most likely, to overuse injury in these athletes.

R. C. Cantu, MD, MA

Arthroscopic Anterior Shoulder Stabilization of Collision and Contact Athletes
Mazzocca AD, Brown FM Jr, Carreira DS, et al (Univ of Connecticut, Farmington; RUSH-Presbyterian–St Luke's Med Ctr, Chicago)
Am J Sports Med 33:52-60, 2005   3–4

Background.—Repair of the anterior labrum (Bankart lesion) with tightening of the ligaments (capsulorrhaphy) is the recommended treatment for recurrent anterior glenohumeral dislocations. Current evidence suggests that arthroscopic anterior stabilization methods yield similar failure rates for resubluxation and redislocation when compared to open techniques.

Study Design.—Case series; Level of evidence, 4

Purpose.—To examine the results of arthroscopic anterior shoulder stabilization of high-demand collision and contact athletes.

Methods.—Thirteen collision and 5 contact athletes were identified from the senior surgeon's case registry. Analysis was limited to patients younger than 20 years who were involved in collision (football) or contact (wrestling, soccer) athletics. Objective testing included preoperative and postoperative range of motion and stability. Outcome measures included the American Shoulder and Elbow Society shoulder score, Simple Shoulder Test, SF-36, and Rowe scores. The surgical procedure was performed in a consistent manner: suture anchor repair of the displaced labrum, capsulorrhaphy with suture placement supplemented with thermal treatment of the capsule when indicated, and occasional rotator interval closure. Average follow-up was 37 months (range, 24-66 months).

Results.—Two of 18 contact and collision athletes (11%) experienced recurrent dislocations after the procedure; both were collision athletes. One returned to play 3 years of high school football but failed after diving into a pool. One patient failed in his second season after his stabilization (>2 years) when making a tackle. None of the contact athletes experienced a recurrent dislocation, with all of them returning to high school or college athletics.

Conclusions.—One hundred percent of all collision and contact athletes returned to organized high school or college sports. Fifteen percent of those collision athletes had a recurrence, which has not required treatment. Participation in collision and contact athletics is not a contraindication for arthroscopic anterior shoulder stabilization using suture anchors, proper suture placement, capsulorrhaphy, and occasional rotator interval plication.

▶ The authors present a case series design (with follow-up between 24 and 66 months) of 18 young athletes involved in collision (football) or contact (wrestling, soccer) sports who underwent arthroscopic surgery for recurrent shoulder dislocation. Results indicated that all patients (mean age, 16.6 years) had improved with respect to various outcome measures after surgery. Two patients in the collision group were characterized as failures since they had resubluxation episodes or pain. All athletes returned to organized sports within 10 months, and more than 50% returned within 6 months. Although the sample is small and included 3 persons who previously had surgery, the results of arthroscopic anterior shoulder stabilization seem promising in a group of young athletes.

D. E. Feldman, PhD, PT

Arthroscopic Bankart Repair Using Suture Anchors in Athletes: Patient Selection and Postoperative Sports Activity
Ide J, Maeda S, Takagi K (Kumamoto Univ, Japan)
Am J Sports Med 32:1899-1905, 2004   3–5

Introduction.—Initial results from arthroscopic procedures in patients with anterior shoulder instability show significantly higher rates of recurrence compared with open repair. Improvements in patient selection and operative technique have steadily reduced recurrence rates to match those of open techniques. Prospective investigation was performed of the arthroscopic Bankart repair by using suture anchors in the treatment of recurrent instability of the shoulder in selected high-risk young athletes.

Methods.—A total of 55 patients were evaluated. The mean follow-up period was 42 months (range, 25-72 months). Thirty-two patients had recurrent dislocations, 14 had recurrent subluxations, and 9 had recurrent subluxations after a single dislocation. The Rowe score, range of motion, recurrence, and sports activities were assessed.

Results.—The mean Rowe score improved from 30.1 to 92.3 points. Of these, 45 scores (82%) were excellent, 5 (9%) were good, 1 (2%) was fair, and 4 (7%) were poor. Patients had a mean loss of 4° of external rotation in adduction. There were 4 (7%) recurrences. The recurrence rate in contact athletes (9.5%; 2 of 21) was similar to that of noncontact athletes (6%; 2 of 34). Forty-four (80%) patients returned at the same level. The complete return rate among overhead-throwing athletes (68%; 17 of 25) was lower compared with nonoverhead throwing athletes (90%; 27 of 30) ($P = .0423$). The results were unsatisfactory in 5 patients.

Conclusion.—Arthroscopic Bankart repair with suture anchor techniques for traumatic anterior instability of the shoulder is reliable in selected high-risk patients. Overhead-throwing athletes need to be warned concerning the probability of restriction in postoperative activities.

▶ These authors have presented a prospective study of 55 patients who underwent arthroscopic stabilization of shoulders with recurrent anterior instability. These were high-risk patients, and the authors determined that arthro-scopic stabilization is a reliable procedure in some high-risk patients.

R. C. Cantu, MD, MA

Traumatic Pseudoaneurysm of the Brachial Artery Caused by an Osteo-chondroma, Mimicking Biceps Rupture in a Weightlifter: A Case Report
Koenig SJ, Toth AP, Martinez S, et al (Duke Univ, Durham, NC)
Am J Sports Med 32:1049-1053, 2004   3–6

Background.—Only 3 cases of pseudoaneurysms caused by osteochon-dromas in the upper extremity have been reported. An acute brachial ar-tery puncture produced by an osteochondroma in a weightlifter initially re-sembled a biceps rupture.

Case Report.—Man, 19, developed pain in his left arm and ante-cubital fossa while doing biceps curls. The pain lasted for 3 days; he then felt a sudden tearing in the midbiceps while extending the elbow and came to the emergency department with swelling and pain. An asymptomatic left humerus osteochondroma had been diagnosed at age 5 years. Swelling and tenderness in the mid and distal left arm and ecchymosis at the antecubital fossa were found on physical examina-tion, as well as pain and some weakness with forearm supination and elbow flexion. An osteochondroma of the medial midshaft humerus was the only abnormal finding on vascular, neurologic, and radio-graphic evaluations, which led to a diagnosis of biceps rupture, for which a sling was prescribed. Two days later the patient's distal and proximal biceps tendons were palpable and taut, and he struggled to generate power for elbow flexion and supination; ecchymosis of the distal arm and a midarm bulge continued. An MRI scan showed a hematoma between the brachialis and biceps muscles, which sug-gested the possibility that the osteochondroma had cut through the biceps muscle belly and caused the bleeding. The patient's pain im-proved with the use of a compression wrap and sling, but 10 days af-ter the initial injury, left elbow pain and anterior interosseous nerve weakness with median nerve paresthesias in the hand occurred. The arm was removed from the sling and elevated to decrease swelling and avoid excessive elbow flexion. Some improvement was noted, but within 2 days, the patient had excruciating pain in the posterior elbow and anterior forearm, increased paresthesia along the median nerve distribution in his left hand, and severe tenderness over the me-dian nerve and brachial artery in the distal third of the arm. MRI then demonstrated a mass at the level of the osteochondroma that had a ring around the periphery, which suggested a pseudoaneurysm; the pseudoaneurysm was confirmed on US and angiography. The mass was then noted retrospectively on the earlier MRI just medial to the osteochondroma. At surgery, the pseudoaneurysm of the brachial artery was in contact with the osteochondroma, and the median nerve was compressed beneath the biceps fascia and lacertus fibrosis. Bleeding from the posterior aspect of the pseudoaneurysm led to the discovery of a small hole in the artery. The osteochondroma was removed, the artery was trimmed to healthy tissue and repaired, and the median nerve was decompressed. The patient's pain was relieved, and paresthesia was reduced; an immediate improvement in strength was noted. Twenty-seven months after surgery, the patient has made a complete recovery and has returned to previous activities.

Conclusions.—A pseudoaneurysm should be included in the differential diagnosis of athletes who have extremity pain, swelling, and nerve compression adjacent to an exostosis, especially when the individual's skeleton is mature. Missing a pseudoaneurysm can lead to the development of a rupture of the aneurysm, hemorrhaging, nerve compression, phlebitis, and the risk of pulmonary emboli.

▶ This is a case study of a 19-year-old male weightlifter with pain after biceps curls. The authors state that the misdiagnosis of a pseudoaneurysm of the brachial artery is common. According to the authors, sports medicine clinicians should consider a pseudoaneurysm in their differential diagnosis when the patient complains of extremity pain, swelling, and nerve compression, particularly in a skeletally mature individual.

R. C. Cantu, MD, MA

Scapular Rotation in Swimmers With and Without Impingement Syndrome: Practice Effects
Su KPE, Johnson MP, Gracely EJ, et al (Drexel Univ, Philadelphia; Univ of the Sciences in Philadelphia; Univ of Oregon, Eugene)
Med Sci Sports Exerc 36:1117-1123, 2004   3–7

Background.—From 10% to 60% of competitive swimmers have shoulder pain, and the incidence increases the longer the athlete competes. Overuse is believed to contribute heavily to these shoulder disorders, referred to as *swimmer's shoulder.* Impingement syndrome is common. Studies of impingement syndrome among the general population have found a link with altered scapular kinematics. An investigation of scapular kinematics in swimmers with no known pathologic shoulder conditions and in those with shoulder impingement syndrome was conducted: whether changes in scapular kinematics caused by swim practice would be greater for swimmers with impingement syndrome than for those without was determined.

Methods.—Participants included 20 swimmers with and 20 swimmers without impingement syndrome. Measurements were made before and after swim practice sessions. A handheld dynamometer was used to determine shoulder strength. An inclinometer measured static scapular upward rotation with the arm at rest and at 45°, 90°, and 135° of humeral elevation.

Results.—During the swim practice training, equal numbers of research subjects selected the 4 swim styles, and all practiced kicking with a kick board and isolated arm motions using a float bell between their legs. The force after swim practice for the shrug and punch was significantly reduced from the values found before practice in both groups. Both the swimmers with impingement and those without impingement had a 14% reduction in shrug strength and a 13% reduction in punch strength. The scapular upward rotation patterns were similar between the 2 groups before swim practice, but after practice, the group with impingement had less upward rotation, especially at the 45°, 90°, and 135° humeral elevations.

Conclusions.—Swimmers who had impingement syndrome experienced a decrease in the amount of scapular upward rotation that they were able to manage after swim practice, and decreases were particularly noted at 45°, 90°, and 135° of humeral elevation. Thus, the scapular kinematics of swimmers with shoulder impingement syndrome changes after they practice and fatigue their shoulder muscles. These abnormalities of scapular kinematics require further evaluation to determine their clinical significance.

▶ These authors studied 20 swimmers with no known shoulder pathology and 20 swimmers with impingement syndrome. The authors determined that shoulder impingement may not be able to be detected until after the swimmer has practiced swimming and has fatigued the shoulder muscles. They caution that these results may not be applicable to all swimmers with shoulder impingement syndrome.

R. C. Cantu, MD, MA

Repetitive Low-Energy Shock Wave Treatment for Chronic Lateral Epicondylitis in Tennis Players
Rompe JD, Decking J, Schoellner C, et al (Johannes Gutenberg Univ, Mainz, Germany)
Am J Sports Med 32:734-743, 2004   3–8

Background.—Lateral epicondylalgia or epicondylitis (tennis elbow) is a repetitive overuse injury that produces microtears in the tendons that attach the extensor muscles to the epicondyle. In tennis players, this most often results from overload during a backhand stroke. Lateral epicondylalgia is more likely to occur in unskilled tennis players who use a racket that is too stiff, who hit the ball late, who frequently "frame" the ball, or whose forearm muscles are weak.

Players over age 40 years have been shown to be more susceptible to lateral elbow epicondylalgia. Extracorporeal shock wave treatment (ESWT) has been used for chronic tennis elbow, but variable results have been reported in several prospective studies. The hypothesis that treatment with repetitive low-energy ESWT is superior to repetitive placebo ESWT was investigated.

Methods.—A total of 78 patients were enrolled in this placebo-controlled trial. All of the patients were tennis players with recalcitrant MRI-confirmed tennis elbow of at least 12 months' duration. The patients were randomly assigned to receive either active low-energy ESWT given weekly for 3 weeks (treatment group) or an identical placebo ESWT (sham group). The main outcome measure was pain during resisted wrist extension at 3 months. The secondary outcome measures were greater than 50% reduction of pain and the Upper Extremity Function Scale.

Results.—At 3 months, there was a significantly higher improvement in pain during resisted wrist extension in the treatment group compared with the sham group (mean [standard deviation] improvement, 3.5 [2.0] vs 2.0 [1.9]) and in the Upper Extremity Function Scale (mean [standard deviation] improvement, 23.4 [14.8] and 10.9 [14.9]). A reduction in pain of at least 50% was achieved by 65% of patients in the treatment group compared with 28% of patients in the sham group.

Conclusion.—Low-energy ESWT was more effective than sham ESWT for treatment of chronic tennis elbow.

▶ This study looked at ESWT for chronic tennis elbow. Seventy-eight patients found those receiving ESWT had less pain than those in the placebo group.

R. C. Cantu, MD, MA

Humeral Torque in Professional Baseball Pitchers

Sabick MB, Torry MR, Kim Y-K, et al (Steadman-Hawkins Sports Medicine Found, Vail, Colo; Gil Med Ctr, Inchon, South Korea)
Am J Sports Med 32:892-898, 2004   3–9

Background.—Spontaneous fractures of the humeral shaft (ball-thrower's fractures) are not common but a well-known occurrence. Recreational athletes are usually involved, but ball-thrower's fractures have also occurred in professional baseball pitchers. Generally, the fracture is spiral, and butterfly fragments may be seen in some cases. It has been hypothesized that the biomechanics of the throw cause these fractures. The torsional stresses acting on the humerus during the pitch were compared with the torsional strength of the humerus, then the biomechanics involved in humeral shaft fractures during a pitch were explored. Finally, evidence was analyzed to pinpoint the phase or phases of the pitching motion during which fractures are more likely to occur.

Methods.—Data were collected from the pitches of 25 professional baseball pitchers throwing in game situations. The torque acting about the long axis of the humerus was calculated then compared with the torsional strength of the humerus.

Results.—Pitches were clocked at a mean of 38.8 m/s (range, 36.2-44.3 m/s). The torque about the shaft of the humerus was 92 Newton-meters approximately 80% through the pitching motion, and its direction tended to rotate the distal end of the humerus externally relative to the proximal end.

The peak of the humeral torque curve was just before maximum shoulder external rotation. After the ball release, the humeral axial torque was essentially 0 during the rest of the pitching movement. Six kinematic variables were significantly linearly related to peak humeral torque, specifically, the elbow extension angular velocity at the maximal internal rotation of the shoulder, the duration of the cocking phase, the stride length, the shoulder abduction angle at stride foot contact (SFC), the shoulder external rotation angle at SFC, and the elbow angle at SFC. The direction of the torque was consistent with the direction of the spiral fractures of the humerus. The average magnitude of the peak humeral torque was 48% of the torsional strength of the humerus. Thus, it is likely that repetitive stress contributes to the development of humeral shaft fractures.

Conclusions.—During the late cocking phase of the pitching motion, a large external rotation torque acts on the shaft of the humerus and is consistent with the mechanism of a humeral shaft fracture during a pitch. This torque exceeds the torsional strength of the humerus. Fractures are more likely to occur at or near the time of maximum shoulder external rotation. If the pitcher extends the elbows more at SFC, the peak humeral torque values are lower.

▶ These authors studied the humeral torque and the resultant spontaneous fracture of the humeral shaft in pitchers. Although rare, it is a well-known occurrence. The authors studied when the fracture may happen during the course of the pitch.

R. C. Cantu, MD, MA

Evidence of Subclinical Medial Collateral Ligament Injury and Postero-medial Impingement in Professional Baseball Players
Kooima CL, Anderson K, Craig JV, et al (Henry Ford Health System, Detroit; Detroit Tigers Baseball, Lakeland, Fla)
Am J Sports Med 32:1602-1606, 2004   3–10

Introduction.—The recognition and treatment of elbow disorders, including medial collateral ligament injury and posteromedial impingement, is increasing in throwing athletes. MRI may offer pivotal information for managing these athletes. Data concerning the frequency and degree of asymptomatic MRI findings in the elbows are lacking. Sixteen professional baseball players with no history of elbow pain or injury underwent MRI to identify abnormalities in the throwing elbows versus nonthrowing elbows.

Methods.—All MRIs were performed by using a standardized sequencing protocol. All images were reviewed in a blinded fashion by 2 musculoskeletal radiologists and 1 orthopedic surgeon.

Results.—Medial collateral ligament abnormalities (including thickening, signal heterogeneity, or discontinuity) were observed in 87% of players' dominant elbows. Findings consistent with posteromedial impingement were observed in 13 of 16 participants ($P = .04$). The throwing elbow was correctly identified in all 16 participants. No significant association between MRI findings and age were identified.

Conclusion.—A high rate of abnormal MRI findings was detected in asymptomatic throwers' elbows. These baseline findings need to be considered when MRI is being used for treatment decisions.

▶ These authors studied 16 asymptomatic professional baseball players who underwent MRI of the elbows Results showed abnormalities present in 87% of those imaged. The authors conclude that imaging of asymptomatic elbows in the professional baseball player can be used as a factor in treatment decisions.

R. C. Cantu, MD, MA

Bilateral Partial Rupture of Triceps Tendon: Case Report and Quantitative Assessment of Recovery
Harris PC, Atkinson D, Moorehead JD (Univ Hosp Aintree, Liverpool, England)
Am J Sports Med 32:787-792, 2004   3–11

Background.—The first report of rupture of the triceps tendon was published in 1868. This is an uncommon injury, although now more than 70 cases have been reported in the literature. Simultaneous bilateral triceps tendon rupture is extremely rare. Presented is the second known case of bilateral triceps tendon rupture.

Case Report.—Man, 39, a body builder with a body mass index of 35, was admitted to the emergency department with acute partial rupture of both triceps tendons. At the time of injury he had performing bench presses with 165 lb in each hand with inclined dumbbells. The patient reported that, while pushing up on the left, his elbow "gave in" without pain He had to lower the left dumbbell quickly while continuing to hold up the right dumbbell. A few seconds later his right elbow gave way, also without pain. Both arms then began to ache. On presentation to the emergency department 3 to 4 hours after injury the patient reported pain in the region of the triceps tendon bilaterally and of numbness in the ulnar nerve distribution of the right hand. He reported the use of anabolic steroids for a short period several years before this injury but denied recent steroid use. The patient also had a history of isolated long head of biceps rupture 3 years previously. This injury had been treated conservatively with full recovery. Clinical findings were similar for both elbows. Fluid collection was noted in the olecranon bursae and tense swellings in the region of the triceps tendons, consistent with hematomata. No palpable gap was present in either triceps tendon. The power of elbow extension was weak, and movement was painful. The range of movement was from 40° to 90°. No sign of neurovascular deficit was present. Extensive bruising developed gradually over the upper and lower arms bilaterally. Plain radiographs demonstrated bilateral bony avulsion fragments proximal to each olecranon. The broadness of the patient's shoulders precluded an MRI scan, so an US scan was performed. US showed severe but incomplete ruptures of both triceps tendons. The patient was treated conservatively with broad arm slings. Clinical assessment was repeated at weekly intervals for 2 weeks because of the risk of progression to complete rupture. The patient ignored medical advice and continuing discomfort in both elbows and returned to weightlifting 4 weeks after injury. He then reported continuing discomfort during weightlifting for 10 weeks after injury. After this, isokinetic strength training was delayed until the 8-week stage. Triceps muscle peak torque and average power were measured on several occasions and the biceps brachii were also assessed, as was the improvement in the patient's weightlifting performance. With conservative management, the patient recovered virtually normal function by 41 weeks.

Conclusions.—Predisposing factors for simultaneous bilateral triceps tendon rupture include renal failure, steroid use, and olecranon bursitis. The only other reported case of this rare injury occurred in a patient undergoing renal dialysis. This is believed to be the only case of simultaneous bilateral triceps tendon rupture in a healthy adult.

▶ This is a case report of a 39-year-old male body builder with acute partial rupture of both triceps tendons, believed to be the only reported case of simultaneous bilateral triceps rupture in a healthy adult. The article discusses operative versus conservative treatment of this rare occurrence.

R. C. Cantu, MD, MA

Ganglion Cyst and Olecranon Physis Nonunion in a Baseball Pitcher: Unique Treatment After Conservative Therapy Failure
Burman ML, Aljassir F, Coughlin LP (Montreal General Hosp; St Mary's Hosp Ctr, Montreal)
Physician Sportsmed 32(6):41-44, 2004   3–12

Background.—Ganglion cysts have been described as a cause of pain and swelling around many joints. Stress fractures through the olecranon physis are rare but have been reported in athletes who participate in throwing sports. The case presented here is a unique one in which ganglion cysts and a stress fracture through the olecranon physis occurred together.

Case Report.—Man, 30, a right-handed pitcher (AA level minor league) was seen for treatment of acute onset of pain in his throwing elbow that occurred after he felt a sudden "pop" while delivering a pitch. He had initial posterior swelling around the bursa, and conservative treatment was used. A period of rest for presumed olecranon bursitis was prescribed, but the patient continued to have posterior elbow pain on terminal extension with throwing. He indicated that he did not have any pain at rest or at night and had no history of fever or drainage from the elbow.

The patient was referred to the authors 6 months after the first report of pain and still had persistent pain and swelling. The physical examination showed swelling posteriorly over the olecranon bursa, mild posterior tenderness to deep palpation, no warmth or erythema, and no crepitation or abnormal motion. The patient had full range of motion without instability. Radiography of the elbow showed an old transverse fracture line through the olecranon without any evidence of healing. The radiographs also showed evidene of posterior soft tissue swelling.

At surgery, a large ganglion cyst was found arising from the fracture site. The stalk of the cyst was dissected from surrounding tissue and found to protrude through the triceps. The fracture site was easily visualized after removal of the ganglion from its base. The patient's elbow was immobilized for 2 weeks, and he began a gradual rehabilitation program. The diagnosis of a ganglion cyst was confirmed with pathologic examination.

At 18 months after surgery, the patient had full range of motion, no pain, full strength, and no recurrence of the ganglion cyst. He was able to return to baseball as a minor league pitching instructor and to throw without pain.

Conclusion.—In a unique case of concurrent ganglion cysts and olecranon physis nonunion in a minor league baseball pitcher, the patient was the first to be treated with fragment excision. He had an excellent result without any compromise of function and stability.

► This is an unusual case of a 30-year-old professional baseball pitcher who sought treatment for the acute onset of pain in his throwing elbow that occurred after feeling a sudden pop during a pitch delivery. After the pitcher failed conservative treatment, additional workup revealed both a ganglion cyst and nonunion stress fracture of the olecranon physis. After excision, the player had a full recovery.

R. C. Cantu, MD, MA

A Comparison of Open and Percutaneous Techniques in the Surgical Treatment of Tennis Elbow
Dunkow PD, Jatti M, Muddu BN (Tameside Hosp, Manchester, England)
J Bone Joint Surg Br 86-B:701-704, 2004   3–13

Background.—The syndrome of pain centered over the common origin of the extensor muscles of the fingers and wrist at the lateral epicondyle, termed *tennis elbow or lateral epicondylitis,* is found more often in nonathletes than in athletes. The peak incidence is the fifth decade. The precise etiology and pathology are unclear, but tennis elbow is usually diagnosed by localizing pain when the patient pinches with the wrist in extension and with resisted extension of the middle finger. Rest, modification of activity, local splinting, and steroid injection are sufficient treatment in 90% of cases. Surgery is needed for up to 8% of patients. Two operative techniques, the open technique and a percutaneous division of the common extensor origin, were compared for their effectiveness in managing tennis elbow.

Methods.—The 45 patients (47 elbows) were assessed preoperatively with the use of the American Academy of Orthopaedic Surgeons Disability of Arm, Shoulder and Hand (DASH) score. Twenty-four patients underwent the open technique, and 23 had the percutaneous operation. Follow-up lasted a minimum of 12 months.

Results.—Both the open and the percutaneous groups had a median preoperative normalized DASH score of 70. Postoperatively, the median normalized DASH scores were 17 for the open group and 20 for the percutaneous group, which was a highly significant difference. On the sport function section of the DASH score, preoperative median scores were 68 and 70 for the open and percutaneous groups, respectively, and the changes in median scores were 11 and 19 for the open and percutaneous groups, respectively. This difference was also highly significant. On the high performance work section of the DASH score, the open group had a median score of 68 preoperatively and 52 postoperatively; these scores for the percutaneous group were 72 and 49, respectively. The change in the median score was 14 for the open group and 24 for the percutaneous group. Significant differences between the groups were also noted with respect to patient satisfaction levels. In the open group, 2 patients were dissatisfied, 16 were satisfied, and 6 were very pleased with the outcome of the surgery. In the percutaneous group, none of the patients were dissatisfied, 9 were satisfied, and 14 were very pleased.

Conclusions.—When surgery is being considered for the management of tennis elbow, the percutaneous procedure may give significantly better results than the open procedure. The percutaneous procedure is accomplished more quickly and can be done under local anesthesia. No significant complications developed in the patients in this study.

▶ This is a study of 45 patients with tennis elbow who underwent surgical treatment of their tennis elbows, either with the open procedure or with a percutaneous technique. Those who underwent the percutaneous technique recovered quicker, and their outcomes were significantly better.

R. C. Cantu, MD, MA

Nerve Conduction Studies of Upper Extremities in Tennis Players

Çolak T, Bamaç B, Özbek A, et al (Kocaeli Univ, Turkey)
Br J Sports Med 38:632-635, 2004   3–14

Objectives.—The influence of regular and intense practice of an asymmetric sport such as tennis on nerves in the elbow region was examined.

Methods.—The study included 21 male elite tennis players with a mean (SD) age of 27.5 (1.7) years and 21 male non-active controls aged 26.4 (1.9) years. Anthropometric measurements (height, weight, limb length, and perimeters of arm and forearm) were determined for each subject, and range of motion assessment and radiographic examination carried out. Standard nerve conduction techniques using constant measured distances were applied to evaluate the median, ulnar, and radial nerves in the dominant and non-dominant limb of each individual.

Results.—The sensory and motor conduction velocities of the radial nerve and the sensory conduction velocity of the ulnar nerve were significantly delayed in the dominant arms of tennis players compared with their non-dominant arms and normal subjects. There were no statistical differences in the latencies, conduction velocities, or amplitudes of the median motor and sensory nerves between controls and tennis players in either the dominant or non-dominant arms. However, the range of motion of the upper extremity was significantly increased in tennis players when compared with control subjects. Tennis players were taller and heavier than control subjects and their dominant upper limb lengths were longer, and arm and forearm circumferences greater, than those of the control subjects.

Conclusions.—Many of the asymptomatic tennis players with abnormal nerve conduction tests in the present study may have presymptomatic or asymptomatic neuropathy similar to subclinical entrapment nerve neuropathy.

▶ This study examines the upper limb electrophysiologic findings in a group of asymptomatic elite tennis players. The authors are to be congratulated for their attention to methodological detail, which is unusual in studies of this nature. Surprisingly, it was noted that radial nerve sensory and motor function was impaired (although not median or ulnar nerve function) in the dominant limb, and speculated that subclinical nerve entrapment was the basis of this finding. I remain unconvinced by the data that a true abnormality exists here, and I also find the electrophysiologic explanation of these changes unconvincing.

P. McCrory, MBBS, PhD

Ulnar Nerve Injury Associated With Trampoline Injuries
Maclin MM II, Novak CB, Mackinnon SE (Washington Univ, St Louis)
South Med J 97:720-723, 2004   3–15

Background.—Trampolines have become extremely popular for both recreation and gymnastics training. This increase in popularity has been accompanied by a significant increase in trampoline injuries in children, usually consisting of soft-tissue injury, fracture or dislocations, and lacerations. No occurrences have been reported in the literature of ulnar nerve neuropathy associated with trampoline-related injuries. Three cases of ulnar neuropathy in children after trampoline-related injuries were described.

Case 1.—Boy, 4 years, fell onto his arm while jumping on a trampoline under supervision and suffered a displaced supracondylar fracture. He was evaluated in the emergency department and subsequently underwent surgery for crossed percutaneous pinning under general anesthesia. He was treated with an above-elbow splint for 2 weeks and was in a cast for 2 weeks. A pin tract infection resolved with oral antibiotics. The child had numbness in the ulnar nerve distribution, with weakness in the right hand for the next month. After 4 months with no improvement, the patient underwent exploration of the ulnar nerve. Significant scarring was observed around the ulnar nerve directly behind the medial condyle in the cubital tunnel region. After intraoperative electrical studies, an anterior submuscular transposition of the ulnar nerve was performed, and the patient experienced recovery of distal sensation and ulnar nerve intrinsic and extrinsic muscle function to his hand.

Case 2.—Girl, 9 years, fell onto her left arm while jumping on a trampoline under supervision and sustained minimally displaced closed proximal radial and ulnar fractures. She was evaluated in the emergency department and received casting only. The girl experienced immediate numbness in the ulnar nerve distribution, with weakness in the left hand. She underwent exploration with intraoperative electrical studies after 5 months without improvement. Significant scarring was present, with the ulnar nerve observed directly adherent to the ulna fracture site. An action potential was obtainable across only 1 fascicle. Internal neurolysis with anterior submuscular transposition of the ulnar nerve was performed with 3 fascicular grafts across a 3-cm gap at the level of the proximal forearm. The patient ultimately experienced recovery of distal sensation and ulnar extrinsic and intrinsic muscle function to her hand.

Case 3.—Boy, 9 years, fell from a trampoline and received a laceration to the proximal forearm. The laceration was repaired in the emergency department. He experienced immediate numbness of the ulnar nerve distribution and weakness in his hand. After 9 months with no improvement, the boy was referred and underwent exploration with intraoperative electrical studies. The ulnar nerve was 90%

transected, and an action potential was obtainable only across 1 uninvolved fascicle. Internal neurolysis with anterior submuscular transposition of the ulnar nerve was performed, along with a nerve transfer of the anterior interosseous branch of the median nerve to the deep motor branch of the distal ulnar nerve. The patient ultimately experienced recovery of distal sensation and ulnar extrinsic and intrinsic muscle function to his hand.

Conclusion.—Children who experience upper-extremity injury should be followed up for possible evolution of ulnar nerve neuropathy with consideration for electrical studies and surgical exploration when no improvement occurs after 3 months.

▶ This article describes 3 cases of ulnar neuropathy in children subsequent to trampoline injuries. Various surgical techniques are described, depending on the problems found. The increasing popularity of trampolines makes it a timely and important article.

The 3 cases that are described are different types of injuries that require different surgical interventions. The strength of the article is that it indicates that these injuries may occur even under adult supervision (2 of the 3 injuries occurred after supervised jumping) and that it is important to evaluate the child with an upper-limb injury for the possibility of ulnar nerve injury. In addition, the authors describe what they feel is an appropriate plan of management for pediatric ulnar nerve injuries.

D. E. Feldman, PhD, PT

Effect of Fluidotherapy on Superficial Radial Nerve Conduction and Skin Temperature
Kelly R, Beehn C, Hansford A, et al (Belmont Univ, Nashville, Tenn)
J Orthop Sports Phys Ther 35:16-23, 2005   3–16

Study Design.—Cross-sectional study.

Objectives.—The purpose of this study was to examine the effects of the superficial heating modality, Fluidotherapy, on skin temperature and on sensory nerve action potential (SNAP) conduction latency and amplitude of the superficial radial nerve in healthy individuals.

Background.—Fluidotherapy is a dry, superficial heating modality, which also provides tactile stimulation through the bombardment of air-fluidized cellulose particles. Previous literature has documented a direct relationship between skin temperature and neural conduction velocity; however, there is an absence of published research examining the effects of Fluidotherapy, and of tactile stimulation specifically, on neural conduction.

Methods and Measures.—Twenty-one subjects between the ages of 22 and 31 years (mean ± SD, 25.5 ± 0.7 years) and without prior history of diabetes, alcoholism, renal or metabolic dysfunction, current pregnancy, or heat sensitivity were invited to participate. Subjects completed an upper quarter screening exam and medical history form prior to participation. One group underwent heat (46.7°-48.9°C) and tactile stimulation, a second group underwent tactile stimulation alone, while a third served as controls. Dependent variables were assessed at 3 intervals: before the intervention, immediately after the intervention, and 20 minutes after the intervention. All interventions were 20 minutes in length.

Results.—A mixed 2-way analysis of variance indicated a significant interaction between time of neural conduction velocity assessment and treatment group for the dependent variables of sensory nerve action potential latency ($P<.001$) and skin temperature ($P<.001$). Appropriate post hoc tests were performed for simple effect comparisons. An inverse linear relationship existed between skin temperature and latency ($r^2 = .65$; Pearson product coefficient, $-.81$).

Conclusions.—Fluidotherapy treatment, which combines the effects of heat and tactile stimulation, significantly elevated superficial skin temperature, while tactile stimulation alone and no treatment (control group) did not bring about a temperature change. As the superficial skin temperature increased, there was a concomitant decrease in the distal sensory latency of the superficial radial sensory nerve action potential. These results should be an important consideration for the clinician using superficial heating modalities.

▶ The goal of this randomized trial was to compare the effects of Fluidotherapy (heat and tactile stimulation), tactile stimulation alone, and placebo on skin temperature and on SNAP conduction latency and amplitude of the superficial radial nerve in healthy adults (aged 22-31 years). The results of the study indicated that Fluidotherapy treatment elevated superficial skin temperature (which remained 20 minutes after treatment was discontinued) and decreased SNAP latencies. These effects support the possible analgesic benefits of Fluidotherapy as well as possible clinical benefits for increasing soft tissue extensibility or reducing joint stiffness with active or passive treatments.

D. E. Feldman, PhD, PT

4 Injuries of the Legs

Effect of Dry Needling of Gluteal Muscles on Straight Leg Raise: A Randomised, Placebo Controlled, Double Blind Trial
Huguenin L, Brukner PD, McCrory P, et al (Australian Inst of Sport, Belconnen, ACT; Univ of Melbourne, Australia; Centre for Sports Medicine Research and Education, Parkville, Victoria, Australia; et al)
Br J Sports Med 39:84-90, 2005   4–1

Objectives.—To use a randomised, double blind, placebo controlled trial to establish the effect on straight leg raise, hip internal rotation, and muscle pain of dry needling treatment to the gluteal muscles in athletes with posterior thigh pain referred from gluteal trigger points.

Methods.—A randomised, double blind, placebo controlled trial of 59 male runners was performed during the 2002 Australian Rules football season. Subjects were thoroughly screened and had magnetic resonance imaging of their hamstring muscles to exclude local pathology. The inclusion criterion was reproduction of recognisable posterior thigh pain with the application of digital pressure to the gluteal trigger points. Subjects randomly received either therapeutic or placebo needle treatment on one occasion at their gluteal trigger points. Range of motion and visual analogue scale data were collected immediately before, immediately after, 24 hours after, and 72 hours after the intervention. Range of motion was measured with passive straight leg raise and hip internal rotation. Visual analogue scales were completed for hamstring and gluteal pain and tightness at rest and during a running task.

Results.—Magnetic resonance imaging scans revealed normal hamstring musculature in most subjects. Straight leg raise and hip internal rotation remained unchanged in both groups at all times. Visual analogue scale assessment of hamstring pain and tightness and gluteal tightness after running showed improvements immediately after the intervention in both groups ($p = 0.001$), which were maintained at 24 and 72 hours. The magnitude of this improvement was the same for therapeutic and placebo interventions. Resting muscle pain and tightness were unaffected.

Conclusions.—Neither dry needling nor placebo needling of the gluteal muscles resulted in any change in straight leg raise or hip internal rotation. Both interventions resulted in subjective improvement in activity related muscle pain and tightness. Despite being commonly used clinical tests in this situation, straight leg raise and hip internal rotation are not likely to help the therapist assess response to treatment. Patient reports of response to such treatment are better indicators of its success. The mechanisms by which these responses occur and the reasons for the success of the placebo needling treatment are areas for further investigation.

▶ Muscular thigh and hamstring pain is a common sports injury presentation. It has been postulated that muscle "trigger points" or areas of local tenderness may have a role in the genesis of such pain in the absence of structural muscular injury. As a result, a variety of different anecdotal treatments are used to treat such trigger points. This study is a randomized controlled trial using dry needling (vs sham needling) to determine the effect on straight leg raise, which is a reproducible outcome measure. The assessment was performed in a double-blinded fashion. This therapeutic modality had no significant effect on straight leg raise; however, subjective muscle pain was significantly reduced by the procedure. This is the first randomized controlled trial that I am aware of that has looked at the therapeutic effectiveness of anecdotal treatment modalities such as dry needling.

P. McCrory, MBBS, PhD

Injury Mechanisms for Anterior Cruciate Ligament Injuries in Team Handball: A Systematic Video Analysis

Olsen O-E, Myklebust G, Engebretsen L, et al (Norwegian Univ of Sport and Physical Education, Oslo)
Am J Sports Med 32:1002-1012, 2004   4–2

Introduction.—The anterior cruciate ligament (ACL) is commonly ruptured during participation in European team handball, United States college and high school sports, and other sports and levels of participation. Few data are available regarding the injury mechanisms of ACL injuries in team sports. A descriptive video analysis was performed to determine the mechanisms of ACL injuries in female team handball participants.

Methods.—Twenty videotapes of ACL injuries from Norwegian or international competition were obtained during 12 seasons (1988-2000). Three physicians and 3 national team coaches systematically evaluated these videos to describe the injury mechanisms and playing situations. Thirty-two players with ACL injuries in the upper 3 divisions in Norwegian team handball were interviewed during the 1998 to 1999 season to compare the injury characteristics between player recall and the video analysis.

Results.—Two important injury mechanisms for ACL injuries in team handball were identified. The most frequent (12/20 injuries) was a plant-and-cut movement that occurred in every case with a forceful valgus and external or internal rotation, with the knee close to full extension. The other injury mechanism (4/20 injuries) was a 1-legged jump shot landing that occurred with a forceful valgus and external rotation with the knee close to full extension. Findings from the video analysis and questionnaire were comparable.

Conclusion.—The injury mechanism for ACL injuries in female team handball was associated with a forceful valgus collapse with the knee close to full extension combined with external or internal rotation of the tibia.

▶ This is a 12-season study of female handballers from Norwegian or international competition. Two main injury mechanisms were identified in this injury: first and most common, a forceful valgus and external or internal rotation with the knee close to full extension and, secondly, a 1-legged jump shot landing. The findings were that the ACL injury in this particular sport resulted from a valgus collapse with the knee close to full extension combined with internal and/or external rotation of the tibia.

R. C. Cantu, MD, MA

The Ottawa Knee Rule: Avoiding Unnecessary Radiographs in Sports
Nugent PJ (Bethesda Hosp, Cincinnati, Ohio)
Physician Sportsmed 32(5):26-32, 2004   4–3

Background.—Few knee plain radiographs are clinically relevant because the structures of the knee most likely to be injured, the menisci and ligaments, are radiolucent. The problem of taking unnecessary knee radiographs was addressed by the development of a set of decision rules known as the Ottawa knee rule to save time and resources.

Ottawa Knee Rule Criteria.—A knee radiograph is indicated after a trauma only when 1 or more of these is present:

• Patient age younger than 18 years or older than 55 years
• Tenderness at fibular head
• Tenderness over patella
• Inability to flex knee to 90°
• Inability to bear weight for 4 steps

Discussion.—The Ottawa knee rule is scientifically validated and easy to use. It uses the results of examinations of injured patients to predict which patients can forgo radiographs. The sensitivity and negative predictive values are 100%, but the specificity is lower; thus, many radiographs will still have normal findings. Injuries that are not fractures must still be diagnosed and treated by the health care provider. The Ottawa knee rule benefits both the patient and the provider.

▶ This article discusses the Ottawa knee rule, developed in the mid 1990s to address the use of unnecessary knee radiographs after injuries. The Ottawa knee rule is a set of clinical criteria for the use of radiographs. The authors validated this rule by showing that no clinically determined injuries were missed using this rule when all the clinical criteria were negative.

R. C. Cantu, MD, MA

99mTc-MDP Bone SPECT in Evaluation of the Knee in Asymptomatic Soccer Players

Yildirim M, Gursoy R, Varoglu E, et al (Ataturk Univ, Erzurum, Turkey; School for Physical Education and Sports, Erzurum, Turkey)

Br J Sports Med 38:15-18, 2004   4–4

Introduction.—Skeletal scintigraphy is usually recognized as the optimal method for assessing suspected stress injuries due to its high sensitivity and ability to demonstrate abnormalities in bone metabolism well before they can be detected radiographically. It is well suited for examination of complex bony structures, such as the knee, in which the ability to separate activity from overlying versus underlying bone and view uptake in all 3 orthogonal planes is useful. Stress fractures in legs (particularly around the knee, tibia, and femur) and knee pathology in active soccer players with no symptoms in the preceding months (defined as asymptomatic) were evaluated.

Methods.—Forty-two asymptomatic soccer players from 7 teams in major female professional and male amateur soccer leagues (21 men, 21 women; age range, 19-31 years) were evaluated by ^{99m}Tc-methylene diphosphonate (MDP) bone scintigraphy during the soccer season. At 4 hours after IV injection of 20 mCi ^{99m}Tc-MDP, standard images—including anterior planar spot images of the legs, lateral images of the knee, and single photon emission CT (SPECT)—were obtained.

Results.—Increased tracer uptake, indicating stress fracture, was observed in 28 (66%) of these asymptomatic players. Most of the stress fractures were identified in the tibia (62%) and femur (5%). In the 42 players (84 legs), 35 sites (42%) showed rupture of the posterior horn of the lateral meniscus and bone bruising of the tibial plateau; there was rupture of the anterior horn of the medial meniscus in 16 sites (19%), bone bruising of the lateral femoral condyle in 11 sites (13%), bone bruising of the medial femoral condyle in 8 sites (10%), and avulsion injury to the infrapatellar tendon insertion in the anterior tibia in 34 sites (40%). Eleven anterior cruciate ligament injuries were observed.

Conclusion.—Bone SPECT is accurate, easy to perform, cost effective, and may provide valuable information before MRI for detecting meniscal tears and may be used successfully when MRI is not available.

▶ This study of asymptomatic soccer players found the use of bone SPECT highly accurate and cost effective in the evaluation of stress fractures.

R. C. Cantu, MD, MA

Subjective Functional Assessments and the Return to Competitive Sport After Anterior Cruciate Ligament Reconstruction
Smith FW, Rosenlund EA, Aune AK, et al (Volvat Med Centre, Oslo, Norway; Univ of Glasgow, Scotland)
Br J Sports Med 38:279-284, 2004   4–5

Background.—When a competitive athlete is given a diagnosis of anterior cruciate ligament (ACL) rupture, the patient's motivation to return to competition at the previous level or to an athletic lifestyle with functionally challenging activities that had been limited by the ACL deficiency generally leads to the choice of reconstructive surgery. To return to competition at the previous level usually means that the patient must be free or nearly free of functional limitations. A disconnection tends to occur between the objective measurements of static stability and the subjective assessment of functional limitations after ACL reconstruction. Tools for assessment should, therefore, be linked to the activities of most interest to patients. The Cincinnati knee rating system assesses functional outcomes after knee ligament surgery. The return to and maintenance of competitive participation as well as the relationship of sports activity and competitive participation to subjective functional assessments at follow-up were investigated with the use of the Cincinnati knee rating system.

Methods.—Seventy-seven of 109 selected patients responded to the questionnaire that was sent a mean of 43 months (range, 24-73 months) after these competitive athletes had ACL reconstruction. The surgical procedure was a transtibial endoscopic technique with either a bone–patellar tendon–bone or a multiple looped hamstring autograft. The questionnaire was based on the Cincinnati sports activity scale (CSAS) and the Cincinnati sports function scales and included questions concerning any changes in competitive level and any complaints.

Results.—Eighty-one percent of the respondents had returned to competition within 12 months of surgery, and 89% of these returned to at least the level at which they were competing before their injuries. Three patients (7%) subsequently had functional problems that led to their retirement from competitive sport. Ninety percent of patients scored themselves at CSAS levels 1 and 2, and 55% of these gave themselves the top score at their level. Sixty-nine percent of men and 41% of women ranked themselves at this level. Competitive patients had significantly higher overall sports function scores than did noncompetitive patients, and male patients had higher scores than female patients. At 12 months, the overall incidence of patients who were competing with a major functional impairment was 21%, whereas the percentage at follow-up was 13%.

Conclusions.—Patients reported a return to competition at their previous level in a high percentage of cases. This result was expected given the standard of treatment, the patient selection, and the study exclusion criteria. Even when competitive participation was discontinued, patients who had few complaints concerning their functional abilities maintained a high level of sporting activity.

▶ These authors studied 109 patients after ACL reconstruction with regard to their return to athletic play. The reported return to competition at the previous level was high; however, the authors state that this was a small study sample, which limited their scope of data analysis.

R. C. Cantu, MD, MA

Effect of Physiotherapy Attendance on Outcome After Anterior Cruciate Ligament Reconstruction: A Pilot Study
Feller JA, Webster KE, Taylor NF, et al (La Trobe Univ, Melbourne, Australia)
Br J Sports Med 38:74-77, 2004   4–6

Introduction.—Physiotherapy-based rehabilitation programs are frequently used after anterior cruciate ligament (ACL) reconstruction, but the role or this therapy and the amount of supervised physiotherapy needed are not clearly defined. The outcome of a group of patients who attended physiotherapy only infrequently was compared in a pilot investigation with that of patients who attended physiotherapy regularly.

Methods.—Ten patients with infrequent physiotherapy attendance (mean, 1.9 visits) during the first 6 months after ACL reconstruction surgery were matched for age, gender, graft type, activity level, and occupation before injury with 10 patients who attended physiotherapy regularly (mean, 26.5 visits). The outcome was evaluated at 12 months by the Cincinnati knee rating system and the International Knee Documentation Committee form.

Results.—Compared with the regular physiotherapy group, the minimal physiotherapy group had fewer symptoms (mean Cincinnati symptom score, 46.2 vs 43.4; P = .045). A trend was observed toward higher overall Cincinnati knee scores in the minimal physiotherapy group (mean, 93.7 vs 87.3; P = .06). There were no between-group differences in International Knee Documentation Committee ratings (Table 2).

Conclusion.—Some patients who choose to attend physiotherapy on an infrequent basis after ACL reconstruction may achieve satisfactory, if not better, outcomes compared with patients who attend physiotherapy regularly.

▶ Although it is a pilot observational study, I chose this article because it is actually supported by several randomized controlled trials on the same subject, and I believe it is important that we begin to question some of our current practices. Attendance at supervised physiotherapy sessions did not improve outcomes in post-ACL reconstruction patients compared with patients who were given a progressive home exercise program.[1,2] Proponents of supervised physiotherapy sessions will likely comment that the therapy in the study didn't include a certain modality or was not provided by therapists with enough experience. Although this may be true, we may also look back 20 years from now

TABLE 2.—Cincinnati Knee Scores and International Knee Documentation Committee Ratings 12 Months After Anterior Cruciate Ligament Reconstruction

	Minimal Attendance	Regular Attendance
Overall Cincinnati (0-100)		
Mean (SD)	93.7 (4.9)	87.3 (5.8)
Median	92	87
Cincinnati symptoms (0-50)		
Mean (SD)	46.2 (2.2)	43.0 (3.2)*
Median	46	44
Cincinnati function (0-50)		
Mean (SD)	47.5 (4.0)	44.3 (3.8)
Median	46	45
Overall IKDC (no of patients)		
A	2	0
B	7	7
C	1	2
D	0	1
IKDC 1 (subjective assessment)		
A	3	0
B	7	10
C	0	0
D	0	0
IKDC 2 (symptoms)		
A	6	2
B	3	5
C	1	2
D	0	1
IKDC 3 (range of motion)		
A	8	6
B	2	4
C	0	0
D	0	0
IKDC 4 (ligament examination)		
A	8	7
B	2	3
C	0	0
D	0	0

*$P < .05$.
Abbreviations: IKDC, International Knee Documentation Committee; *SD*, standard deviation.
(Courtesy of Feller JA, Webster KE, Taylor NF, et al: Effect of physiotherapy attendance on outcome after anterior cruciate ligament reconstruction: A pilot study. *Br J Sports Med* 38:74-77, 2004, with permission from the BMJ Publishing Group.)

and comment about how we continued to use treatments despite mounting evidence to the contrary.

I. Shrier, MD, PhD

References

1. Schenck RC Jr, Blaschak MU, Lance ED, et al: A prospective outcome study of rehabilitation programs and anterior cruciate ligament reconstruction. *Arthroscopy* 13:285-290, 1997.
2. Fischer DA, Tewes DP, Boyd JL, et al: Home based rehabilitation for anterior cruciate ligament reconstruction. *Clin Orthop* 347:194-199, 1998.

Lower Body Positive-pressure Exercise After Knee Surgery

Eastlack RK, Hargens AR, Groppo ER, et al (Univ of California, San Diego)
Clin Orthop 431:213-219, 2005   4–7

Introduction.—Lower body positive pressure allows unloading of the lower extremities during exercise in a pressurized treadmill chamber. This study assessed the preliminary feasibility of lower body positive pressure exercise as a rehabilitation technique by examining its effects on gait mechanics and pain, postoperatively. Fifteen patients who had arthroscopic meniscectomy or anterior cruciate ligament reconstruction participated in this study. Patients exercised for 5 minutes at 2.0 mph under three body weight conditions (normal body weight, 60% body weight, and 20% body weight) in random order. Bilateral ground reaction force, electromyographs, and dynamic knee range of motion were collected, and pain was assessed using a visual analog scale. Ground reaction forces for surgically treated and contralateral extremities were reduced 42% and 79% from normal body weight conditions when ambulating at 60% and 20% body weight, respectively. After meniscectomy, ambulatory knee range of motion decreased only at 20% body weight (37°), compared with normal body weight conditions (49°). Peak electromyographic activity of the biceps was maintained at all body weight conditions, whereas that of the vastus medialis was reduced at 20% body weight. Pain relief was significant with lower body positive pressure ambulation after anterior cruciate ligament reconstruction. This study showed that lower body positive pressure exercise is effective at reducing ground reaction forces, while safely facilitating gait postoperatively.

Level of Evidence.—Therapeutic study, Level II-1 (study of untreated controls from a previous randomized controlled trial.)

▶ The fascination of some doctors with wonder devices never seems to cease. Here, a treadmill is encased inside a pressure chamber with a kayak-like seal, and upward pressure at the waist is intended to lift the patient, reducing ground-reaction forces on the lower limbs after surgical treatment of the knee. The cost of the device is not specified, although, not surprisingly, it is said to be cheaper than a submersible treadmill (where there are grave dangers of electrocution!). One would suspect that on top of the capital cost of the pressurizing device, there is a need for a specialized operating crew, and a power supply with 3-phase wiring. The reduction in ground reaction force achieved by the equipment is likely to vary substantially from 1 person to another, depending on the fit of the kayak "skirt." Moreover, the application of positive pressure to the lower half of the body positive pressure is likely to increase cardiac loading substantially, a significant consideration for older patients. There must be many simpler ways of exercising with reduced gravitational forces—exercising on a cycle ergometer while lying down, taking the weight off the legs during treadmill exercise by means of the hand-rail supports or a waist harness, and walking in a pool once the wound has healed, to name but a few options. I suspect that the pressurized treadmill will have only a brief blaze of glory!

R. J. Shephard, MD, PhD, DPE

Interlimb Asymmetry in Persons With and Without an Anterior Cruciate Ligament Deficiency During Stationary Cycling

Hunt MA, Sanderson DJ, Moffet H, et al (Univ of British Columbia, Vancouver, Canada; Intl Collaboration on Repair Discoveries, Vancouver, BC, Canada; Laval Univ, Quebec City, Canada; et al)
Arch Phys Med Rehabil 85:1475-1478, 2004   4–8

Introduction.—The anterior cruciate ligament (ACL) is the most frequently injured ligament in the human body. Goals for rehabilitation for an ACL injury include restoration of knee joint range of motion, lower-limb muscular strength, and cardiovascular fitness. A reduction in muscular output in the injured limb would be undesirable. No trial has assessed the level of asymmetry in measures of force production in ACL-deficient patients during stationary cycling. The power output generation from ACL-injured and noninjured limbs during stationary cycling was examined.

Methods.—Ten patients with unilateral ACL deficiency and 10 uninjured control subjects matched for age and gender performed 6 randomized bouts of stationary cycling at intensities of 2 cadences (60, 90 rpm) and 3 power outputs (75, 125, 175 W) for approximately 2 minutes for each bout during a single laboratory visit. The primary effective component of force (perpendicular to the crank) was measured and used to determine the power output contribution from each limb to the total power output.

Results.—Participants with ACL injury generated significantly more power from uninjured limbs compared with injured limbs. Injured limbs also differed significantly from limbs of control subjects. For all riding conditions evaluated, participants with ACL injury exhibited significantly greater interlimb asymmetry than control subjects ($P < .001$). A trend toward greater asymmetry was observed within both groups as cadence was increased or power output was diminished; changes in cadence or power output did not significantly affect interlimb asymmetry ($P < .05$).

Conclusion.—Individuals with ACL injury have a decreased total output from the injured limb and rely on the uninjured limb for most of the power output. This may compromise the ability to restore lower-limb muscle strength after injury.

▶ These authors studied 10 people with ACL deficiency and 10 uninjured people in their control group. The purpose of this study was to look at injured versus noninjured ACL limbs and the power output during stationary cycling. These authors concluded, not surprisingly, that people with ACL injuries generate significantly more power output from uninjured limbs than injured limbs.

R. C. Cantu, MD, MA

A Cross-Sectional Analysis of Sagittal Knee Laxity and Isokinetic Muscle Strength in Soccer Players

Ergün M, Işlegen Ç, Taşkiran E (Ege Univ, Izmir, Turkey)

Int J Sports Med 25:594-598, 2004   4–9

Background.—Several studies have shown that uninjured knee laxity in patients with injuries to the anterior cruciate ligament (ACL) is greater than the average knee laxity in normal subjects. These findings prompted speculation about a possible association between ligamentous injury and previous joint laxity. However, conclusions thus far regarding such an association are controversial. Sagittal knee laxity and isokinetic strength of knee extensor and flexor muscle groups were measured, and differences related to leg dominance were evaluated.

Methods.—This cross-sectional study included 44 healthy male soccer players and 44 sedentary persons (control group). All the participants were tested with a KT-1000 knee arthrometer for knee laxity.

Results.—Posterior laxity in the nondominant side of soccer players was significantly higher than in the dominant side, whereas no significant differences occurred in anterior and total anteroposterior laxity in both groups. The soccer players had significantly lower anterior and total anteroposterior laxity values than control subjects, although no significant difference occurred between posterior laxity values on both sides. The dominant extremity in soccer players demonstrated significantly higher knee flexor peak torque and hamstring/quadriceps (H/Q) ratio at 180°/s in soccer players. In the sedentary control subjects, H/Q ratio at 60°/s of the dominant side was significantly higher than that of the nondominant side. No significant correlations between knee laxity and isokinetic knee extensor and flexor strength and H/Q ratios occurred in either group, with the exception of a weak negative correlation between posterior knee laxity and isokinetic extensor peak torque at 60°/s, 180°/s, and 300°/s on the nondominant side of soccer players and at 300°/s on the nondominant side of control subjects.

Conclusions.—Soccer players were found to have significantly less sagittal knee laxity and higher isokinetic strength of the knee flexors and extensors compared with sedentary control subjects. The difference in isokinetic strength was found to be greater for the flexor muscle group. More studies are needed to determine whether the increased H/Q ratio decreases the risk of ligamentous injury.

▶ These authors studied 44 male soccer players and 44 sedentary people to determine posterior laxity in dominant versus nondominant sides. The outcome for these authors was that soccer players had significantly higher laxity on their nondominant side compared with their dominant side, with no significant differences in the control group.

R. C. Cantu, MD, MA

Immediate Effects of a Knee Brace With a Constraint to Knee Extension on Knee Kinematics and Group Reaction Forces in a Stop-Jump Task

Yu B, Herman D, Preston J, et al (Univ of North Carolina at Chapel Hill; Univ of Hong Kong)

Am J Sports Med 32:1136-1143, 2004   4–10

Introduction.—The noncontact nature of most anterior cruciate ligament (ACL) injuries indicates that the intrinsic forces produced by athletes themselves are likely to be an important cause of injury. A small knee flexion angle in landing tasks has been identified as a possible risk factor for the frequent noncontact ACL injuries that occur in sports. A newly designed knee brace with a constraint to knee extension was constructed with the use of an existing functional knee brace (4titude; dj Orthopedics, LLC, Vista, California). This knee brace fabricated with a constraint to knee extension was evaluated by means of repeated measure design for brace effects to determine whether it would significantly increase the knee flexion angle at the landing of the stop-jump task and whether the maximum ground reaction forces would be decreased as the knee flexion angle at landing increased.

Methods.—Three-dimensional videographic and force plate data were obtained from 10 male and 10 female healthy recreational athletes, aged 18 to 28 years, with no known knee disorders. All participants performed a stop-jump task with and without the specially designed brace. The knee flexion angle at landing, maximum knee flexion angle, and peak ground reaction forces during the stance phase of the stop-jump task were ascertained for each participant with and without the knee brace.

Results.—The specially designed knee brace significantly increased the knee flexion angle at the landing in the stop-jump task (average, from 27.4°-32.5° in men and from 22.3°-27.6° in women [$P = .001$]). Female participants had significantly smaller knee flexion angles at the landing ($P = .003$) and the stop-jump task ($P = .001$), compared to men in both brace and nonbrace conditions.

No significant effect on the maximum posterior or ground reaction force ($P = .588$), the maximum medial ground reaction force ($P = .708$), or the maximum knee flexion angle ($P = .508$) was observed in the stop-jump task in the knee brace condition.

Conclusion.—The specially designed knee brace did not significantly impact participants' performances in the stop-jump tasks. Further investigation is needed to determined the effects of the knee brace on lower extremity kinematics and kinetics of patients with ACL injuries.

▶ This study showed that this particular knee brace did not significantly affect the subjects' performance in stop-jump tasks or consistently affect the subjects' running and jumping performance in a positive or negative way.

R. C. Cantu, MD, MA

The Complete Type of Suprapatellar Plica in a Professional Baseball Pitcher: Consideration of a Cause of Anterior Knee Pain

Adachi N, Ochi M, Uchio Y, et al (Hiroshima Univ, Japan; Shimane Med Univ, Izumo, Japan)
Arthroscopy 20:987-991, 2004   4–11

Introduction.—Synovial plicae are the intra-articular remnants present in the early fetal stages. They may be classified as infrapatellar, suprapatellar, and mediopatellar, depending on the membrane from which they arise. Medial plicae are regarded as a source of anterior knee pain; few reports have addressed symptomatic suprapatellar plicae. Described is the case of a professional baseball pitcher with a complete type of suprapatellar plica who was successfully treated by resecting the plica under arthroscopy.

> *Case Report.*—Man, 27, a professional baseball pitcher, was seen for increasing right anterior knee pain while pitching for more than a 2-year period. He was right-hand dominant. Several conservative treatments were not able to diminish the anterior knee pain. On physical examination, he had no swelling or ballottement of his affected knee joint and no limitation in range of motion of the femorotibial joint. Patellar mobility was limited. Tracking of the patella on the patellar groove was normal He reported tenderness along the joint line of his lateral patellofemoral joint. Flexion of his right knee joint more than 70° during the early cocking phase of the throwing motion induced the right anterior knee pain. Preoperative radiograph revealed an osteophyte formation on the lateral edge of the patella. Preoperative sagittal MRI showed a suprapatellar plica in the suprapatellar pouch as if it were dividing the suprapatellar pouch into 2 cavities. On MRI, the cartilage surface of the patella appeared slightly irregular. No patellar malalignment was observed on plain radiographs or MRI. Isokinetic muscle strength test revealed that the side-to-side ratio of the peak torque was 69%. The peak torque curve of the injured knee was not smooth; it had remarkable loss of peak torque at around 70° to 80° of flexion, which was the ankle in which the patient reported knee pain. Arthroscopic examination showed obvious cartilaginous damage on the lateral facet of the patella and facing trochlea of the femoral condyle. This complete suprapatellar plica appeared to be anchoring the patella, which decreased mobility of the patella. After resecting the complete type of suprapatellar plica, mobility of the patella improved The patient had rapid reduction of anterior knee pain and was able to return to pitching.

Conclusion.—The primary cause of this patient's anterior knee pain was cartilaginous damage on the patella and the trochlea; this may have been accelerated by the existence of the suprapatellar plica that decreased the mobility of the patella.

▶ This is a case report of a 27-year-old baseball pitcher who underwent an arthroscopic suprapatellar plica resection for relief of anterior knee pain. The authors discuss evaluation, diagnosis, and treatment of this condition.

R. C. Cantu, MD, MA

Open Versus Closed Kinetic Chain Exercises in Patellofemoral Pain: A 5-Year Prospective Randomized Study
Witvrouw E, Danneels L, Van Tiggelen D, et al (Ghent Univ, Belgium)
Am J Sports Med 32:1122-1130, 2004   4–12

Background.—The management of patellofemoral pain syndrome (PFPS) is usually conservative initially. Usually, open kinetic chain (OKC) leg extension exercises are used to strengthen the quadriceps, but symptoms may be exacerbated with these movements. Closed kinetic chain (CKC) exercises are being used more often because they simulate and replicate many functional movements. CKC exercises produce lower patellofemoral joint stresses and may be better tolerated by patients with PFPS. An investigation determined the long-term outcomes with both exercise protocols and whether the short-term positive results were maintained at long-term follow-up.

Methods.—The 49 patients were randomly assigned to a 5-week program of purely CKC (25 patients) or purely OKC (24 patients) exercises for their PFPS. Evaluations included muscular characteristics, subjective symptoms, and functional performance at the initial physical examination, 3 months after treatment, and after 5 years.

Results.—After 5 years, 9 patients in the OKC group and 10 patients in the CKC group were pain free. Thirty-seven patients (75%) participated actively in sports, 22 of whom had OKC treatment and 15 of whom had CKC treatment. All patients were instructed to continue their exercises at home, but after 5 years, 66% of the OKC group and 35% of the CKC group did not do so. Four patients in the OKC group and 10 patients in the CKC group were still doing their exercises weekly at 5 years. Subjectively, the OKC group had significantly less swelling of the knee joint, less pain while descending stairs, and less pain at night than did the CKC group. The Kujala score and 18 visual analog scale scores were used to document subjective outcomes (Fig 1). No statistical differences were found between the groups with respect to functional assessment or muscle strength measurements. At 5 years, patients in the OKC group experienced significantly more pain during sitting with the knees bent than they had at 3 months. However, no significant difference in the Kujala score was found. On functional assessment of the patients in the OKC group at 5 years, pain-free maximal knee bending was significantly improved, but the patients' performance during the triple-jump test was significantly worse for both the injured and the uninjured legs. At 5 years, the results of the 45-cm step-up test were significantly better than at 3 months, and 92% of patients were free of pain during its performance compared with only 73% earlier. Neither hamstring nor quadriceps strength

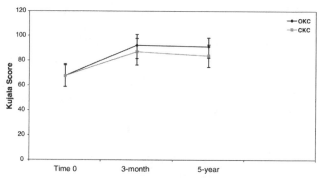

FIGURE 1.—Mean values of both groups on the Kujala scale at the different evaluation periods. *Abbreviations: OKC*, Open kinetic chain; *CKC*, closed kinetic chain. (Courtesy of Witvrouw E, Danneels L, Van Tiggelen D, et al: Open versus closed kinetic chain exercises in patellofemoral pain: A 5-year prospective randomized study. *Am J Sports Med* 32:1122-1130, 2004.)

measurements improved between the 3-month and the 5-year assessments. Compared with the pain felt at 3 months, the pain was significantly more for patients in the CKC group after 5 years while descending the stairs, when jumping, during sports activities, and with prolonged sitting with flexed knees. More clicking sensations were noted also. The Kujala score did not change significantly between the 3-month and 5-year assessments. Seventy-three percent of patients performed the 45-cm step-up test pain free at 3 months and 80% performed it pain free at 5 years, which was not a significant increase. Pain-free maximal knee bending and the triple-jump performance showed no significant change over time for the CKC group. Quadriceps strength was not significantly different at the 2 assessment points, but hamstring strength was significantly decreased after 5 years compared with the values at 3 months.

Conclusions.—After 5 years, both groups had good maintenance of positive subjective and functional outcomes. Most variables showed no differences between the CKC and OKC groups. Combining the 2 approaches may be the optimal choice.

▶ We continue to search for the most appropriate rehabilitation exercise program. CKC exercises are partially based on the principle of specific adaptations to imposed demand (SAID principle). Although some studies have shown them to be superior to OKC exercises, this study suggests that still more needs to be learned. Fundamentally, one might theoretically suggest that the relative efficacy of each would depend on the cause of the problem. For example, according to the SAID principle, OKC exercises should be more beneficial in breaststrokers with patellofemoral pain because it simulates their offending activity more than does CKC exercises.

I. Shrier, MD, PhD

Effects of Taping on Pain and Function in Patellofemoral Pain Syndrome: A Randomized Controlled Trial

Whittingham M, Palmer S, Macmillan F (Army Training Regiment Bassingbourn, Royston, Hertfordshire, England; Queen Margaret Univ College, Edinburgh, Scotland)
J Orthop Sports Phys Ther 34:504-510, 2004   4–13

Background.—The causes of patellofemoral pain syndrome (PFPS) are likely to be multifactorial. The effects of PFPS on daily life include all activities that load the patellofemoral joint. Conservative management with physical therapy is advocated for pain control and muscle strengthening. Taping to promote patellar alignment and performing exercises to activate and strengthen the vascus medialis obliquus (VMO) are the primary approaches used. The effectiveness of patella taping and exercise with respect to reducing pain and increasing function in individuals with PFPS was assessed.

Methods.—The 30 participants (24 men, 6 women; ages 17-25 years; mean age, 18.7 years) were split into 3 equal groups of 10 each and randomly assigned to 1 of 3 programs: patella taping combined with a standardized exercise program (group 1), placebo-patella taping-and-exercise program (group 2), or an exercise program alone (group 3). The taping and exercises were performed daily for 4 weeks. Weekly visual analog scale (VAS) scores were used to indicate pain, and completion of a functional index questionnaire (FIQ) assessed function.

Results.—All 3 groups had a progressive decline in pain during the 4-week assessment period. Those having taping plus exercise (group 1) were pain free after 4 weeks, reflecting a statistically significant change from baseline. The experimental groups 2 and 3 differed significantly in their outcomes. No differences were noted between these 2 groups for the first week, but the group following the taping-and-exercise combination treatment had significantly lower VAS ratings than the other groups at weeks 2, 3, and 4. The placebo taping-and-exercise and the exercise-alone groups did not differ significantly in VAS scores at any point. FIQ scores changed significantly with

TABLE 5.—Mean (±SD) Functional Index Questionnaire (FIQ) Scores (Normal Function is 16/16)

Time Period	Taping and Exercise	Placebo Taping and Exercise	Exercise Alone
Initial	7.6 ± 1.0	7.8 ± 0.8	7.7 ± 0.8
Week 1	11.3 ± 1.2*	10.3 ± 1.1	10.0 ± 0.8
Week 2	14.0 ± 0.8†	11.6 ± 1.0	11.3 ± 0.8
Week 3	15.5 ± 0.7†	12.5 ± 1.3	12.7 ± 0.9
Week 4	16.0 ± 0.0†	13.5 ± 1.1	13.5 ± 1.0

*Significantly better than exercise-alone group (*P* < .01).
†Significantly better than placebo-taping-and-exercise and exercise-alone groups (*P* < .01).
(Reprinted from Whittingham M, Palmer S, Macmillan F: Effects of taping on pain and function in patellofemoral pain syndrome: A randomized controlled trial. *J Orthop Sports Phys Ther* 34:504-510, 2004. Copyright 2004 with permission of the Orthopaedic and Sports Sections of the American Physical Therapy Association.)

time, with significantly better FIQ scores at weeks 2, 3, and 4 for the taping-and-exercise group compared to the placebo taping-and-exercise group and significantly better scores for the taping-and-exercise group at weeks 1 through 4 compared to the exercise-alone group (Table 5). Groups 2 and 3 did not differ significantly with respect to FIQ outcomes at any point.

Conclusions.—Combining daily patella taping with an exercise program for 4 weeks was more effective than placebo taping-and-exercise or exercise only in reducing the pain and improving the function of patients with PFPS. Patella taping plus muscle-strengthening exercises would be an appropriate choice for PFPS patients and should enhance the speed of recovery.

▶ Patellofemoral taping continues to be promoted as an effective treatment, and studies such as the current one are partly the reason. The results of this randomized controlled trial suggest that taping is superior to a home exercise program. Although taping is effective, readers should be cautious in interpreting that exercises are inferior. As in all exercise studies, only 1 type of exercise program was used; the exercise program included both stretching and strengthening, but a different choice of exercises may achieve superior or inferior results.

I. Shrier, MD, PhD

Relation Between Running Injury and Static Lower Limb Alignment in Recreational Runners
Lun V, Meeuwisse WH, Stergiou P, et al (Univ of Calgary, Canada)
Br J Sports Med 38:576-580, 2004   4–14

Objectives.—To determine if measurements of static lower limb alignment are related to lower limb injury in recreational runners.

Methods.—Static lower limb alignment was prospectively measured in 87 recreational runners. They were observed for the following six months for any running related musculoskeletal injuries of the lower limb. Injuries were defined according to six types: R1, R2, and R3 injuries caused a reduction in running mileage for one day, two to seven days, or more than seven days respectively; S1, S2, and S3 injuries caused stoppage of running for one day, two to seven days, or more than seven days respectively.

Results.—At least one lower limb injury was suffered by 79% of the runners during the observation period. When the data for all runners were pooled, 95% confidence intervals calculated for the differences in the measurements of lower limb alignment between the injured and non-injured runners suggested that there were no differences. However, when only runners diagnosed with patellofemoral pain syndrome (n = 6) were compared with non-injured runners, differences were found in right ankle dorsiflexion (0.3 to 6.1), right knee genu varum (-0.9 to -0.3), and left forefoot varus (-0.5 to -0.4).

Conclusions.—In recreational runners, there is no evidence that static biomechanical alignment measurements of the lower limbs are related to lower limb injury except patellofemoral pain syndrome. However, the effect of static lower limb alignment may be injury specific.

▶ The evidence that biomechanical misalignments in the lower limb may be related to injuries has received much interest over the years. This study in a group of 87 recreational runners found no differences in pooled static limb measurements when comparing injured with noninjured runners. The only significant finding was when data from runners with patellofemoral pain syndrome were analyzed separately, differences were found in ankle dorsiflexion, knee genu varum, and forefoot varus in the injured group, suggesting that biomechanical alignment may be injury specific. The overall finding is in keeping with other prospective studies in this area.

P. McCrory, MBBS, PhD

Similar Histopathological Picture in Males With Achilles and Patellar Tendinopathy
Maffulli N, Testa V, Capasso G, et al (Keele Univ, Stoke-on-Trent, England; Dynamic Ctr, Angri, Italy; Second Univ of Naples, Italy; et al)
Med Sci Sports Exerc 36:1470-1475, 2004   4–15

Background.—Disorders of the Achilles tendon and patellar tendons are major problems for competitive and recreational athletes. Achilles tendinopathy and patellar tendinopathy occur in athletic patients of similar age groups. Achilles tendinopathy occurs in the main body of the tendon, whereas patellar tendinopathy occurs adjacent to the bone-tendon interface. Whether the pathologic processes of these tendinopathies are similar is unclear. Whether differences in the histopathologic appearance of tendinopathic Achilles and patellar tendons exist was determined.

Methods.—Biopsy specimens were obtained from tendinopathic Achilles tendons in men with an average age of 34 years (21 biopsies) and from tendinopathic patellar tendons in men with an average age of 32 years (28 biopsies). These biopsies were compared with biopsies of Achilles and patellar tendons obtained from deceased patients with known tendon pathologic conditions and patellar tendons from patients undergoing reconstruction of the anterior cruciate ligament. Hematoxylin-stained slides were interpreted by using a semiquantitative grading scale (0, normal, to 3, maximally abnormal) for fiber structure, fiber arrangement, rounding of the nuclei, regional variations in cellularity, increased vascularity, decreased collagen stainability, and hyalinization.

Results.—The highest mean score of tendinopathic Achilles tendons did not differ significantly from that of tendinopathic patellar tendons. The ability to differentiate between an Achilles tendon and a patellar tendon was low.

Conclusions.—The histologic aspects of Achilles and patellar tendons are similar. In this study, determining whether a specimen was harvested from an Achilles or a patellar tendon was not possible on the basis of histologic examination. The general pattern of degeneration was common to both tendinopathic Achilles and patellar tendons. A common, as yet unidentified, etiopathologic mechanism may act on both of the tendon populations in this study.

▶ These authors studied both the Achilles and patellar tendon problems in both recreational and competitive sports to attempt to determine the histologic components of both and determined that these 2 tendon groups have similar histopathologic components.

R. C. Cantu, MD, MA

Eccentric Decline Squat Protocol Offers Superior Results at 12 Months Compared With Traditional Eccentric Protocol for Patellar Tendinopathy in Volleyball Players
Young MA, Cook JL, Purdam CR, et al (La Trobe Univ, Bundoora, Victoria, Australia; Australian Inst of Sport, Bruce, ACT, Australia; Univ of Umea, Sweden)
Br J Sports Med 39:102-105, 2005   4–16

Background.—Conservative treatment of patellar tendinopathy has been minimally investigated. Effective validated treatment protocols are required.

Objectives.—To investigate the immediate (12 weeks) and long term (12 months) efficacy of two eccentric exercise programmes for the treatment of patellar tendinopathy.

Methods.—This was a prospective randomised controlled trial of 17 elite volleyball players with clinically diagnosed and imaging confirmed patellar tendinopathy. Participants were randomly assigned to one of two treatment groups: a decline group and a step group. The decline group were required to perform single leg squats on a 25 degrees decline board, exercising into tendon pain and progressing their exercises with load. The step group performed single leg squats on a 10 cm step, exercising without tendon pain and progressing their exercises with speed then load. All participants completed a 12 week intervention programme during their preseason. Outcome measures used were the Victorian Institute of Sport Assessment (VISA) score for knee function and 100 mm visual analogue scale (VAS) for tendon pain with activity. Measures were taken throughout the intervention period and at 12 months.

Results.—Both groups had improved significantly from baseline at 12 weeks and 12 months (Fig 3). Analysis of the likelihood of a 20 point improvement in VISA score at 12 months revealed a greater likelihood of clinical improvements in the decline group than the step group. VAS scores at 12 months did not differ between the groups.

Conclusions.—Both exercise protocols improved pain and sporting function in volleyball players over 12 months. This study indicates that the decline squat protocol offers greater clinical gains during a rehabilitation programme for patellar tendinopathy in athletes who continue to train and play with pain.

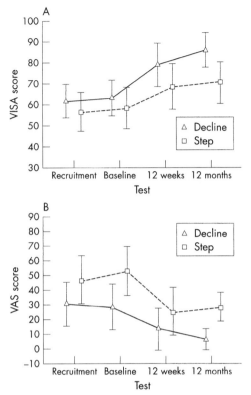

FIGURE 3.—Mean (SD) change in (A) Victorian Institute of Sport Assessment (VISA) scores and (B) visual analogue scale (VAS) scores over 12 months. (Courtesy of Young MA, Cook JL, Purdam CR, et al: Eccentric decline squat protocol offers superior results at 12 months compared with traditional eccentric protocol for patellar tendinopathy in volleyball players. *Br J Sports Med* 39:102-105, 2005. Reprinted with permission from the BMJ Publishing Group.)

▶ As the field of sport medicine grows, it is encouraging to see more and more studies evaluating different exercise programs for different conditions. This study was well conducted, but strength coaches may note that the technique used in the step protocol did not match with basic strength training principles. During a squat, most people advocate that the weight should be centered over the hind to mid foot, with little to no weight over the toes. In the photo shown in the article, it appears that there is substantial body weight over the toes. Interestingly, if one tries the decline apparatus that was used, it is necessary to shift the weight posteriorly to maintain balance on the decline. Therefore, the mechanism of action for the apparatus may be through forcing the subject to use the correct posture for a squat. If true, the benefit of making it easier to teach proper technique would need to be balanced against the added cost, difficulty in travel situations, and so on.

I. Shrier, MD, PhD

Patellar Tendinosis: Acute Patellar Tendon Rupture and Jumper's Knee
DePalma MJ, Perkins RH (Ohio State Univ, Columbus)
Physician Sportsmed 32(5):41-45, 2004   4–17

Background.—Patellar tendinopathy, so-called jumper's knee, is common among those who play sports that involve explosive lower-limb movements. It is characterized by collagen degeneration followed by fibrosis of the bone-tendon junction of the inferior patella. Acute patella ligament rupture usually affects male athletes younger than 40. A case of stage 4 tendinopathy, with complete rupture of the patellar ligament was discussed.

Case Report.—Man, 34, recreational athlete, landed hard after a layup during a basketball game. He heard a popping sound and felt a left knee cramp. He was unable to bear weight or actively extend the left knee. He was taken to the emergency department. The patient said that he had experienced intermittent anterior knee pain with squatting and climbing stairs over the previous month. The patella was located proximal to the tibiofemoral joint with a large effusion. The inferior patellar pole was tender, and there was a palpable gap. Plain radiographs revealed patella alta with avulsed bone fragments. The distal patella was elongated with induration and effusion. The Insall-Salvati ratio and Caton ratio were abnormal. The patient underwent surgical repair with reinforcement on day 6 after injury. Initial postoperative rehabilitation included weight bearing, isometric knee extension, and active knee flexion. At 6 weeks, active knee extension was added. By 3 months, closed-chain activities for strength and flexibility were included in his regimen. At 9 months, the athlete reported mild swelling but no pain on athletic activity.

Conclusions.—Jumper's knee can occur in athletes who engage in explosive lower-limb actions. The end-stage of patellar tendinopathy is an acute patellar tendon rupture. Postoperative rehabilitation must address the abnormalities that may have predisposed the patient to disruptive patellar tendon strain. Counseling patients with early stage tendinopathy with appropriate flexibility and plyometric exercises may prevent development of end-stage tendinopathy.

► This study looks at the athlete who uses explosive lower-limb movements, such as in sports using jumping. This jumping motion causes a contraction of the quadriceps when landing and may lead to acute patellar tendon rupture. The study focuses on treatment and prevention of these injuries.

R. C. Cantu, MD, MA

The Appearance of Kissing Contusion in the Acutely Injured Knee in the Athletes

Terzidis IP, Christodoulou AG, Ploumis AL, et al (Thessaloniki, Greece)
Br J Sports Med 38:592-596, 2004   4–18

Background.—MRI can be used to confirm a diagnosis of bone contusion. Kissing contusion refers to a bone contusion on both surfaces of the knee. The frequency, type, and distribution of kissing contusions of the knee in young athletes were assessed.

Study Design.—The study included 197 male and 58 female athletes, 16 to 32 years old, who had MRI examinations for acute knee injuries from April 1996 to December 2000. The examinations were reviewed by 2 independent examiners. Bone contusions were classified as follows: Type I lesions had a loss of signal intensity on T1 W or proton density sequences and increased signal on T2. Type II and type III lesions had the same signal characteristics as type I, but type II had an interruption of the black cortical line, and type III lesions were located in the bone region immediately adjacent to the cortex without a definite cortical interruption.

Findings.—Bone contusions were diagnosed in 71 (28%) of the 255 injured athletes. Of these, 16 (6.3%) were kissing contusions. Of the kissing contusions, 8 were associated with anterior cruciate ligament tears, 3 with meniscal tears, 4 were isolated lesions, and 1 was delayed after a meniscal tear. Type I lesions were more common on the lateral femoral condyle, whereas type III were more common on the lateral tibial condyle. Of the 16 patients diagnosed with kissing contusions, 12 had arthroscopy and were followed up for an average of 31 months. Recovery time averaged approximately 5 months overall.

Conclusions.—The diagnosis of bone contusion of the knee can be confirmed with MRI before arthroscopy. Kissing contusions are rare and are often associated with ligamentous or meniscal tears. After arthroscopy, recovery times were prolonged for patients with kissing contusions.

▶ These authors looked at multiple knee joint diagnosis, one being kissing contusion. They found that kissing contusion is rare, with single bone contusions being seen more often. Although kissing injuries are rare, when they are seen, they are significant and are often associated with ligamentous or meniscal tears.

R. C. Cantu, MD, MA

Local Corticosteroid Injection in Iliotibial Band Friction Syndrome in Runners: A Randomised Controlled Trial

Gunter P, Schwellnus MP (Univ of Cape Town, Newlands, South Africa)
Br J Sports Med 38:269-272, 2004   4–19

Background.—Iliotibial band friction syndrome (ITBFS) is a common running injury that involves an inflammation of the lateral aspect of the knee caused by repetitive friction between the iliotibial band and the lateral femoral condyle. Initial treatment includes management of local inflammation and pain and often includes corticosteroid injection. The efficacy of corticosteroid injection for early phase treatment of ITBFS was investigated in a randomized, placebo-controlled, blinded study.

Study Design.—The study group included 18 runners (ages 20-50 years) who were clinically diagnosed with ITBFS. After a complete clinical evaluation, a treadmill running test was used to assess pain. The 18 participants were then selected randomly to an injection of either 40-mg methylprednisolone acetate mixed with 10-mg lignocaine (EXP group) or lignocaine alone (CON group) into the space between the lateral femoral condyle and iliotibial band. Participants were not allowed to exercise for the 14-day study period. They were allowed to ice twice a day. They kept a daily diary of pain and adverse events. At day 7 and 14, the treadmill running assessment was repeated and pain perception was compared between these 2 groups.

Findings.—A significant decrease was noted in the total pain experienced during running on the treadmill in the EXP group compared with that of the CON group by day 14. No adverse events occurred.

Conclusions.—Corticosteroid injection is both safe and effective for the early-phase treatment of ITBFS. The next phase of treatment must include identification and correction of the underlying cause of ITBFS in these patients.

▶ These authors studied 18 runners with iliotibial band friction syndrome to see whether an injection of 40-mg methylprednisone acetate was effective in decreasing pain while running. They concluded that this injection effectively decreases pain during running in the first 2 weeks of treatment.

R. C. Cantu, MD, MA

Asymptomatic Tibial Stress Reactions: MRI Detection and Clinical Follow-up in Distance Runners
Bergman AG, Fredericson M, Ho C, et al (Stanford Univ, Calif; Sand Hill Imaging, Menlo Park, Calif)
AJR 183:635-638, 2004   4–20

Background.—Stress reactions of both bone and soft tissue are common among athletes. MRI is a sensitive method for the detection of bone stress reactions. Previous articles have described incidental MRI findings of bone stress reactions in athletes. The incidence of MRI findings of tibial stress among asymptomatic distance runners and whether this predicts the development of subsequent symptomatic tibial stress injuries were examined.

Study Design.—The study group consisted of 21 athletes on a long-distance university running team. MRI examinations were performed within 1 week of completion of training. All athletes were asymptomatic. All were followed up for clinical signs of lower leg pain as long as they remained on the team.

Findings.—Of the 21 asymptomatic long distance runners, 43% had MRI abnormalities indicative of tibial stress injuries; these were bilateral in 5 of the 9 athletes. During follow-up of their college running career, none had signs of a tibial stress injury.

Conclusions.—MRI signs of tibial stress reactions are common among young, asymptomatic distance runners. These MRI findings were not associated with symptomatic tibial stress reactions during these athletes' college careers but probably reflected their high training load. These findings also emphasize the importance of correlating sensitive MRI findings with clinical results before making therapeutic decisions.

▶ These authors found that MRI scanning of asymptomatic distance runners for tibial stress reactions revealed MRI abnormalities indicating stress injuries in 43%. The runners in this study were found to have unilateral as well as bilateral stress injuries. The authors attribute these findings to the high training load to which elite distance runners are subjected.

R. C. Cantu, MD, MA

Acute Fracture Through an Intramedullary Stabilized Chronic Tibial Stress Fracture in a Basketball Player: A Case Report and Literature Review
Baublitz SD, Shaffer BS (DC Sportsmedicine Inst, Washington DC)
Am J Sports Med 32:1968-1972, 2004   4–21

Background.—Stress fractures in athletes are most commonly located in the shaft of the tibia. Most tibial stress fractures, particularly those of the posteromedial cortex, can be treated with rest with or without immobilization. However, lesions located in the anterior cortex of the central tibia have been found to have a poor tendency to heal. Several treatment strategies exist for these fractures, and surgical intervention is often necessary for fractures that do not respond to conservative measures Intramedullary nailing is an established approach for the treatment of delayed or nonunited tibial stress fracture. Described was a fracture after intramedullary rodding of a chronic tibial stress fracture.

Case Report.—Man, 19, an NCAA Division I basketball player, was evaluated after several weeks of physical activity–related pain in his left leg. He reported no specific episode of trauma but had had similar intermittent symptoms over the previous 1.5 years. Examination revealed focal tenderness and swelling at the junction of the middle and distal third of the anterior tibia. Radiographs showed a subtle radiolucency at the junction of the middle and distal third of the anterior tibia, with accompanying cortical thickening. The patient was treated with temporary activity modifications, including transient nonweightbearing. Initial improvement occurred, and the patient was able to play in the next season. However, symptoms recurred, and the patient was reevaluated 10 months later. Focal tenderness and swelling were present, and a defect of the anterior tibial cortex (the "dreaded black line") was seen on radiographs. Surgical treatment was chosen by the patient. A reamed, unlocked, intramedullary rod was placed uneventfully in the left tibia. The patient initially responded well, but at 8 weeks after surgery he drove for a layup, torqued his leg, and felt a "pop" and acute pain in the mid left leg. Radiographic evaluation revealed a radiolucency of the midtibia with a spiral fracture centered at the site of the anterior tibial cortical debridement. The tibial fracture was nondisplaced. The patient was diagnosed with an acute fracture through a chronic tibial stress fracture after intramedullary rodding. The patient was treated with a period of nonweightbearing, followed by weightbearing with a Cam walker. By 12 months the patient returned to symptom-free full physical activity, including collegiate basketball. The most recent anteroposterior and lateral radiographs showed perseverance of the anterior cortical lucency, although the patient remained asymptomatic.

Conclusions.—Intramedullary nailing is an established approach for the treatment of delayed or nonunited tibial stress fracture. However, a possibility of fracture exists after stabilization, which may justify a more cautious approach in terms of a return to activity.

▶ These authors looked at a 19-year-old NCAA Division I basketball player with a several-week history of physical activity–related leg pain. This study looked at a fracture after intramedullary rodding of a chronic stress fracture that had not been previously reported.

R. C. Cantu, MD, MA

The Effect of Pulsed Ultrasound in the Treatment of Tibial Stress Fractures
Rue J-PH, Armstrong DW III, Frassica FJ, et al (Johns Hopkins Univ, Baltimore, Md; Natl Naval Med Ctr, Bethesda, Md; United States Naval Academy, Annapolis, Md)
Orthopedics 27:1192-1195, 2004   4–22

Introduction.—Tibial stress fractures commonly occur in athletes and military recruits. This prospective, randomized, double-blind clinical study sought to determine whether pulsed ultrasound reduces tibial stress fracture healing time. Twenty-six midshipmen (43 tibial stress fractures) were randomized to pulsed ultrasound or placebo treatment. Twenty-minute daily treatments continued until patients were asymptomatic with signs of healing on plain radiographs. The groups were not significantly different in demographics, delay from symptom onset to diagnosis, missed treatment days, total number of treatments, or time to return to duty. Pulsed ultrasound did not significantly reduce the healing time for tibial stress fractures.

▶ This randomized clinical trial of pulsed US indicated no difference in healing time for tibial stress fractures among midshipmen in the United States Navy. Although a previous case report may have been encouraging for this type of treatment, the present study provides evidence of no benefit for using low-intensity pulsed US for tibial stress fractures.

D. E. Feldman, PhD, PT

A Successful Conservative Approach to Managing Lower Leg Pain in a University Sports Injury Clinic: A Two Patient Case Study
Cunningham A, Spears IR (Univ of Teesside, Middlesbrough, England)
Br J Sports Med 38:233-234, 2004   4–23

Introduction.—Information is lacking concerning the conservative treatment of lower leg pain caused by running. The noninvasive treatment based on change of footwear was described in 2 case reports.

Case 1.—Woman, 28, was a healthy recreational runner with bilateral lower leg pain. She had no history or trauma or illness. The patient exercised 3 times a week (4 miles twice weekly and 6 miles once weekly) after a standard warm-up protocol. Her lower leg pain was more intense on the left; it had gradually increased during the preceding 4 months. She ceased running when pain started, which was within 10 minutes of activity. The woman stopped running completely on recommendation of her physician. Pain recurred upon return to activity.

Case 2.—Man, 20, was a sprinter who was experiencing symptoms in both legs, especially on the right. A clinical diagnosis of probable anterior compartment syndrome was made. The man was inactive at the time of referral.

Diagnosis and Treatment.—Both patients underwent video assessment of gait, then ran on a powered treadmill at their usual running speeds on 2 separate occasions (first in their normal running shoes, then unshod). This protocol was repeated outside when wearing footwear with harder, thinner soles.

"No pain" scores were documented throughout the evaluations. The first patient was started on a progressive 5-week training program while using the harder and thinner-soled training shoes. The second patient was advised to return immediately to normal training while wearing the harder, thinner-soled shoes. Both patients returned to a pain-free training schedule.

Conclusion.—The use of video analysis during running may emphasize changes in dorsiflexor angle at heel strike. Changing footwear to diminish dorsiflexor activity may be beneficial in cases of lower leg pain.

▶ This is a case study of 2 university clinic patients, the first a recreational runner and the second a sprinter, both with lower leg pain as a result of their respective sports. This article looks at chronic exertional compartment syndrome as an overuse injury in these 2 athletes, which was successfully treated with a change in footwear.

R. C. Cantu, MD, MA

Exercise Induced Compartment Syndrome in a Professional Footballer
Cetinus E, Uzel M, Bilgiç E, et al (Univ of Kahramanmaras, Turkey; Univ of Çukurova, Adana, Turkey)
Br J Sports Med 38:227-229, 2004   4–24

Introduction.—Major causes of recurrent pain in the lower leg in persons who exercise regularly include exercise-induced compartment syndrome (EICS), periostitis of the tibia, stress fracture, venous disease, obliterative arterial diseases, and shin splints. The least common of these is EICS. The treatment and outcome of a professional footballer with EICS were described.

Case Report.—Man, 20, was a professional footballer with an 18-month history of pain in the left leg precipitated by running. The time before the onset of pain while running had dropped from 30 minutes to 10 minutes. He described the pain as a tightening over the postero-medial aspect of the lower leg. Symptoms were relieved with rest.

The patient had not been able to play football in the preceding 6 months. Initially, he was treated by the team physiotherapist. He was treated in an orthopedic outpatient clinic where he received no relief from massage and oral anti-inflammatory agents. One year later, he was seen in an outpatient department where physical examination of the lower leg demonstrated nothing remarkable at rest. Immediately after exercise, marked tenseness over the posteromedial aspect of the lower leg was visible. Passive dorsiflexion of the left foot produced pain in the calf.

Plain radiography and MRI of the left cruris showed no evidence of stress fracture or any soft tissue pathology. Doppler US of the lower leg demonstrated no evidence of either venous or obliterative arterial disease. Compartment pressure was measured before and after treadmill exercise for suspected EICS. A diagnosis was made of exercise-induced left chronic posterior compartment syndrome. The patient underwent left posterior deep and superficial compartment fasciotomies. He was allowed to run 6 weeks postoperatively and return to football in the second national league without any restrictions. He expressed no difficulties at 8-month follow-up.

Conclusion.—The diagnosis of EICS can be established by history and physical examination after measurement of intracompartmental pressure. In most patients, definitive treatment is surgical fasciotomy. Patients can typically return to full activity shortly after surgery.

▶ This is a case study of a 20-year-old professional footballer with a history of pain in the left lower leg brought on by running. This is a good discussion of the diagnosis and treatment of EICS.

R. C. Cantu, MD, MA

Histology of the Fascial-Periosteal Interface in Lower Limb Chronic Deep Posterior Compartment Syndrome
Barbour TDA, Briggs CA, Bell SN, et al (Univ of Melbourne, Australia; Olympic Park Sports Medicine Centre, Melbourne, Australia)
Br J Sports Med 38:709-717, 2004   4–25

Objective.—To describe the histological features of the fascial-periosteal interface at the medial tibial border of patients surgically treated for chronic deep posterior compartment syndrome and to make statistical comparisons with control tissue.

Methods.—Nineteen subjects and 11 controls were recruited. Subject tissue was obtained at operation, and control tissue from autopsy cases. Tissue samples underwent histological preparation and then examination by an independent pathologist. Samples were analysed with regard to six histological variables: fibroblastic activity, chronic inflammatory cells, vascularity, collagen regularity, mononuclear cells, and ground substance. Collagen regularity was measured with respect to collagen density, fibre arrangement, orientation, and spacing. The observed changes were graded from 1 to 4 in terms of abnormality. Mann-Whitney U test, Spearman correlation coefficients, and intraobserver reliability scores were used.

Results.—With regard to collagen arrangement, control tissue showed greater degrees of irregularity than subject tissue ($P = 0.01$) (Fig 3). Subjects with a symptom duration of greater than 12 months (as opposed to less than 12 months) showed greater degrees of collagen irregularity ($P = 0.043$). Vas-

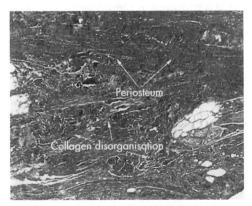

FIGURE 3.—Periosteum is seen at the top of the slide, and disorganized collagen is present throughout the lower part. 10 × magnification, Masson's trichrome stain. (Courtesy of Barbour TDA, Briggs CA, Bell SN, et al: Histology of the fascial-periosteal interface in lower limb chronic deep posterior compartment syndrome. *Br J Sports Med* 38:709-717, 2004. Reprinted with permission from the BMJ Publishing Group.)

cular changes approached significance ($P = 0.077$). With regard to the amount of fibrocyte activity, chronic inflammatory cell activity, mononuclear cells, or ground substance, there were no significant differences between controls and subjects. Good correlation was seen in scores measuring chronic inflammatory cell activity and mononuclear cells ($r = 0.649$), and moderate correlation was seen between fibrocyte activity and vascular changes ($r = 0.574$). Intraobserver reliability scores were good for chronic inflammatory cell activity and moderate for vascular changes, but were poor for collagen and fibrocyte variables. Individual cases showed varying degrees of fibrocyte activity, chronic inflammatory cellular infiltration, vascular abnormalities, and collagen fibre disruption.

Conclusions.—Statistical analysis showed no histological differences at the fascial-periosteal interface in cases of chronic deep posterior compartment syndrome, except for collagen, which showed less irregularity in subject samples. The latter may indicate a remodeling process, and this is supported by greater collagen irregularity in subjects with longer duration of symptoms.

▶ Compartment syndromes are common in running and jumping athletes, and the causes of the pain include stress fracture, medial tibia periostalgia, popliteal artery entrapment, and chronic exertional compartment syndrome (CECS). CECS is characterized by exercise-induced, inflammatory medial tibial pain with palpable tenderness over the medial tibial border. Tissue biopsies of subjects with this injury indicated that the major differences were in the structure of collagen in the injured subjects. The collagen structure was much more irregular in the injured subjects; in addition, vascularity was less well developed in the injured group. The end result is lack of fascial compliance during exercise and pain at the interface of the fascia and the periosteum.

M. J. L. Alexander, PhD

Acute Compartment Syndrome of the Anterior Thigh Following Quadriceps Strain in a Footballer
Burns BJ, Sproule J, Smyth H (St Vincent's Univ, Dublin; St James's Hosp, Dublin)
Br J Sports Med 38:218-220, 2004   4–26

Introduction.—Acute anterior compartment syndrome of the thigh in an athlete can be limb threatening and life threatening. It necessitates urgent diagnosis. Reported was a rare case of acute anterior compartment syndrome in the thigh of a footballer precipitated by an acute quadriceps strain that was exacerbated by poor first aid and alcohol consumption.

> *Case Report.*—Man, 21, was seen in the emergency department for severe constant pain in the right thigh 17 hours after participating in a game of soccer in which he jumped vertically upwards from standing to compete for a header when he experienced acute pain in

his right thigh. He continued to play for an additional 10 minutes before limping off the pitch. He did not receive any treatment and took no analgesics. He consumed about 8 units of alcohol during that evening.

He was not able to bear weight on the right leg by the time he was seen in the emergency department. He had a small area of ecchymosis on the anterolateral aspect of the distal thigh. The thigh circumference at 10 cm proximal to insertion of the quadriceps tendon was 52 cm on the right and 46 cm on the left. The right quadriceps muscle was tense and exquisitely tender. A straight leg raise was restricted and painful. Anterior, medial, and posterior compartment pressures were 29, 25, and 27 mm Hg, respectively. Radiographs showed no fracture.

A diagnosis of acute anterior compartment syndrome was made and the patient underwent immediate fasciotomy. The wound was packed open and covered with a sterile dressing. Four days postoperatively, the defect underwent placement of a split skin graft and the patient was immobilized. There were no complications.

Rehabilitation involved initially passive, then gradual active, motion exercises. At 3-month follow-up, the patient was fully mobile and had full range of motion. He was able to return to playing soccer at 5 months after the injury.

Conclusion.—Acute quadriceps strain causing inflammation and edema in the muscle is a common and usually nonthreatening injury. In the patient described, this injury progressed into a compartment syndrome due to increased capillary pressure and increased surface area caused by acute muscle strain, aggravated by the vasodilatory effects of alcohol coupled with the effect of gravity that reduced venous return. The clinician needs a high index of suspicion to not overlook acute compartment syndrome.

▶ A case of acute anterior thigh compartment syndrome following a quadriceps strain in a 21-year-old soccer player serves to discuss the evaluation and treatment of this uncommon compartment syndrome.

R. C. Cantu, MD, MA

Acute Peroneal Compartment Syndrome Following Ankle Inversion Injury: A Case Report
Gabisan GG, Gentile DR (Monmouth Med Ctr, Long Branch, NJ)
Am J Sports Med 32:1059-1061, 2004   4–27

Background.—Acute peroneal compartment syndrome is a relatively rare injury. Minor athletic trauma may produce a rupture of the peroneus longus muscle, with development of a tense intracompartmental hematoma. Presented is a case that underscores the importance of awareness of the possibility of acute peroneal compartment syndrome in patients with ankle inversion injuries.

> *Case Report.*—Man, 23, sustained a noncontact inversion injury to his left ankle while playing flag football. The patient reported feeling a "pop" in his left lower leg, followed immediately by pain and a subsequent limp. The anterolateral left leg became increasingly painful 8 hours after injury. Radiographs at a local emergency department were negative, and the patient was discharged with a diagnosis of ankle sprain. However, he continued to have increasing pain in the anterolateral leg, which was not relieved by Percocet. At 24 hours after injury, the patient was referred to another emergency department. Examination showed tenseness in the anterior and lateral compartments of the left leg. He had decreased sensation on the dorsum and in the first web space of his foot, and he could not actively evert his foot. Radiographs of the tibia and fibula showed no fractures. Compartment pressures measured 130 mm Hg in the lateral compartment and 60 mm Hg in the anterior compartment. The superficial and deep posterior compartment pressures were less than 20 mm Hg. The patient's blood pressure was 127/74 mm Hg. Fasciotomies of the anterior and lateral compartments were performed. The anterior compartment muscles appeared normal, but the lateral compartment was tense with hematoma, and a tear in the peroneus longus muscle belly was found. The patient had immediate relief of pain in the recovery room after evacuation of the hematoma. Examination at 10 days showed normal sensation, active foot eversion, and no evidence of wound infection or drainage. The patient used a lace-up ankle brace for 2 months. Examination at 12 months after surgery revealed full active range of motion, full eversion and dorsiflexion strength, and no sensory deficits.

Conclusions.—Peroneal compartment syndrome should be considered in the differential diagnosis of a patient with a painful inversion injury. A tear in the peroneus longus muscle may result in a compressive hematoma in the lateral compartment, leading to delayed development of compartment syndrome.

▶ This is a case study of a 23-year-old man who had a peroneal compartment syndrome after sustaining an inversion injury during a flag football competition. The authors discuss diagnosis and treatment of this rare occurrence and bring to the attention of medical personnel treating ankle inversions to keep this differential diagnosis in mind when evaluating these patients.

R. C. Cantu, MD, MA

Popliteal Artery Entrapment Syndrome in an Elite Rower: Sonographic Appearances

Rey IA, Rey GA, Cruz JRA, et al (Virgen de la Victoria Univ, Malaga, Spain; Vimac Rehabilitation Ctr, Malaga, Spain; Malaga Univ, Spain; et al)
J Ultrasound Med 23:1667-1674, 2004   4–28

Background.—In popliteal artery entrapment syndrome (PAES), the popliteal artery and surrounding musculotendinous structures have an abnormal anatomic relation that compresses the artery during exercise. Young sports participants or athletes lacking any cardiovascular risk factors are primarily affected, with symptoms such as transient tingling or coldness in the foot and intermittent claudication. Irreversible arterial damage risking the limb's viability can develop if treatment is delayed. The case of a young rower with PAES was reported.

Case Report.—Man, 22, an Olympic rower, had sharp pain in the right calf and a brief experience of paleness and paresthesia of the first toe during training, then noted pain in the right calf while walking. Some relief came with running, but the patient also began walking with a pigeon-toed gait. After a month, the rower was diagnosed with possible fibrillary tear of the gastrocnemius muscle. Physical examination found no palpable pedal or right posterior tibial pulses, but the rest of the evaluation was normal. Duplex color Doppler sonography of the arterial system of the right lower leg revealed an absence of signal at the level of the pedal artery. Further Doppler studies showed continuous color flow and monophasic curves with low systolic-diastolic velocity, indicating severe stenosis or obstruction in the most proximal areas. Probable thrombus or intramural hematoma of 50% of the arterial lumen was diagnosed from B-scan images showing reduced echogenicity of the musculotendinous area of the gastrocnemius muscle in front of the anterior wall of the popliteal artery and a solid hypoechoic 2-cm lesion growing toward the interior of the lumen. Another solid intraluminal lesion was adhering to the posterior wall, nearly occluding the distal popliteal artery. The patient was given subcutaneous heparin with the presumptive diagnosis of a thrombus or intramural hematoma in the context of PAES. On an MRI scan of the popliteal fossa with longitudinal relaxation time sequences, a high anomalous insertion of the gastrocnemius tendon was noted. An axial T1 projection revealed the anomaly and compression of the popliteal artery by the gastrocnemius muscle. The patient had paresthesias develop in the same leg after 24 hours on heparin. Duplex color Doppler sonography revealed the thrombus had enlarged slightly; B-scan images showed the thrombus had a double lumen with a central wall. Arterial dissection was diagnosed. Sonography performed after the patient had sudden, intense paleness and coldness of the extremity showed complete arterial dissection of the distal popliteal artery, which was confirmed on arteriography. The patient had intra-arterial thrombolysis for 48 hours; arteriography then revealed complete patency of the popliteal artery and its distal branches. The patient underwent deinsertion of a large tendon of the medial head of the gastrocnemius, excision of the troublesome segment of the artery, and insertion of an autogenous vein graft from the internal saphenous vein.

Conclusions.—Patients suspected to have PAES should undergo duplex color Doppler sonography with high-frequency transducers to visualize the 3 segments of the popliteal artery, flow at that point, and the status of more distal pedal and posterior tibial arteries. Studies are performed at rest and with exercise to reveal functional compression. When evidence of possible PAES is found, MRI studies are the diagnostic method of choice. Treatment depends on symptom severity and imaging findings.

▶ This is a case report of a 22-year-old Olympic rower with sharp pain in the right calf and a fleeting episode of paleness and paresthesias of the first toe while training. The authors discuss evaluation, diagnosis, and treatment of this condition.

R. C. Cantu, MD, MA

Identification of a Fibular Fracture in an Intercollegiate Football Player in a Physical Therapy Setting
Goss DL, Moore JH, Thomas DB, et al (Patch Health Clinic, Stuttgart, Germany; US Army-Baylor Univ, Fort Sam Houston, Tex; Brooke Army Med Ctr, Fort Sam Houston, Tex; et al)
J Orthop Sports Phys Ther 34:182-186, 2004   4–29

Background.—A physical therapist is sometimes the first health care professional to evaluate a patient with an ankle injury. Therefore, it is important for a physical therapist to be able to distinguish between ankle sprains and fractures and to determine when radiographs are necessary. The Ottawa Ankle Rules (OAR) were developed to aid such clinical decision making. According to the OAR, ankle radiographs are only required under the following circumstances: (1) pain in the malleolar zone; (2) bone tenderness over the posterior edges or tips of the medial or lateral malleoli; or (3) inability to bear weight. The Buffalo modification moves the area of palpitation over the crests of the malleoli and away from ligamentous attachments. A case in which a physical therapist used the OAR to diagnose probable ankle fracture was described.

Case Report.—Man, 20, intercollegiate football player, reported to physical therapy clinic during walk-in hours complaining of ankle pain. He had sustained a forced-dorsiflexion and external-rotation injury to his left ankle during a game. His gait was antalgic, with extremely rotated lower-left extremity. Left- leg stance time and stride were decreased approximately 50%. The left ankle was swollen, and active range of motion was limited. The patient was tender to palpation over the posterior and middle of the lateral malleolus and up the distal fibula. A raised palpable defect with crepitation was observed on the distal fibula. The patient was given crutches and plain radiographs were ordered on the basis of the OAR. Radiographs revealed a fibular fracture. Patient had open-reduction internal-fixation surgery that afternoon. By 26 weeks, the patient had returned to athletic activity.

Conclusions.—The OAR are effective clinical guidelines to assist physical therapists in determining whether radiographs are necessary for the diagnosis of acute ankle injuries.

▶ This is a case study of a 20-year-old intercollegiate football player seen in the physical therapy clinic for left ankle pain. The authors discuss the use of the OAR used for determining whether radiographs are necessary in ankle injuries. The rules supply a set of criteria for determining use of radiographs in diagnosing these injuries. These authors discuss the beneficial use of these rules in aiding physical therapists' treatment of athletes with ankle injuries.

R. C. Cantu, MD, MA

Predicting Hamstring Strain Injury in Elite Athletes
Brockett CL, Morgan DL, Proske U (Monash Univ, Melbourne, Australia)
Med Sci Sports Exerc 36:379-387, 2004   4–30

Introduction.—Hamstring strains are often associated with eccentric contractions. These contractions produce microscopic muscle damage, indicating a causal relationship between the 2 processes. It may be that the initial event, which produces microscopic damage from eccentric exercise, is nonuniform lengthening of sarcomeres. Athletes with a prior history of hamstring injuries have a higher incidence of hamstring strains, compared with other athletes. Angle-torque curves were constructed for previously injured muscles with the use of isokinetic dynamometry and compared with uninjured muscles of the other leg in athletes with a history of hamstring strains in 1 leg only. The data were also compared with those of uninjured athletes.

Results.—In previously injured muscles, torque peaked at significantly shorter lengths, compared with those of uninjured muscles. Peak torque and quadriceps/hamstrings torque ratios did not differ significantly.

Conclusion.—The shorter optimum of previously injured muscles makes them more susceptible to damage from eccentric exercise, compared to uninjured muscles. This may explain the high reinjury rate. The shorter optimum may reflect the muscle's preinjury state or be a consequence of the healing process. To decrease the incidence of strain injuries, it is recommended that a combined program of eccentric exercise and muscle testing be performed.

▶ Many clinicians believe that the most important predictor of injury is the history of a previous injury to the same area. Other studies have suggested that weakness/fatigability following an injury is the important mechanistic variable (either agonist/antagonist or side-to-side differences). Instead, this study suggests that the problem may be a left shift in the torque-versus-angle relationship, ie, eccentric contractions are more likely to occur while the muscles are on the descending part of the curve.

Although the current results might be interpreted to mean that stretching should be the most effective intervention, both Svernlov[1] and Holmich[2] found that strengthening was considerably more effective than stretching. There are 2 obvious explanations for the apparent contradiction. First, the current study did not correlate the shift in torque-versus-angle relationship with reinjury rate, and therefore the shift may be an incidental finding and not a causally related factor. Second, the effect of strengthening post injury may have an effect on the torque-versus-angle relationship that we are not aware of.

I. Shrier, MD, PhD

References

1. Svernlov B, Adolfsson L: Non-operative treatment regime including eccentric training for lateral humeral epicondylalgia. *Scand J Med Sci Sports* 11:328-334, 2001.
2. Holmich P, Uhrskou P, Ulnits L, et al: Effectiveness of active physical training as treatment for long-standing adductor-related groin pain in athletes: Randomised trial. *Lancet* 353:439-443, 1999.

A Comparison of 2 Rehabilitation Programs in the Treatment of Acute Hamstring Strains
Sherry MA, Best TM (Univ of Wisconsin, Madison)
J Orthop Sports Phys Ther 34:116-125, 2004   4–31

Background.—Hamstring strains are common athletic injuries that take significant time for recovery and are prone to reinjury. The effectiveness of rehabilitation programs for hamstring injuries has not been well studied. This prospective randomized study compared the efficacy of 2 rehabilitation programs by assessing time needed before return to sport and the reinjury rate during the first 2 weeks and the first year after return to the sport.

Study Design.—The study group consisted of 24 athletes, aged 14 to 49 years, with recent (3-4 days) acute hamstring injuries. These injured athletes were then randomly assigned, with stratification for age and sex, to either static stretching, isolated progressive hamstring resistance exercise, and icing (STST) or progressive agility and trunk stabilization and icing (PATS).

Study participants could return to sports when they demonstrated 5/5 strength on manually resisting knee flexion, had no palpable tenderness, and felt ready to return. However, they were encouraged to continue the rehabilitation program for 2 months after their return to sports. They were called at 2 weeks and at 1 year after return to sports to report any injury recurrence.

Findings.—The average time required to return to sports was 37.4 days in the STST group and 22.2 days in the PATS group. The reinjury rate at both 2 weeks and 1 year was significantly greater in the STST group.

Conclusion.—An acute hamstring injury rehabilitation program consisting of progressive agility and trunk stabilization was more effective in promoting return to sport and in preventing reinjury than a traditional isolated stretching and strengthening program. Future trials should analyze the use of PATS programs for prevention of hamstring injury.

▶ This randomized trial found that a "progressive agility and trunk stabilization" program prevented reinjury more effectively than a combined stretching and strengthening program. Whether it was the section on (1) progressive agility, (2) trunk stabilization, or (3) a combination of both should be the subject of future experiments. That being said, 6 reinjuries in the stretch/strengthen program occurred in the first 2 weeks after returning to sport. On closer examination, the progressive agility part of the trunk stabilization program included activities closely related to running, but the stretch/strengthening did not have a similar section. Therefore, it seems that subjects went from no activity to full activity once they passed functional tests. Whether adding a progressive increase in activity section to the stretch/strengthen program would have changed the results should also be the subject of future research.

I. Shrier, MD, PhD

Factors Associated With Recurrent Hamstring Injuries
Croisier J-L (Univ of Liege, Belgium)
Sports Med 34:681-695, 2004   4–32

Background.—Athletes returning to activity after a hamstring strain are at a high risk of reinjury and persistent pain. Some of the risk factors associated with the possible recurrence of this injury are likely already implicated in the initial injury. The factors associated with recurrent hamstring injuries were reviewed, with emphasis on the role of questionable approaches to the diagnostic process, drug treatment, or rehabilitation design and presentation of a model for effective management of hamstring strain.

Overview.—The factors associated with recurrent hamstring strain can be grouped as extrinsic factors (those peculiar to a specific sporting activity) and intrinsic factors (other contributing factors based on the athlete's individual features). For both categories, the persistence of mistakes or abnormalities in action are unquestionably contributing factors to the reinjury cycle. Among the most significant extrinsic factors involved in hamstring strain are inadequate warm-up, fatigue, and inadequate training, resulting in low fitness levels. It is crucial for trainers to have scientific knowledge and qualifications, particularly in the area of exercise physiology. Intrinsic factors associated with recurrent hamstring strain included eccentric deficits, a lack of flexibility, age-related factors, joint dysfunction, and hormonal status. In addition, structural modifications in the muscle can be the result of muscle strain, and some of these modifications, if not treated, will promote persistent reports of chronic injury. Among the questionable options in treatment are incorrect initial diagnosis, the use of nonsteroidal anti-inflammatory medications, and the administration of glucocorticoids and local anesthetics. Finally, a premature return to competition can result in recurrent injury after hamstring strain. A management model for hamstring strain is proposed and includes guidelines for treatment in 5 phases of recovery, including the acute phase (48-72 hours), subacute phase (days 2-4 to day 8), remodeling phase (2 to 4 weeks after injury), recovering phase (week 4 to weeks 6-8), and transition phase (week 6 to the athlete's return to competition).

Conclusions.—A multifactorial cause is apparently at work in hamstring reinjuries. One current difficulty is the lack of valid objective measures for identifying the factor or combination of factors responsible for strain recurrence. The most likely factors are presented in this report, along with a management model that can facilitate the return of the athlete to full fitness and prevent recurrence of the hamstring strain. An increased emphasis on the knowledge of therapists and trainers involved in the rehabilitation process is also needed.

▶ The author did a prospective study of 2376 English professional football players over 2 competitive seasons looking at recurrent hamstring injuries after returning to competitive sport. He determined that hamstring injuries have the highest recurrence rate of all injuries seen in these football players.

R. C. Cantu, MD, MA

Immediate Achilles Tendon Response After Strength Training Evaluated by MRI

Shalabi A, Kristoffersen-Wiberg M, Aspelin P, et al (Huddinge Univ Hosp, Stockholm)
Med Sci Sports Exerc 36:1841-1846, 2004   4-33

Background.—There has been a dramatic increase in the incidence of overuse injury in sports in the last 30 years. One of the most common injuries among athletes is Achilles tendinopathy. However, the causes of this tendinopathy are unclear. Several theories have associated tendinopathies with overuse stresses, poor vascularity, lack of flexibility in genetic makeup, sex, and endocrine or metabolic factors. Excessive repetitive overload, or overuse, is thought to be the main pathological stimulus leading to tendinopathy. Chronic pain in the Achilles tendon region, or achillodynia, is a common condition not only in athletes but also in persons with low activity levels. In response to repetitive overload, the Achilles tendon may respond with either inflammation of its sheath or degeneration of its body, or by a combination of these two responses. A recent study has reported that daily eccentric calf muscle strength training in patients with chronic Achilles tendinosis resulted in both decreased tendon volume and intratendinous MR signal and improved clinical outcome. The tendon response after acute strength training in chronic Achilles tendinosis using MRI was evaluated.

Methods.—The study group was composed of 22 patients (15 men, 7 women) with bilateral symptoms. The median age of the patients was 45 years (range, 28-57 years). Both Achilles tendons in all patients were examined with MRI before and immediately after a standardized training program. The most painful sides were loaded with 6 sets and 15 repetitions of heavy-loaded eccentric training. The contralateral tendons were subjected to concentric loading only. The tendon volume and the intratendinous signal were evaluated and calculated by MRI using a seed-growing technique.

Results.—The immediate response of eccentric loading on the symptomatic tendons resulted in a 12% increase in tendon volume and a 31% increase in the intratendinous signal evident on proton-density weighted imaging. In corresponding sequences on the contralateral, concentrically loaded tendons demonstrated a 17% increase in tendon volume and an increase of 27% of the intratendinous signal. There was no significant difference of the mean of the increased tendon volume and the intratendinous signal between the eccentrically heavily loaded symptomatic tendons and the concentrically loaded contralateral tendons.

Conclusions.—Total tendon volume and intratendinous signal were increased in the Achilles tendon after both eccentric and concentric loading. This increase may be attributed to a higher water content and/or hyperemia in the Achilles tendon during and/or immediately after strength training of the gastrocnemius-soleus complex.

▶ These authors looked at 22 patients with the clinical diagnosis of chronic Achilles tendinosis. They looked at excessive, repetitive use of the Achilles tendon and subsequent tendinopathy and chronic pain, and evaluated each with MRI studies. These studies were done in conjunction with a standardized training program.

R. C. Cantu, MD, MA

The Role of Stretching in Rehabilitation of Hamstring Injuries: 80 Athletes Follow-up
Malliaropoulos N, Papalexandris S, Papalada A, et al (SEGAS, Thessaloniki, Greece)
Med Sci Sports Exerc 36:756-759, 2004   4–34

Background.—Hamstring injuries are very common among athletes. Rehabilitation includes stretching, but the effect of stretching on injured muscles has not been well documented. In the current randomized study, the influence of stretching on second-degree hamstring injuries was examined among training athletes.

Study Design.—The study group consisted of 80 Greek athletes who had second-degree strains of the hamstring muscles from 1996 through 2001. During the first 48 hours, all athletes underwent the PRICE protocol (ie, protection, rest, ice compression, elevation). Then the athletes were randomly assigned to a rehabilitation program that included 1 stretching session per day or 4 stretching sessions per day. The time needed to equalize active knee extension between the 2 sides and the time required for full rehabilitation were compared between these 2 groups.

Findings.—Both the time to equalize active knee extension and the time for full rehabilitation were significantly shorter in the group with a rehabilitation program that included more stretching.

Conclusions.—A rehabilitation program that included an increased frequency of stretching exercises is superior to one with less stretching and increases the speed of recovery for athletes with second-degree hamstring strains.

▶ These authors studied 80 male and female Greek athletes who presented with a second-degree strain of the hamstring muscles. The study concentrated on whether the role of stretching had an effect on injuries to the hamstring muscles. The authors found that stretching led to faster rehabilitation without compromising the overall results. They recommend further studies that examine the effect of different stretching programs.

R. C. Cantu, MD, MA

The Effects of Fatigue and Chronic Ankle Instability on Dynamic Postural Control

Gribble PA, Hertel J, Denegar CR, et al (Univ of Toledo, Ohio; Univ of Virginia, Charlottesville; Pennsylvania State Univ, University Park)
J Athl Train 39:321-329, 2004   4–35

Objective.—Deficits in static postural control related to chronic ankle instability (CAI) and fatigue have been investigated separately, but little evidence links these factors to performance of dynamic postural control. Our purpose was to investigate the effects of fatigue and CAI on performance measures of a dynamic postural-control task, the Star Excursion Balance Test.

Design and Setting.—For each of the 3 designated reaching directions, 4 separate 5 (condition) × 2 (time) × 2 (side) analyses of variance with a between factor of group (CAI, healthy) were calculated for normalized reach distance and maximal ankle-dorsiflexion, knee-flexion, and hip-flexion angles. All data were collected in the Athletic Training Research Laboratory.

Subjects.—Thirty subjects (16 healthy, 14 CAI) participated.

Measurements.—All subjects completed 5 testing sessions, during which sagittal-plane kinematics and reaching distances were recorded while they performed 3 reaching directions (anterior, medial, and posterior) of the Star Excursion Balance Test, with the same stance leg before and after different fatiguing conditions. The procedure was repeated for both legs during each session.

Results.—The involved side of the CAI subjects displayed significantly smaller reach distance values and knee-flexion angles for all 3 reaching directions compared with the uninjured side and the healthy group. The effects of fatigue amplified this trend (Fig 6).

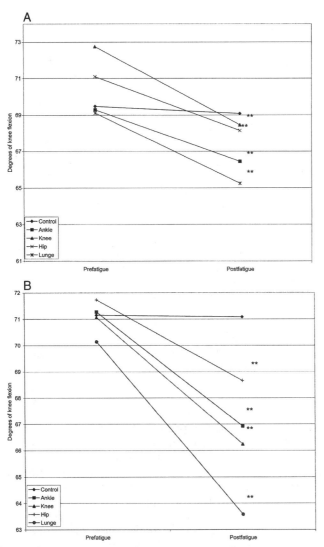

FIGURE 6.—Group × day × time interaction for knee flexion in the medial direction (**$P < .01$). A, Healthy subjects. B, Chronic ankle instability subjects. (Reprinted from Gribble PA, Hertel J, Denegar CR, et al: The effects of fatigue and chronic ankle instability on dynamic postural control. *J Athl Train* 39:321-329, 2004. Copyright 2004, with permission from The National Athletic Trainers' Association.)

Conclusions.—Chronic ankle instability and fatigue disrupted dynamic postural control, most notably by altering control of sagittal-plane joint angles proximal to the ankle.

▶ The results of this study support the hypothesis that previous injury is associated with decreased performance on tests of balance. In this study, fatigue increased the magnitude of the deficits. Similar to the study by Tripp et al (Abstract 5–33) in this issue of the YEAR BOOK OF SPORTS MEDICINE, there remain questions of whether strength, endurance, or proprioceptive training is most likely to minimize the effect observed.

I. Shrier, MD, PhD

High Ankle Sprains: Minimizing the Frustration of a Prolonged Recovery
Smith AH, Bach BR Jr (Rush Univ, Chicago)
Physician Sportsmed 32(12):39-43, 2004   4–36

Background.—Ankle sprains occur more often than any other sports injury and range in severity from minor ligamentous injury to complete ligament rupture with joint dislocation. From 1% to 15% of ankle sprains are syndesmotic injuries, or high ankle sprains. The mechanisms of injury are dorsiflexion of the ankle, external rotation of the leg, or a combination of both, which disrupts the syndesmotic ligament complex, including the anterior and posterior tibiofibular ligaments. The diagnosis, assessment, treatment, and prognosis for athletes with ankle sprains were outlined.

Diagnosis and Assessment.—Injured athletes often give a history of twisting on a planted foot, which is common for football linemen, downhill skiers, and hockey players. Point tenderness over the anterolateral tibiofibular joint where the fibers of the anterior tibiofibular ligament are usually disrupted is a common symptom, along with pain on passive dorsiflexion of the ankle. The injury is evaluated by the external rotation stress test and the squeeze test. More severe injuries cause pain closer to the knee during the squeeze test. Level of injury can be determined by further testing. Patients often have pain too severe to permit squatting with the feet flat. Sport-specific activities may also elicit pain. The results of standard anteroposterior, lateral, and mortise radiographs may be within normal limits. When a high ankle sprain is suspected, the entire tibia and fibula should be viewed on anteroposterior and lateral radiographs to find any associated proximal fibular fracture. Syndesmotic injuries may be present if radiographs reveal abnormal anatomic relations. Dynamic radiographs can demonstrate instability more accurately, as can stress radiographs. MRI scans can detect the zone of soft-tissue injury, talar bone bruises, and injuries to anterior and posterior tibiofibular ligaments. If syndesmotic injuries with concomitant lateral talar shift are overlooked, the tibial talar joint is at increased risk for developing posttraumatic arthritis. Ossification of the interosseous ligament and potential tibiofibular synostosis may also develop.

Treatment and Prognosis.—Treatment for grade 1 high ankle sprains is the same as for a typical inversion ankle sprain, including rest, ice, compression, elevation, and refraining from athletic participation. Some patients benefit from immobilization by using a long, semirigid pneumatic stirrup brace extending to just below the knee. Up to 3 weeks of protected weight bearing is needed. Protective taping and a heel lift may permit the athlete to return to play more quickly. Treatment of grade 2 syndesmotic injuries is also nonoperative, with extended restrictions on weight bearing (3-6 weeks). Grade 3 injuries require surgical anatomic reduction of the syndesmotic joint and stabilization with screws. The screws can be permanent but are usually removed in 3 to 6 months.

Recovery from high ankle sprains takes longer than from inversion ankle sprains, with a minimum of 3 to 6 weeks of inactivity. With more proximal tenderness, recovery time is increased. Distal progression of local fibular tenderness is assessed over the recovery period. The athlete must be evaluated in a sport-specific simulation before being released to competition.

Conclusions.—Syndesmotic injuries occur less often than inversion sprains and require specific diagnosis and treatment. Recovery time is extensive compared with the time for a simpler ankle injury. Realistic expectations for a return to sports must be maintained.

▶ These authors looked at ankle sprains, the most common of all sports injuries. They discuss the diagnosis, evaluation, treatment, and return to sports for all grades of ankle sprains and realistic expectations for return to sports after these injuries.

R. C. Cantu, MD, MA

Stress Fracture Nonunion at the Base of the Second Metatarsal in a Ballet Dancer: A Case Report
Muscolo L, Migues A, Slullitel G, et al (Hosp Italiano de Buenos Aires, Argentina)
Am J Sports Med 32:1535-1537, 2004   4–37

Background.—Repetitive stresses that are in and of themselves harmless may precipitate a spontaneous stress fracture, usually located in the metatarsal shaft in the general population. Ballet dancers tend to have stress fractures at the base of the second metatarsal. A ballet dancer with nonunion at the base of the second metatarsal secondary to a stress fracture was managed surgically.

> *Case Report.*—Man, 24, was a professional ballet dancer and reported pain on the dorsum of the foot at the base of the second metatarsal position. The demipointe position tended to exacerbate the pain, which had begun 2 months previously with no causative trauma. The second tarsometatarsal joint was tender, but plain radiographs showed only the cortical thickening of the second metatarsal

shaft typical of ballet dancers. Increased uptake of technetium-99m was found in this area on a bone scan, but only on MRI were the stress fractures at the proximal metaphyseal–diaphyseal junction and bone marrow edema revealed. All balletic activities were suspended for 6 weeks, after which a gradual return to dancing was permitted; however, the patient had only transient relief after 6 months. CT showed a fracture line, sclerotic and hypertrophic changes, and obliteration of the medullary canal, which was interpreted as nonunion. Ten months after the patient first came for treatment, surgery was undertaken. The fracture line and mobility of the fragments were identified, sclerotic bone was removed, and an autogenous corticocancellous inlay bone graft was placed at the site of the nonunion. A 5-hole 3.5-narrow low-contact dynamic compression plate with 4 screws was used to fix the fragments in place. The patient wore a short-leg non–weight-bearing cast for 4 weeks after the operation, and active range of motion exercises were begun 1 month after surgery. Weight-bearing was permitted as tolerated 2 weeks later. The patient began a progressive return to dancing after 3 months and had no symptoms. Complete healing was noted at 1 year after surgery, and the plate did not need to be removed.

Conclusions.—Generally, stress fractures heal with rest and nonoperative measures; however, in this case, nonunion persisted and required surgery. Stress fractures should be closely monitored to ensure that adequate primary healing occurs.

▶ These authors discuss the case of a 24-year-old ballet dancer with a nonunion stress fracture at the base of the second metatarsal. This is an uncommon fracture. The article discusses the successful outcome after surgical treatment.

R. C. Cantu, MD, MA

Shoe Rim and Shoe Buckle Pseudotumor of the Ankle in Elite and Professional Figure Skaters and Snowboarders: MR Imaging Findings
Anderson SE, Weber M, Steinbach LS, et al (Univ Hosp of Bern, Switzerland; Univ of California, San Francisco; Lindenhofspital, Bern, Switzerland)
Skeletal Radiol 33:325-329, 2004   4–38

Background.—Elite figure skaters and professional snowboarders are at significant risk for serious ankle injuries and overuse syndromes. There have been several descriptions of overuse syndromes of the ankle joint region, including tendinitis and malleolar bursitis. However, no MRI or clinical descriptions have been given of subcutaneous impingement of the ankle region by the shoe rim or shoe buckle with formation of a pseudotumor in elite figure skaters or professional snowboarders. The MRI findings in figure skaters and snowboarders with painful soft tissue swelling of the lateral supramalleolar region with a clinical provisional diagnosis of soft tissue tumor were reviewed.

Methods.—MR images in 4 female athletes engaged in heavy training regimens were prospectively reviewed by 2 specialized musculoskeletal radiologists. The findings were correlated with a second clinical review and examination of the shoe wear. The athletes included 2 figure skaters and 2 professional snowboarders ranging in age from 16 to 25 years. Three of the 4 patients had unilateral masses with pain, and 1 patient had bilateral clinical findings.

Results.—MR imaging showed subcutaneous, focal soft tissue masses of the supramalleolar region in 5 ankles at the same level above the ankle joint. On the basis of these findings, a second clinical review was conducted along with correlation of the shoe wear. The MRI findings correlated with the level of the shoe rim or shoe buckle in all patients, confirming the suspected MRI diagnosis of an impingement syndrome. All the athletes were found to be training excessively and were ignoring safety advice regarding the duration of training, timing of breaks, and shoe wear rotation.

Conclusions.—Ice skaters and snowboarders are at risk for persistent and disabling pain, which on MRI correspond to a focal soft tissue abnormality. This abnormality may result from impingement of subcutaneous fat between the fibula and the shoe rim or shoe buckle.

▶ These authors studied 4 female patients, 2 elite figure skaters and 2 professional snowboarders, presenting with unilateral or bilateral masses with pain. MRI studies showed a diagnosis of impingement syndrome corresponding to soft tissue abnormalities that could be caused by impingement between the fibula and the shoe rim or shoe buckle. This is a limited study.

R. C. Cantu, MD, MA

Ankle Syndesmosis Sprains in National Hockey League Players
Wright RW, Barile RJ, Surprenant DA, et al (Washington Univ, St Louis; St Louis Blues Hockey Club; Dallas Stars Hockey Club)
Am J Sports Med 32:1941-1945, 2004   4–39

Introduction.—Syndesmosis sprains are less common than lateral ligament ankle sprains (1%-20% vs 30%-45%) and are reported to have a prolonged recovery time. No previous trial has described these injuries in hockey players. Ice hockey has unique features that places players at increased risk for ankle trauma; the foot is immobilized in a skate on an ice surface that is surrounded by rigid boards in this high-speed contact sport. A retrospective review was conducted of syndesmosis ankle sprains in members of 2 National Hockey League franchises.

Methods.—The medical records of the St Louis Blues (1994-2001) and Dallas Stars (1991-2001) National Hockey League teams were reviewed by the head athletic trainers according to an injury surveillance system. Ankle sprains were identified and placed in 1 of 2 groups: syndesmosis and lateral sprains. Player demographics, treatment, and time lost to play were documented for both injuries.

Results.—Fourteen players were diagnosed with syndesmosis sprains and 5 had lateral sprains during the evaluation period. The mean time to return to game play was 45 days (range, 6-137 days) for syndesmosis sprains versus 1.4 days (range, 0-6 days) for lateral sprains.

Conclusion.—Compared with athletes in other sports, hockey players with syndesmosis sprains require a prolonged recovery time. Despite the rigidity of the skate and the diminished impact loading with skating versus running, no advantage is gained by participating in hockey compared with other sports.

▶ These authors looked at syndesmosis sprains in National Hockey League players, specifically the St Louis Blues and the Dallas Stars teams, and found that even though in other types of sports lateral sprains are more common, syndesmosis sprains are more common in hockey players, leading to the need for extended time off. They looked at evaluation, diagnosis, and treatment of this injury in these players.

R. C. Cantu, MD, MA

Navicular Stress Fractures in Identical Twin Runners
Murray SR, Reeder M, Ward T, et al (Mesa State College, Grand Junction, Colo; Univ of Wisconsin, La Crosse)
Physician Sportsmed 33(1):28-33, 2005   4–40

Background.—Stress fractures are common overuse injuries in athletes and account for about 10% of all athletic injuries. Most of these fractures are characterized by insidious onset of localized pain that worsens with repetitive activity and are classified as low risk. However, some stress fractures are accompanied by vague pain and may be difficult to diagnose. These fractures can lead to complications and a prolonged recovery and are described as high risk. Tarsal navicular fractures are an example of such a high-risk stress fracture. A case of high-risk stress fractures in the tarsal navicular bones of identical twin girls participating in high school distance running was reported.

> *Case Report.*—The patients were 17-year-old identical twin, female distance runners who presented 3 weeks apart with recurring foot pain of several weeks' duration. Both patients related an insidious onset of foot pain after they added speed work to their normal training schedule of 50 miles of distance running per week during the spring track season. Neither girl had a history of swelling, bruising, neurologic symptoms, or night pain. Most of the symptoms occurred only during running but could be elicited with palpation. Physical examinations showed minimal bilateral pronation in both patients. Gait analysis was otherwise unremarkable. There was no evidence of

other pathologic processes or instability in the foot or ankle. Range of motion was symmetric, with no increase in pain with resisted dorsiflexion of the foot. Initial plain radiographs were normal in both patients. The initial bone scan in the first patient showed diffuse uptake in the talonavicular area. MRI of the first patient showed a nondisplaced stress fracture of the navicular bone of the left foot and a stress reaction in the navicular bone of the right foot. MRI of the second patient showed a nondisplaced navicular stress fracture. Neither patient showed evidence of a complete fracture through both the dorsal and plantar cortices. In both patients, the injured feet were immobilized in non–weight-bearing casts for 6 weeks. After cast removal, the patients were fitted with semi-rigid molded orthoses and allowed to gradually return to training over 8 weeks. After a period of rehabilitation, training counseling, and nutrition counseling, the patients were able to compete successfully during the fall cross-country season with no recurring injuries.

Conclusions.—The patients in this case represented classic examples of runners who experience stress fractures. The treatment of low-risk fractures involves relative rest and cessation of the activity that caused the fracture. However, high-risk fractures such as those presented in this report often require non–weight-bearing immobilization combined with therapy, and surgery may also be required.

▶ These authors report a case study of two 17-year-old identical twin girls who were high school long-distance runners and who both suffered from tarsal navicular stress fractures. The authors look at evaluation and diagnosis modalities, as well as treatment of these fractures. They also recommend further study of predisposing genetic and nutrition factors.

R. C. Cantu, MD, MA

The Effect of Sesamoid Mobilization, Flexor Hallucis Strengthening, and Gait Training on Reducing Pain and Restoring Function in Individuals With Hallux Limitus: A Clinical Trial
Shamus J, Shamus E, Gugel RN, et al (Healthsouth Sports Medicine and Rehabilitation Ctr, Pembroke Pines, Fla; Nova Southeastern Univ, Fort Lauderdale, Fla; Lynn Univ, Boca Raton, Fla; et al)
J Orthop Sports Phys Ther 34:368-376, 2004   4–41

Introduction.—Metatarsophalangeal joint (MPJ) sprains occur frequently and can produce long-term sequelae, including persistent pain and loss of range of motion (ROM) secondary to bony proliferation and articular degeneration. It is important to ascertain the most effective intervention for functional hallux limitus to reduce pain and to restore functioning. The effect of 2 conservative interventions for functional hallux limitus was examined in 20 patients with newly acquired MPJ pain, loss of motion, and weakness.

Methods.—All patients were treated with the following modalities: whirl-pool, US, first-time MPJ mobilization, calf and hamstring stretching, marble pick-up exercise, cold packs, and electric stimulation. Ten patients (experimental group) also received sesamoid mobilizations, flexor hallucis strengthening exercises, and gait training. Patients were treated 3 times weekly for 4 weeks. Measurements of first-time MPJ extension ROM, flexor hallucis strength, and subjective pain level were conducted on first and last visits.

Results.—After 12 therapy sessions, the experimental group experienced significantly greater MPJ extension, ROM, and flexor hallucis strength and significantly lower pain levels than did control subjects ($P < .001$).

Conclusion.—Sesamoid mobilization, flexor hallucis strengthening, and gait training should be included in the treatment strategy for patients with functional hallux limitus.

▶ Clinical trials in rehabilitation are becoming ever more important. This study suggests that a combination of sesamoid mobilization, flexor hallucis strengthening, and gait training for hallux limitus (rigidus) is superior to a traditional rehabilitation program. Of note, the patients were given the strengthening exercises as a home program, and it would also have been possible to teach them self-mobilizations. Which of the 3 interventions is most important for rehabilitation should be the subject of future research.

I. Shrier, MD, PhD

Disabling Foot Cramping in a Runner Secondary to Paramyotonia Congenita: A Case Report
Fredericson M, Kim B-J, Date ES (Stanford Univ, Calif)
Foot Ankle Int 25:510-512, 2004   4–42

Background.—Athletes commonly experience muscle cramps and stiffness. Among the causes of these symptoms are myotonic syndromes, which involve abnormally slow relaxation after voluntary muscle contraction because of a muscle membrane abnormality. These relatively rare syndromes vary in expression among patients and involve symptoms that can be difficult to describe. A runner was given a diagnosis of paramyotonia congenita after experiencing cramping foot pain when he increased his training intensity.

    Case Report.—Man, 18, had a 1-year history of cramping pain in his left foot. The symptoms developed insidiously after he increased his speed work training. Severe pain and tightness developed in his left foot about 20 minutes into exercising; in addition, he had occasional calf cramping after excessive exercise. He maintained a high competitive level even with these symptoms. He had been treated with physical therapy, interdigital nerve blockade, and immobilization in a walking cast for more than 1 month for a suspected stress fracture, but none of these had been successful. No abnormalities were found on 2 MRI scans, nor were his blood studies abnormal. A detailed history revealed cramping of his hands, feet, or jaw related to cold weather or on immersing himself in cold water. His sister and maternal uncle had similar symptoms, and his mother had a milder variant. His physical examination was unremarkable, but neurologic testing found mild proximal muscle weakness at the deltoid and triceps. He demonstrated his symptoms by running: cramping began after 20 minutes and started with a feeling of tightness on the plantar surface of the left foot; it then grew worse with continued running. Symptoms resolved 10 minutes after he stopped running. Compartment syndrome was ruled out, but a needle electromyelographic study at rest revealed abnormal sustained runs of positive sharp waves at nearly every needle site in each of his limbs. When it was repeated after he had immersed his hands in cold water for 4 to 5 minutes, many myotonic discharges were found in the first dorsal interossei in the hand. However, muscle biopsy results were normal. Based on all the evaluations, the diagnosis of paramyotonia congenita was made. Treatment with carbamazepine and mexiletine was begun but was discontinued because of adverse effects. Doses of 400 mg/h phenytoin minimized his symptoms and permitted him to run with fewer symptoms if he limited himself to running less than 50 miles per week, running on softer surfaces, and modifying his workouts during colder weather. The medication has permitted him to function well, although he gave up running because he could not maintain enough mileage to compete successfully at the elite college level.

Conclusions.—The clinical and electrodiagnostic findings in this case were consistent with paramyotonia congenita. The patient had exercise-induced cramping and stiffness of his left foot along with muscle tightness related to exposure to cold. The possibility of myotonia should be considered in such patients to avoid costly and unneeded testing and to make an appropriate referral to a neurologic specialist.

▶ This article is a case study of an 18-year-old runner with a differential diagnosis of paramyotonia congenita. This brings to light a diagnosis to be considered when working up athletes who complain of exercise-induced muscle stiffness or cramping.

R. C. Cantu, MD, MA

Plantar Fascia Ruptures in Athletes

Saxena A, Fullem B (Palo Alto Med Found, Calif)
Am J Sports Med 32:662-665, 2004   4–43

Background.—The plantar fascia is one of the most important supportive structures for maintenance of plantar arch integrity in the foot. Plantar fasciitis is a well-known condition in athletes, particularly runners. Rupture of the fascia may occur spontaneously during athletic activity but is not a commonly reported injury. Rupture of the plantar fascia is often described as an intense tearing sensation on the bottom of the foot.

Previous studies have focused on the association of prior corticosteroid injection for treatment of plantar fasciitis. This study attempted to educate sports medicine practitioners in regard to the length of time for an athlete to return to activity after suffering a plantar fascia rupture.

Methods.—A review was conducted of patients treated from 1990 to 2000 for plantar fascia ruptures associated with athletic activity. The diagnosis was based on clinical findings, although radiographic studies were done. The patients were treated for 2 to 3 weeks with a below-knee or high-top boot, non–weight-bearing, with an additional 2 to 3 weeks of weight-bearing in the boot. All of the patients underwent physical therapy.

Results.—A total of 18 athletes (12 men and 6 women), including 6 elite athletes, were evaluated. The mean age of the patients was 40.9 ± 13.2 years. The duration of prior plantar fascia symptoms ranged from 0 to 52 weeks. All but 2 ruptures were of the medial portion. Four of the patients had injections prior to rupture, and 5 patients wore orthoses before injury; 14 patients wore orthoses after injury. All of the patients returned to activity after 2 to 26 weeks (mean 9.1 ± 6.0 weeks). The mean post injury follow-up was 42 months. Most of the athletes (12 of 18) were runners; the remaining injuries involved hiking, basketball, tennis, and soccer.

Conclusion.—A postinjury protocol that includes the use of a cast-boot, a period of non–weight-bearing, physical therapy, and appropriate use of foot orthoses can facilitate complete recovery from rupture of the plantar fascia with complete return to activity. In contrast to findings in other studies, none of the 18 patients in this study experienced reinjury or postinjury sequelae or needed surgery.

▶ These authors studied 18 athletes with plantar fascial ruptures, including 6 elite athletes. These athletes consisted of runners, tennis players, and volleyball and basketball players. The focus of this article is to educate sports medicine practitioners as to the length of time for return to play of an athlete with plantar fascial rupture and treatment modalities such as non–weight-bearing in a boot, weight-bearing in a boot, and physical therapy.

R. C. Cantu, MD, MA

Intra-articular Hyaluronic Acid Treatment for Golfer's Toe: Keeping Older Golfers on Course

Petrella RJ, Cogliano A (Univ of Western Ontario, London, Canada)
Physician Sportsmed 32(7):41-45, 2004   4–44

Background.—Both walking and recreational activity can be hampered by osteoarthritis of the first metatarsophalangeal (MTP) joint, or great toe. The range of motion (ROM) is progressively limited and activity elicits pain. Older golfers appear to be particularly susceptible to this condition. For treatment, nonpharmacologic approaches are followed by oral analgesic medication and nonsteroidal anti-inflammatory drugs, then intra-articular corticosteroid injections, and finally surgical manipulation. Intra-articular hyaluronic acid (HA) injections have been used for progressive osteoarthritis in the knee and offer the advantages of a low incidence of systemic adverse effects, the absence of drug interactions, and a nearly unlimited frequency of use. The efficacy of using intra-articular HA for the first MTP joint was investigated.

Methods.—Efficacy, safety, and patient satisfaction were measured for 47 older men (mean age, 71 years) who had intra-articular injections of HA into the first MTP joint. The patients all reported having osteoarthritis-associated pain, loss of ROM of the MTP joint, and disability that limited their participation in golf. Injections were given weekly for 8 weeks. Measures of MTP joint ROM, pain at rest and immediately after walking tiptoe for 10 m, and global patient satisfaction were obtained at baseline, after 9 weeks, after 16 weeks, and when the patient received a second course of injections.

Results.—Grade 1 osteoarthritis was found in the first MTP joint of 36% of patients, grade 2 in 42%, and grade 3 in 22%. After 9 and 16 weeks as well as at final follow-up, the pain at rest and with tiptoe walking was significantly improved for all but 2 subjects. Global patient satisfaction was also significantly improved from the sixth visit through the follow-up period. ROM increased by 16° of flexion after 9 weeks, 22° after 16 weeks, and 18° at final follow-up. Three patients requested injection with intra-articular corticosteroid over the 16-week follow-up period to manage pain at rest. Two patients had no improvement in their pain and were considered treatment failures. None of the patients had local or systemic adverse events develop. Gastrointestinal pain from nonsteroidal anti-inflammatory medications required 2 patients to discontinue these drugs.

Conclusions.—HA injections into the first MTP joint improved the pain level and function of older patients with osteoarthritis of this joint. No local or systemic adverse effects developed in any patients. Patient satisfaction was high, with few patients requesting concomitant therapy during follow-up.

▶ These authors studied 47 male golfers who complained of osteoarthritis-associated pain, loss of joint ROM, and disability that interfered with their participation in golf. After patients received HA injections, there was significant improvement in pain tolerance at rest and exertion with very few adverse reactions.

R. C. Cantu, MD, MA

5 Muscle and Biomechanics

Reliability of Motor-Evoked Potentials During Resting and Active Contraction Conditions
Kamen G (Univ of Massachusetts, Amherst)
Med Sci Sports Exerc 36:1574-1579, 2004   5–1

Purpose.—To determine the reliability of motor-evoked potentials (MEP) obtained using transcranial magnetic stimulation (TMS) in the first dorsal interosseous (FDI) and biceps brachii muscles.

Methods.—Fourteen college subjects attended the laboratory on three separate days. TMS was used to obtain MEP with the subject relaxed (resting condition) at stimulation intensities of 70%, 85%, and 100% of maximal stimulator output. MEP were also obtained during four active contraction conditions involving contractions of 25%, 50%, 75%, and 100% of maximal effort (MVC). Reliability was measured using an intraclass correlation analysis of variance (ANOVA) design.

Results.—In the resting condition, substantial increases in MEP amplitude were observed for both muscles from day 1 to day 2. Intraclass reliability estimates were higher for the biceps muscle (ICC = 0.95-0.99) than for the FDI muscle (ICC = 0.60-0.81). During the active conditions, the greatest MEP were observed at 25% and 50% MVC, with smaller MEP at 75% and 100% MVC. Intraclass correlations in the active condition were approximately 0.63-0.73.

Conclusions.—Moderate to good reliability of MEP amplitude in the biceps and FDI muscles can be obtained using TMS in both resting and active contraction conditions.

▶ This is a methodological article discussing the reliability of TMS in producing reproducible peripheral MEPs. TMS is an experimental electrophysiologic technique that allows direct stimulation of the interneurons in the motor cortex of the brain. This, in turn, activates the descending corticospinal neurons with a resulting motor response in the peripheral muscles that can be recorded with a conventional electromyogram. Given that there are more than 500 articles published on this topic each year, the reliability of the method becomes crucial. This study shows a 0.7 correlation between studies performed on sequential days in the same patient. The clinical usefulness of this technology is not established at this time.

P. McCrory, MBBS, PhD

Effect of Sex on Preactivation of the Gastrocnemius and Hamstring Muscles
DeMont RG, Lephart SM (Univ of Pittsburgh, Pa)
Br J Sports Med 38:120-124, 2004   5–2

Introduction.—Strain placed on the anterior cruciate ligament results from the knee joint angle, the compressive forces on the joint, and the function of the muscles crossing the joint. Muscle preactivation (preactivity) is less prevalent in the literature than reactive or postloading responses, but it may influence these responses.

There are no data on sex differences regarding the normal preactivation of the hamstrings and gastrocnemius or preactivation during dynamic activities in healthy research subjects. Thirty-four healthy research subjects (17 male, 17 female) were evaluated to ascertain whether there is a level of preactivation of the gastrocnemius and hamstring muscles during dynamic activity that is affected by sex.

Methods.—Maximum voluntary contraction normalized electromyographic (EMG) activity of the quadriceps, hamstrings, and gastrocnemius muscles was documented during downhill walking (0.92 m/s) and running (2.08 m/s) on a 15° declined treadmill. Preactivation of the EMG signal was determined by setting a mark 150 ms before foot strike, as indicated by a footswitch. Multiple t tests for sex differences of preactivity mean percentage EMG during the downhill activities were conducted.

Results.—Female participants had a higher mean percentage EMG for the medial hamstrings, compared with males (31.73 and 23.04, respectively; $t_{[2,32]} = 2.732$; $P = .01$) during walking. No other muscles demonstrated a sex difference in M-EMG% during either activity.

Conclusion.—Women had higher medial hamstring preactivation than men. This may be because they were not injured, indicating a propensity for joint stabilization. No sex difference in gastrocnemius preactivation was observed, adding to the controversy concerning whether this muscle contributes to forward joint stability.

▶ In a study of 34 healthy adults, 17 males and 17 females, the correlation between sex and preactivation of the medial hamstring muscles was seen in females, but no sex difference was seen in preactivation of the gastrocnemius muscle. Further long-term study of muscle preactivation in males and females is needed.

R. C. Cantu, MD, MA

Average Versus Maximum Grip Strength: Which Is More Consistent?

Haidar SG, Kumar D, Bassi RS, et al (City Hosp, Birmingham, England)

J Hand Surg [Br] 29B:82-84, 2004   5–3

Introduction.—The American Society of Hand Therapists recommends using the average of 3 consecutive measurements of handgrip force. The American Society for Surgery of the Hand recommends documenting all 3 measurements for determination of handgrip force. The consistency of the maximum value versus the average value of 3 consecutive measurements of handgrip force was evaluated in 100 healthy volunteer hospital workers (50 women; 50 men) with no upper extremity disability.

Methods.—The average participant age was 34 years (range, 21-58 years) for women and 37 years (range, 23-63 years) for men. Three measurements of handgrip force were obtained on 2 occasions separated by a 2-week interval. For each hand, 2 average values and 2 maximum values were recorded (Table 1).

Results.—Ninety-five percent limits of agreement for the method in which values were averaged was $-$ 81.3 N to 70.6 N (-8.3 to $+7.2$ kg); for the maximum handgrip force method, these values were -87.3 N to 78.5 N (-8.9 to $+8$ kg).

Conclusion.—Both average and maximum handgrip force methods have high repeatability and the small difference between them is negligible.

▶ I was surprised to read the results of this study and find out that the average of several values was no more reliable than the peak value for any given measurement. In certain studies, an author may now prefer to report one or the other, depending on the objective. Unfortunately, the methodology for the experiments is unchanged; the subjects must still repeat the trials several times.

I. Shrier, MD, PhD

TABLE 1.—The Means of the Averages and the Maximums of Both Men and Women in Kilograms (1 kg force = 9.81 N)

| | Dominant Hand | | | | Non-Dominant Hand | | | |
| | Men | | Women | | Men | | Women | |
	Mean	SD	Mean	SD	Mean	SD	Mean	SD
Average								
Right hand	46	9.9	29	7.8	42	9.8	26	7.5
Left hand	42	10.7	26	6.5	41	12.3	27	6.7
Maximum								
Right hand	49	9.9	31	8.3	44	11.1	28	7.7
Left hand	45	12.4	28	6.9	46	11.4	30	7.4

Abbreviation: SD, Standard deviation.

(Reprinted from Haider SG, Kumar D, Bassi RS, et al: Average versus maximum grip strength: Which is more consistent? *J Hand Surg [Br]* 29B:82-84, 2004. Copyright 2004, with permission from The British Society for Surgery of the Hand.)

Effect of Self-selected Handgrip Position On Maximal Handgrip Strength
Boadella JM, Kuijer PP, Sluiter JK, et al (Univ of Amsterdam)
Arch Phys Med Rehabil 86:328-331, 2005   5–4

Objective.—To assess whether participants were able to select the hand-grip position on a Jamar hand dynamometer with which the maximal hand-grip strength could be delivered, while sitting and while standing.

Design.—A criterion standard comparison study.

Setting.—A university campus in the Netherlands.

Participants.—Fifty-six healthy subjects (30 men, 26 women; mean age, 30 y; range, 19-60 y) voluntarily participated.

Interventions.—Not applicable.

Main Outcome Measures.—Maximal handgrip strength for the self-selected and non-self-selected handgrip position of the hand dynamometer (positions 2 or 3), while sitting and while standing.

Results.—The self-selected handgrip position resulted in the highest mean maximal grip strength compared with the non-self-selected handgrip strength, both for sitting (mean difference, 2.3 kg; $P \leq .001$) and for stand-ing (mean difference, 2.1 kg; $P \leq .001$) (Table 1).

Conclusions.—Both in sitting and in standing, participants were able to self-select the handgrip position on the hand dynamometer with which the maximal handgrip strength could be delivered. Therefore, it may be useful to introduce self-selection of the handgrip position in protocols to assess the maximal handgrip strength.

▶ Because body position affects the results on clinical and biomechanical muscle function tests, investigators usually set the body position to a prede-termined setting. However, as this study suggests, the investigator-chosen standardized position may put some people at a disadvantage and others at an advantage, and this too could affect the results. The important principle in a pre-post test is that each subject is measured using the same conditions. Therefore, although it requires extra time, it is possible to allow subject-selected postures, record the posture, and ensure the same posture is used by

TABLE 1.—Mean and SD of Maximal Handgrip Force for the Self-Selected and Non–Self-Selected Handgrip Position While Sitting and Standing

Handgrip Strength	N	Mean ± SD (kg)	P
Sitting			
Self-selected	56	39.7 ± 12.1	
Non–self-selected	56	37.4 ± 12.7	.000
Standing			
Self-selected	56	40.8 ± 12.5	
Non–self-selected	56	38.7 ± 11.9	.001

that individual on the subsequent trial. Multiple regression techniques could be used to investigate a potential effect of body position. Of course, studies could be done in which all subjects are always tested in a variety of body positions, but this is not feasible for most studies.

I. Shrier, MD, PhD

The Supine Hip Extensor Manual Muscle Test: A Reliability and Validity Study

Perry J, Weiss WB, Burnfield JM, et al (Rancho Los Amigos Natl Rehabilitation Ctr, Downey, Calif)
Arch Phys Med Rehabil 85:1345-1350, 2004   5–5

Background.—Hip extensor muscle torque is seldom evaluated even though it is an important predictor of walking ability. Hip extensor function during walking is subtle, and an assessment in the prone position, which is required for conventional manual muscle testing (MMT), is inconvenient. A reliable supine testing technique able to differentiate at least 4 levels of hip extensor muscle torque comparable with those assessed in prone MMT was developed. Values were compared with those obtained in the traditional prone test.

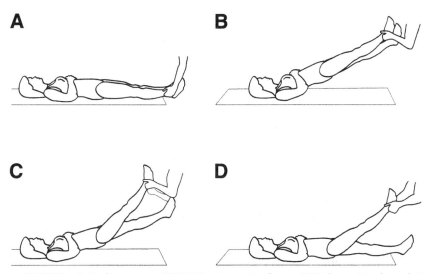

FIGURE 2.—Supine hip extensor MMT. (A) Starting position for test. (B) Ending position for grade 5 (normal). Pelvis and back elevate as a locked unit while the leg is raised by the examiner. The hip maintains the fully extended, neutral position throughout the test. (C) Ending position for grade 4 (good). Hip flexion occurs before pelvis elevates while the examiner raises the leg. (D) Ending position for grades 3 (fair) and 2 (poor). Full elevation of the limb to the end of the straight-leg raising range with no elevation of the pelvis. Examiner feels "good" resistance for grade 3, little resistance for grade 2, and no active resistance for grade 0. (Reprinted from Perry J, Weiss WB, Burnfield JM, et al: The supine hip extensor manual muscle test: A reliability and validity study. *Arch Phys Med Rehabil* 85:1345-1350, 2004. Copyright 2004 with permission from The American Congress of Rehabilitation Medicine and the American Academy of Physical Medicine.)

Methods.—The participants were adult volunteers recruited from the community and outpatient clinics. Sixteen adults (31 limbs) with postpolio syndrome were assessed for reliability tests. Validity testing used 2 groups, 1 comprising 18 subjects (18 limbs) without pathologic conditions and 1 comprising 26 individuals (51 limbs) with clinical signs of hip extensor weakness. Four manual supine torque grades were compared with isometric hip extension joint torque (Fig 2).

Results.—Reliability testing revealed an excellent level of agreement in grade for the 31 limbs tested, with identical grades for 27 limbs and a discrepancy of only 1 level for 4 limbs. The healthy limbs group had grade 5 (normal torque) for 16 limbs and grade 4 (good torque) in 2 limbs. Mean hip extension torque was 212 Nm for the grade 5 limbs and 120 Nm for the grade 4 limbs. A statistically significant difference was found between the mean peak torque of these 2 torque levels. Four grade levels were identified in the 51 limbs with hip extensor weakness: normal (grade 5), good, (grade 4), fair (grade 3), and poor (grade 2). Five participants had grade 5 torque, 14 had grade 4 torque, 22 had grade 3 torque, and 10 had poor torque. For grades 5, 4, 3, and 2, the mean hip extension torques were 176, 103, 67, and 19 Nm, respectively. Significant differences in the mean torque levels of these 4 grades were found ($P < .01$). The mean torques for the grade 4 and grade 5 limbs were less than those of the volunteers without pathologic conditions, but the difference was not statistically significant.

Conclusions.—The torque levels of the supine MMT test were comparable to those of the prone test. Four grades of torque levels were identified. The supine muscle grading postures reflected patients' use of hip flexion to compensate for hip extensor weakness. The supine hip extensor test avoided the effect produced by lumbar spine extension that occurred in the prone test.

▶ Manual muscle testing is popular among clinicians because it is inexpensive and quick to perform in the office setting. However, it is important for all tests to be both valid and reliable. The results of this study suggest that hamstring torque can be tested in the supine position, but some limitations need to be noted. For interrater reliability from 2 raters, one is normally presented with the raw data rather than simply the kappa statistic as reported here. Because there were several categories, it is possible for the kappa statistic to be high and yet there may still be disagreement in certain areas. Another important aspect of a test is for it to be able to discriminate between subjects and to measure change over time. In this study, 16 (88.9%) of 18 subjects without pathology had "excellent" torque, and as such, this aspect of the test could not be tested. Despite the limitations, this is a good first step to create a more clinically relevant hip extensor torque measure. The supine test avoids the unnatural lumbar lordosis that occurs during hip extension in the prone position.

I. Shrier, MD, PhD

Manual Strength Testing in 14 Upper Limb Muscles: A Study on Inter-rater Reliability

Jepsen JR, Laursen LH, Larsen AI, et al (Central Hosp, Esbjerg, Denmark; Novozymes, Bagsvaerd, Denmark; Univ of Pittsburgh, Pa)
Acta Orthop Scand 75:442-448, 2004   5–6

Background.—Manual muscle testing has been termed a " "lost art" " and is often considered to be of minor value. The aim of this investigation was to study the inter-rater reliability of manual examination of the maximal voluntary strength in a sample of upper limb muscles.

Patients and Methods.—The material consisted of a series of 41 consecutive patients (82 limbs) who had been referred to a clinic of occupational medicine for various reasons. Two examiners who were blinded as to patient-related information classified 14 muscles in terms of normal or reduced strength. In order to optimize the evaluation, the individual strength was assessed simultaneously on the right and left sides with the limbs in standardized positions that were specific for each muscle (Figs 1, 2, and 3). Information on upper limb complaints (pain, weakness and/or numbness/tingling) collected by two other examiners resulted in 38 limbs being classified as symptomatic and 44 as asymptomatic. For each muscle the inter-rater reliability of the assessment of strength into normal or reduced was estimated by κ-statistics. In addition, the odds ratio for the relation to symptoms of the definition in agreement of strength was calculated.

Results.—The median κ-value for strength in the muscles examined was 0.54 (0.25-0.72). With a median odds ratio of 4.0 (2.5-7.7), reduced strength was significantly associated with the presence of symptoms.

Interpretation.—This study suggests that manual muscle testing in upper limb disorders has diagnostic potential.

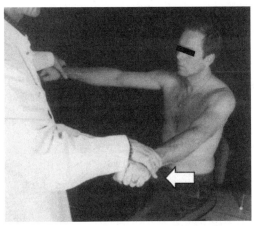

FIGURE 1.—Standard posture I. Testing of the posterior deltoid muscle. The *arrow* indicates the direction of the examiner's force against the patient's resistance. (Courtesy of Jepsen JR, Laursen LH, Larsen AI, et al: Manual strength testing in 14 upper limb muscles: A study on inter-rater reliability. *Acta Orthop Scand* 75:442-448, 2004.)

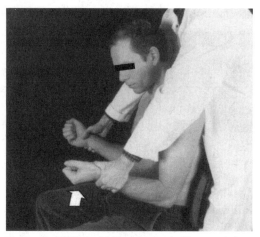

FIGURE 2.—Standard posture II. Testing of the triceps muscle. The *arrow* indicates the direction of the examiner's force against the patient's resistance. (Courtesy of Jepsen JR, Laursen LH, Larsen AI, et al: Manual strength testing in 14 upper limb muscles: A study on inter-rater reliability. *Acta Orthop Scand* 75:442-448, 2004.)

▶ Manual strength testing is used extensively by rehabilitation professionals, such as physical therapists, athletic therapists, and orthopedists to examine muscle strength in injured patients. However, its value has been questioned because of the lack of reliability and validity that is perceived for the modality. This study examined the ability of 2 examiners to determine whether 14 muscles were of normal or reduced strength (only muscles of 4 or 5 on a 5-point scale were examined). They found the inter-rater reliability was moderate to good in 11 of 14 upper- limb muscles, and the remaining 3 muscles had only fair reliability. There appears to be some diagnostic value in the use of manual strength testing for patients with mild upper-limb disorders.

M. J. L. Alexander, PhD

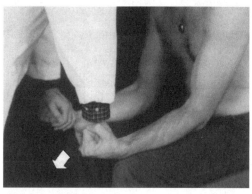

FIGURE 3.—Standard posture III. Testing the flexor carpi radialis muscle. The *arrow* indicates the direction of the examiner's force against the patient's resistance. (Courtesy of Jepsen JR, Laursen LH, Larsen AI, et al: Manual strength testing in 14 upper limb muscles: A study on inter-rater reliability. *Acta Orthop Scand* 75:442-448, 2004.)

Upper and Lower Extremity Muscle Fatigue After a Baseball Pitching Performance

Mullaney MJ, McHugh MP, Donofrio TM, et al (Lenox Hill Hosp, New York)
Am J Sports Med 33:108-113, 2005   5–7

Background.—Fatigue may be the most important factor in the risk of injury when pitching a baseball because it may lead to a loss of proper mechanics. The influence of extended pitching (fatigue) on kinematic and kinetic parameters has been evaluated in previous studies, but no quantification of the fatigue associated with a pitching performance has been performed. Muscle fatigue in upper and lower extremity muscle groups was determined after a pitching performance.

Methods.—A group of 13 baseball pitchers from 4 universities and 1 independent minor league team were tested before and after 19 games. The pitchers threw an average of 99 pitches during an average of 7 innings per game. Shoulder, scapular, and lower extremity muscle force were assessed by a handheld dynamometer before and after the pitching performance.

Results.—Baseline force measurements showed that the pitching arm was 12% weaker in the empty can test (supraspinatus) compared with the contralateral side. Postgame shoulder strength tests indicated selective fatigue of 15% in shoulder flexion, 18% in internal rotation, and 11% in shoulder adduction. Minimal fatigue was noted in empty can test, scapular stabilizers, and hip musculature.

Conclusions.—A trend was present toward significant baseline force in internal rotation and selective postgame fatigue on internal rotation of the dominant upper extremity, which indicated that a high performance demand is placed on the internal rotators during pitching. Weakness in the empty can test on the dominant arm was combined with minimal postgame fatigue; these findings were surprising because previous studies and injury patterns have indicated a high performance demand on the supraspinatus during pitching.

▶ These authors studied 13 baseball players to determine the fatigue associated with a pitching performance. Findings showed that internal rotators experience a high performance demand during pitching and that the muscle fatigue was minimal in the scapular and hip muscles of these pitchers.

R. C. Cantu, MD, MA

Skeletal Muscle Adaptation: Training Twice Every Second Day vs. Training Once Daily

Hansen AK, Fischer CP, Plomgaard P, et al (Univ of Copenhagen)
J Appl Physiol 98:93-99, 2005   5–8

Background.—Low muscle glycogen content has been demonstrated to enhance transcription of a number of genes involved in training adaptation. These results made us speculate that training at a low muscle glycogen con-

TABLE 1.—Maximal Power Output and Time Until Exhaustion at 90% of Maximal Power Output Before and After 10 Weeks of Training and Total Work Before and After 10 Weeks of Training

Parameter	Pretraining		Posttraining	
	Low	High	Low	High
P_{max}, W	74 ± 7	77 ± 6	107 ± 7*	106 ± 6†
T_{exh}, min	5.0 ± 0.7	5.6 ± 1.2	19.7 ± 2.4*‡	11.9 ± 1.3†
Total work, kJ	22 ± 5	25 ± 7	114 ± 14*‡	69 ± 8†

Note: Values are means ± SE. Low, leg trained with low muscle glycogen protocol; High, leg trained with high muscle glycogen protocol.
*Significant difference ($P < 0.05$) from pretraining in Low.
†Significant difference ($P < 0.05$) from pretraining in High.
‡Significant difference ($P < 0.05$) between Low and High.
Abbreviations: P_{max}, Maximal power output; T_{exh}, time until exhaustion; Total work, $P_{max} \times T_{exh}$.
(Courtesy of Hansen AK, Fischer CP, Plomgaard P, et al: Skeletal muscle adaptation: Training twice every second day vs. training once daily. J Appl Physiol 98:93-99, 2005. Copyright The American Physiological Society.)

tent would enhance training adaptation. We therefore performed a study in which seven healthy untrained men performed knee extensor exercise with one leg trained in a low-glycogen (Low) protocol and the other leg trained at a high-glycogen (High) protocol. Both legs were trained equally regarding workload and training amount. On *day 1*, both legs (Low and High) were trained for 1 h followed by 2 h of rest at a fasting state, after which one leg (Low) was trained for an additional 1 h. On *day 2*, only one leg (High) trained for 1 h. *Days 1* and *2* were repeated for 10 wk. As an effect of training, the increase in maximal workload was identical for the two legs. However, time until exhaustion at 90% was markedly more increased in the Low leg compared with the High leg (Table 1). Resting muscle glycogen and the activity of the mitochondrial enzyme 3-hydroxyacyl-CoA dehydrogenase increased with training, but only significantly so in Low, whereas citrate synthase activity increased in both Low and High. There was a more pronounced increase in citrate synthase activity when Low was compared with High. In conclusion, the present study suggests that training twice every second day may be superior to daily training.

▶ An important question in training is whether the body's adaptation to training occurs in response to a lack of carbohydrate during exercise or to a surplus from intake following training. By training twice a day, the body is training at a low muscle glycogen content and a low substrate level that may increase the activity of glycolytic enzymes. In this study, both legs were trained with the same volume, 1 leg was trained every day, the other trained with 2 training periods every other day. This study concluded that aerobic training on a cycle ergometer twice every second day was superior to daily training, likely because of the greater depletion of substrate during the twice-each-day regimen.

M. J. L. Alexander, PhD

Transferability of Strength Gains From Limited to Full Range of Motion
Barak Y, Ayalon M, Dvir Z (Wingate Inst, Netanya, Israel; Tel Aviv Univ, Israel)
Med Sci Sports Exerc 36:1413-1420, 2004   5–9

Background.—Rehabilitation of joint injuries focuses on regaining full range of motion (ROM) and recovering muscle performance. Prescribing an optimal rehabilitation protocol to achieve these goals can be challenging. Among the factors that must be considered are the specificity of training and the transfer of training, or the effect of training on muscle performance outside the trained ROM. Whether isokinetic conditioning that uses the short ROM of the quadriceps transfers to muscles outside the trained range was evaluated. It was hypothesized that some gains in strength values would occur at both the inner and outer range and that gains of work in the trained ROM would exceed those in the untrained ROM.

Methods.—Four groups were randomly determined from a group of 55 women. Fourteen trained concentrically at 30°/s (G1); 14 trained concentrically at 90°/s (G2); 13 trained similarly but used the eccentric mode at 30°/s (G3); and 14 trained similarly but used the eccentric mode at 90°/s (G4). Knee flexion was maintained within 30° to 60°. The participants did 4 sets of 10 maximal repetitions 3 times a week for 6 weeks. Assessments included isokinetic power output (W_{isk}) (obtained within 3 angular ROMs [85° to 60°, 60° to 30°, and 30° to 5°, designated R1, R2, and R3, respectively] before training and 2 days after it was completed), the isometric peak extension moment (PM), and the rate of force development (RFD) at 10°, 45°, and 80°.

Results.—The power output at ROM R1 and R2 did not differ. However, a general but nonsignificant increase in power was noted at ROM R3. A significantly greater gain in power values was achieved at ROM R1 and R2 than at R3, and no advantage was seen in concentric or eccentric testing. Thus, training transfers from the middle ROM toward the outer ROM but not to the inner ROM. All knee extension PMs showed a significant increase in most testing modes. When the testing and training conditions were similar, a higher increase occurred. All joint angles showed a significant increase in isometric PM between pretraining and posttraining measurements. Uniform and significant increases in RFD occurred at 45° for all groups, and a significantly greater increase occurred in RFD at this angle than at 10°. Groups 3 and 4 differed significantly in increased isokinetic PM between the different testing modes, and a greater increase occurred in the eccentric than the concentric PM values. The various groups exhibited different gains in isokinetic PM as a result of the greater increase in eccentric PM in groups 3 and 4 compared with groups 1 and 2. The various joint angles in experimental groups 1, 3, and 4 had significantly different gains in isometric PM. The isometric PM increased significantly more at 45° than at 80° and 10°.

Conclusions.—Whether concentric or eccentric conditioning was used, with relatively short or long movement durations, the power output increased significantly outside the trained ROM. Therefore, isokinetic conditioning within a restricted ROM translated to functional value both inside and outside that ROM and was seen as a significant increase in power values.

Most changes occurred in the trained ROM and when the muscle was lengthened (outer ROM) rather than when the muscle was shortened.

▶ This study has important implications for rehabilitation. Many therapists insist on obtaining close to full ROM after an injury before beginning a strengthening program. The rationale often used is that strength gains only occur in the range trained; therefore, strength training early in rehabilitation is of limited usefulness. Although strength gains decrease as one moves away from the trained range, significant gains are still made when the muscle is tested at longer lengths, and nonstatistical gains are made at shorter muscle lengths.

I. Shrier, MD, PhD

Skeletal Muscle Pathology in Endurance Athletes With Acquired Training Intolerance
Grobler LA, Collins M, Lambert MI, et al (Univ of Cape Town, Newlands, South Africa; Med Research Council of South Africa, Tygerberg)
Br J Sports Med 38:697-703, 2004   5–10

Background.—It is well established that prolonged, exhaustive endurance exercise is capable of inducing skeletal muscle damage and temporary impairment of muscle function. Although skeletal muscle has a remarkable capacity for repair and adaptation, this may be limited, ultimately resulting in an accumulation of chronic skeletal muscle pathology. Case studies have alluded to an association between long term, high volume endurance training and racing, acquired training intolerance, and chronic skeletal muscle pathology.

Objective.—To systematically compare the skeletal muscle structural and ultrastructural status of endurance athletes with acquired training intolerance (ATI group) with asymptomatic endurance athletes matched for age and years of endurance training (CON group).

Methods.—Histological and electron microscopic analyses were carried out on a biopsy sample of the vastus lateralis from 18 ATI and 17 CON endurance athletes. The presence of structural and ultrastructural disruptions was compared between the two groups of athletes.

Results.—Significantly more athletes in the ATI group than in the CON group presented with fibre size variation (15 vs 6; $P = 0.006$), internal nuclei (9 vs 2; $P = 0.03$), and z disc streaming (6 vs 0; $P = 0.02$).

Conclusions.—There is an association between increased skeletal muscle disruptions and acquired training intolerance in endurance athletes. Further studies are required to determine the nature of this association and the possible mechanisms involved.

▶ Highly trained endurance athletes may suffer from ATI because of skeletal muscle damage and temporary impairment of muscle function. There appears to be an association between long-term high-volume endurance training and racing and chronic skeletal muscle damage. More athletes with ATI in this study presented with structural and ultrastructural skeletal muscle pathology. The z disk appears to be the structure most often injured in exercise-induced muscle damage. Prolonged strenuous endurance exercise may restrict the ability of skeletal muscle to adapt and regenerate. This will result in an accumulation of chronic skeletal muscle damage that will lead to impaired training and racing performance. There may be a limit to the ability of muscle to adapt and regenerate, and beyond this limit, muscle damage is irreversible and irreparable.

M. J. L. Alexander, PhD

Sensory Level Electrical Muscle Stimulation: Effect on Markers of Muscle Injury
McLoughlin TJ, Snyder AR, Brolinson PG, et al (Univ of Toledo, Ohio; Northwest Ohio Ctr for Sports Medicine)
Br J Sports Med 38:725-729, 2004   5–11

Background.—Monophasic high voltage stimulation (MHVS) is widely prescribed for the treatment of inflammation associated with muscle injury. However, limited scientific evidence exists to support its purported benefits in humans.

Objective.—To examine the efficacy of early initiation of MHVS treatment after muscle injury.

Methods.—In a randomised, cross over design, 14 men performed repetitive eccentric contractions of the elbow flexor muscles followed by either MHVS or control treatment. MHVS treatments were applied five minutes and 3, 6, 24, 48, 72, 96, and 120 hours after eccentric contractions.

Results.—MHVS resulted in a significant reduction ($P < 0.05$) in delayed onset muscle soreness 24 hours after eccentric exercise compared with controls (Fig 2). Elbow extension was significantly increased immediately after administration of MHVS compared with controls. No significant differences were observed between MHVS treatment and controls for maximal isometric strength, flexed arm angle, or arm volume.

Conclusions.—Early and frequent application of MHVS may provide transient relief from delayed onset muscle soreness and short term improvements in range of motion after injurious exercise. However, MHVS treatment may not enhance recovery after muscle injury because of lack of improvements in strength and active range of motion.

▶ Delayed onset muscle soreness results from unaccustomed eccentric contractions that produce microscopic muscle injury, usually affecting the actin and myosin filaments and the z-line of the sarcomere. This muscle injury produces decreased range of motion, decreased force production, and muscle soreness. MHVS has been used to treat muscle injury associated with strenuous exercise. In this study, subjects were treated with MHVS following strenuous eccentric exercise, and this treatment was found to be effective in reducing delayed-onset muscle soreness and increasing elbow flexibility. However,

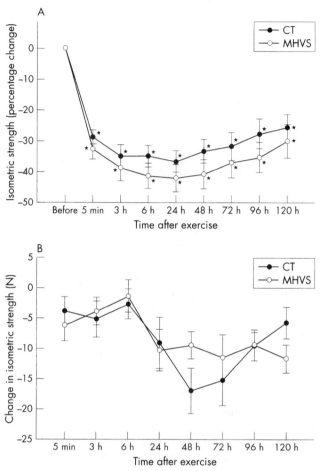

FIGURE 2.—Effect of monophasic high voltage stimulation (MHVS) on maximal isometric strength after eccentric contractions. **A** Long-term effect. Measurements were taken before the control (CT) or MHVS treatments at rhe respective time points (expressed as percentage change relative to measurement before the exercise (baseline measurement). *Significantly different from the baseline measurement (*P* < .05). **B** Short-term effect. Measurements were taken approximately 15 minutes after the CT or MHVS treatments and subtracted from the measurement before the treatment at the respective time points. All values are mean (SEM) (n = 14). (Courtesy of McLoughlin TJ, Snyder AR, Brolinson PG, et al: Sensory level electrical muscle stimulation: Effect on markers of muscle injury. 38:725-729, 2004. Reprinted with permission from the BMJ Publishing Group.)

there were no changes in arm volume or isometric strength. Since the effects of using MHVS were not widespread or universal in all subjects, it was suggested that there is presently no indication that this treatment should be used regularly or systematically in subjects with muscle injury.

M. J. L. Alexander, PhD

Influence of Pre-exercise Muscle Temperature on Responses to Eccentric Exercise

Nosaka K, Sakamoto K, Newton M, et al (Edith Cowan Univ, Joondalup, Western Australia; Yokohama City Univ, Japan)
J Athl Train 39:132-137, 2004   5–12

Background.—Warm-up exercises used to prevent injury may also reduce the severity of eccentric exercise-induced muscle damage and delayed-onset muscle soreness (DOMS). The mechanism by which this is accomplished has been believed to relate to changes in muscle temperature. The increased muscle temperature produced by the warm-up exercises could increase muscle and connective tissue extensibility, which would make these structures less susceptible to muscle damage. If this is true, the opposite effect would hold if muscle temperatures were lowered. The effect of altering the pre-exercise muscle temperature on muscle damage indicators was investigated.

Methods.—Twenty female students who had not participated in resistance training were assigned to receive either a passive warming (microwave) treatment (10 students) or a cooling (icing) treatment (10 students). The deep muscle temperature increased by about 3°C by the microwave treatment and declined about 5°C with the icing. After the treatment, each participant performed 12 maximal eccentric actions of the forearm flexors of each arm twice; 4 weeks separated the 2 occasions. The opposite, untreated arm served as a control. Changes were noted in maximal isometric force, and indirect markers of muscle damage (ie, range of motion, upper arm circumference, muscle soreness, and plasma creatine kinase [CK] activity) were assessed.

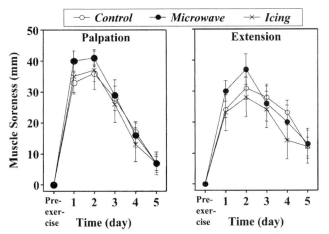

FIGURE 4.—Changes in muscle soreness with palpation (**A**) and extension (**B**) before (pre-exercise) and 1 to 5 days after eccentric exercise in the treatment (microwave, icing) and control conditions. No significant differences were noted among conditions. (Reprinted from Nosaka K, Sakamoto K, Newton M, et al: Influence of pre-exercise muscle temperature on responses to eccentric exercise. *J Athletic Train* 39:132-137, 2004. Copyright 2004, with permission from The National Athletic Trainers' Association.)

Results.—The treatments produced no significant difference in muscle force during exercise, maximal isometric force, upper arm circumference, severity of DOMS (Fig 4), or plasma CK activity. Two to 3 days after exercise, the microwave treatment produced a significantly larger decline in the relaxed angle. In addition, the flexed elbow angle was significantly greater immediately after completing the exercise, increased more in the first day after exercise, and gradually declined over the subsequent 4 days. Range of motion decreased significantly more with the microwave treatment than with icing or in the control condition. Significant differences between the result with microwave treatment and that for the icing and control groups were noted 2 to 5 days after exercise.

Conclusions.—Changing muscle temperature by giving heating or cooling treatments before exercise did not change the maximal isometric force, the upper arm circumference, DOMS, or the plasma CK activity. Relaxed and flexed elbow angles and range of motion were altered significantly more with the microwave treatment than with icing or under control conditions. It was believed that the microwave treatment would attenuate the response to eccentric exercise, but the opposite proved true. Neither heat nor cold increased the severity of the muscle-damage response under these conditions.

▶ Several studies have suggested that pre-exercise muscle activity at a low intensity will prevent injury when exercise is then performed at higher intensities. Traditionally, this has been called a warm-up, and many people believe that the mechanism is an increase in temperature. However, an increase in temperature caused by passive warming in this study was associated with a nonsignificant decrease in muscle force, range of motion, and muscle soreness. Along with studies on the effects of stretching and studies on the effects of fatigue, these results suggest that the mechanism behind warm-up is not muscle temperature. A greater understanding of the basic science in this field may lead to improved injury prevention programs.

I. Shrier, MD, PhD

Improving Golf Performance With a Warm Up Conditioning Programme
Fradkin AJ, Sherman CA, Finch CF (Australian Inst of Sport, Leverrier Crescent, Bruce, ACT, Australia)
Br J Sports Med 38:762-765, 2004   5–13

Background.—A warm-up is a period of preparatory exercise to enhance subsequent competition or training performance. The purpose of a warm-up is to prepare the body both physiologically and psychologically and to reduce the risk of injury. Studies conducted in the 1950s to 1970s produced contradictory results regarding the benefits of a warm-up period versus no warm-up. However, most of these studies had major faults. Despite the questions surrounding these studies, the preponderance of evidence suggests that a warm-up period before play will improve performance compared with no warm-up. Warming up has been widely promoted as an

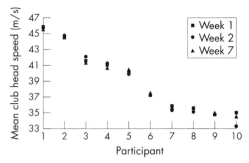

FIGURE 1.—Control group mean club head speeds over testing period (n = 10). (Courtesy of Fradkin AJ, Sherman CA, Finch CF: Improving golf performance with a warm up conditioning programme. *Br J Sports Med* 38:762-765, 2004. Reprinted with permission from the BMJ Publishing Group.)

important performance-enhancing and injury-prevention measure for both amateur and professional golfers, but this approach has not been formally evaluated. This study sought to determine whether a golf-specific warm-up program, performed 5 times a week for 5 weeks, would improve performance in golfers.

Methods.—A cohort of 20 male golfers were matched for age and handicap and divided into an exercise group and a control group. Club head speed was assessed by 2-dimensional video analysis in a laboratory setting. In the first week, all golfers performed 10 strokes. In weeks 2 and 7, the control group performed the same procedure as in the first week, while the exercise group performed a specially designed warm-up, 5 times per week for 5 weeks, during weeks 2 through 7.

Results.—The mean club head speeds in the exercise group were improved at each testing week. Between weeks 1 and 2, the club head speeds in the exercise group were improved by an average of 3 to 6 m/s (12.8%), and between weeks 1 and 7, club head speeds were increased by 7 to 10 m/s (24%). With one exception, the mean club head speeds of the golfers in the

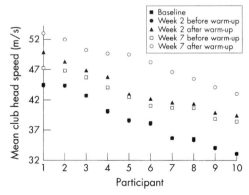

FIGURE 2.—Exercise group mean club head speeds over testing period (n = 10). (Courtesy of Fradkin AJ, Sherman CA, Finch CF: Improving golf performance with a warm up conditioning programme. *Br J Sports Med* 38:762-765, 2004. Reprinted with permission from the BMJ Publishing Group.)

control group showed little variation over the testing period (Fig 1). There was a significant difference between the mean club head speeds of the exercise and control groups over the duration of the study, and a significant interaction over time (Fig 2).

Conclusions.—The performance of golfers was significantly improved by participation in a golf-specific warm-up program compared with golfers who did not perform the warm-up activities.

▶ The effect of warm-up on injury prevention and performance continues to be of interest to many readers. This study is consistent with previous findings in other activities—force and power are increased with an acute warm-up and with regular warm-up/training. The authors correctly acknowledge that golf accuracy was not tested in this study. One issue not raised in this study is the differential effects of stretching versus prior activity on performance. In this study, the intervention was a combination of brisk movements, stretching, and air swings with the club. For the acute effects of the intervention, there is a substantial body of research suggesting stretching immediately prior to activity impairs performance, and there is some evidence that light muscle contractions prior to activity improve performance (which may or may not be temperature related). It would be interesting for future studies to separate the interventions from each other. Although stretching regularly over weeks improves performance in other activities, the authors may still want to separate the components of their intervention in future studies to determine which effect predominates.

I. Shrier, MD, PhD

Treatment of Muscle Injuries by Local Administration of Autologous Conditioned Serum: A Pilot Study on Sportsmen With Muscle Strains
Wright-Carpenter T, Klein P, Schäferhoff P (Institut Gustave-Roussy, Villejuif, France; MediaPark Clin for Sports Medicine & Orthopaedics, Köln, Germany; German Sport Univ, Köln, Germany; et al)
Int J Sports Med 25:588-593, 2004   5–14

Background.—A number of growth factors play a role in muscle regeneration. A previously described method of physical and chemical stimulation of autologous whole blood was tested under specific conditions (autologous conditioned serum) for a number of growth factors and cytokines.

Methods.—A preliminary study was conducted of muscle strain injuries in professional athletes receiving either autologous conditioned serum (ACS) or Actovegin/Traumeel treatment as control. Recovery from injury was assessed by the ability of the athlete to participate fully (100%) under competitive conditions in his respective sport and by MRI analysis.

Results.—A significant difference in recovery time from injury was noted in the ACS group (16.6 ± 0.9 days) compared with the control group (22.3 ± 1.2 days). Analysis of MRI findings was supportive of the observed acceleration of the lesion recovery time.

Conclusion.—ACS injection is a promising method for reducing time to recovery from muscle injury.

▶ These authors studied professional sportsmen with muscle strain to determine whether ACS treatment accelerated the recovery time of these athletes. Their study determined that the injection of ACS is a promising approach to a more rapid recovery and return to full activity from muscle strain in these athletes.

R. C. Cantu, MD, MA

Cryotherapy Does Not Impair Shoulder Joint Position Sense
Dover G, Powers ME (Univ of Florida, Gainesville; Shenandoah Univ, Winchester, Va)
Arch Phys Med Rehabil 85:1241-1246, 2004   5–15

Background.—The glenohumeral joint relies on dynamic restraint by the rotator cuff to maintain stability, which makes shoulder proprioception an important consideration. Fatigue, injury, and overhand athletic activities may impair shoulder proprioception. Rehabilitation of the shoulder usually includes proprioception exercises. During injury management, cryotherapy is often used to diminish pain and inflammation. Muscle electrophysiologic activity can be changed by cryotherapy, which can be used to disrupt afferent signals and modify neuromuscular control during a proprioception assessment. Shoulder joint position sense (JPS) was evaluated after a 30-minute cryotherapy session in healthy individuals to determine the effects of cryotherapy on shoulder proprioception.

Methods.—A total of 15 men and 15 women participated in this crossover design study with repeated measures. All were healthy, with a mean age of 23.7 years for the men and 20.7 years for the women. Thirty-minute cryotherapy treatments were given to the dominant shoulder. JPS was determined with the patient in standing position and concentrated on the dominant shoulder. An inclinometer was used before and after the 30-minute application of no ice or a 1-kg ice bag (Fig 2). Total internal rotation and external rotation range of motion were measured while the shoulder was maintained in 90° of abduction and the elbow in 90° of flexion. Skin temperature measurements below the tip of the acromion process were obtained every 5 minutes over the 30-minute therapy session and immediately after it was completed.

Results.—Skin surface temperatures did not differ significantly between the men and women during or after cryotherapy, nor were other gender differences noted; thus, the male and female error scores were combined in the remainder of the analyses. Temperatures decreased significantly during cryotherapy. Measures of shoulder JPS (ie, absolute error after the cryotherapy session, constant error after the cryotherapy session, and the variable error score) indicated that the 30 minutes of cryotherapy had no adverse effect on proprioception.

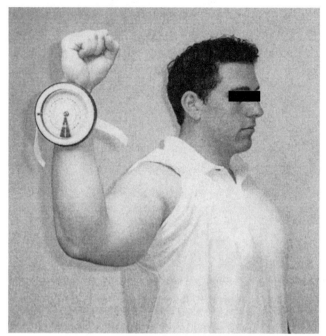

FIGURE 2.—Subject position during joint position sense testing. (Courtesy of Dover G, Powers ME: Cryotherapy does not impair shoulder joint position sense. *Arch Phys Med Rehabil* 85:1241-1246, 2004. Copyright 2004 with permission from The American Congress of Rehabilitation Medicine and the American Academy of Physical Medicine and Rehabilitation.)

Conclusions.—Cryotherapy did not impair shoulder JPS. Rehabilitation considerations should include this observation in the management of shoulder injuries.

▶ These results conflict with studies on the ankle and knee. Although the different results may reflect differences due to the joint being studied, it may also reflect an increased variability of the measure in the shoulder. This would lead to a decreased chance of showing statistically significant results. For example, both external and internal rotation in the current study were measured with the shoulder in the 90° abducted position. However, the shoulder was not fixed in this position. Therefore, slight changes in glenohumeral abduction and scapular rotation might also affect position sense for external and internal rotation of the glenohumeral joint. This study represents a good start toward addressing the effects of cryotherapy on the shoulder joint, but more research is needed.

I. Shrier, MD, PhD

Shoulder Rotation Characteristics in Professional Tennis Players

Schmidt-Wiethoff R, Rapp W, Mauch F, et al (Dreifaltigkeits-Krankenhaus, Cologne, Germany; Catholic Univ Leuven, Belgium; Orthopädische Klinik im Olgahospital, Stuttgart, Germany; et al)
Int J Sports Med 25:154-158, 2004   5–16

Introduction.—Chronic shoulder pain in overhead athletes is commonly caused by a failure within the kinematic chain. Objective measurement of the glenohumeral joint motion is challenging due to the multijoint nature of the total shoulder movements and the intricate interplay with the scapulothoracic joint. Glenohumeral joint internal and external rotational range of motion were evaluated with a US-based kinematic measurement device.

Methods.—Twenty-seven male professional tennis players underwent bilateral measurement of internal and external rotation at 90° of shoulder abduction while avoiding scapulothoracic motion. Twenty asymptomatic control subjects not involved in overhead sports activities were also evaluated.

Results.—The dominant arm (playing arm) had a significantly greater range of external rotation compared to the nondominant arm. There was a significant deficit in internal rotation in the dominant versus the nondominant arm. The total rotational range of motion in the dominant arm was significantly decreased compared to that of the nondominant arm and to the control subjects. No significant differences were observed between the dominant and nondominant extremity in control subjects.

Conclusion.—US-based real time motion analysis may have clinical application in the development of rehabilitation and preventive programs.

▶ A study of 27 male professional tennis players using a US-based kinematic device to measure their internal and external shoulder rotation was found useful in rehabilitation and preventive programs for these athletes.

R. C. Cantu, MD, MA

Relative Balance of Serratus Anterior and Upper Trapezius Muscle Activity During Push-Up Exercises

Ludewig PM, Hoff MS, Osowski EE, et al (Univ of Minnesota, Minneapolis)
Am J Sports Med 32:484-493, 2004   5–17

Introduction.—The lower and middle divisions of the serratus anterior (SA) muscle are important contributors to normal and abnormal scapular motion and control. The SA is considered a prime mover of the scapula. It is unique among the scapulothoracic muscles in that it has the ability to augment all components of the 3-dimensional movement of the scapula on the thorax during elevation of the arm. SA strengthening is used to prevent and treat poor scapular control. Push-up exercises were evaluated for their ability to maximally activate the SA, while minimally activating the upper trapezius (UT).

Methods.—Thirty research subjects aged 18 to 50 years performed standard push-up plus exercises and modifications on elbows, knees, and against a wall. Surface electromyography of the SA and UT was performed. Group 1 (19 participants) had normal, healthy shoulders and had no history of shoulder pain, trauma, fracture, dislocation, or surgical procedure. Group 2 (11 participants) had shoulder pain or dysfunction for which SA-strengthening exercises would be advocated clinically.

Results.—Both groups had similar responses to the exercises. The standard push-up plus had the highest activation of the serratus (to 123%) and lowest trapezius/serratus ratios (less than 0.2) during plus phases. The wall push-up plus and phases of other exercises had higher UT/SA ratios (to 2.0).

Conclusion.—In clinical situations in which UT activation or imbalance of serratus and trapezius activation occurs, the push-up plus is an optimal exercise. Some patients may benefit from a progression of modified push-up exercises.

▶ This is a study of 30 subjects either healthy or with mild shoulder dysfunction and use of standard push-ups as well as modified push-up exercises.

R. C. Cantu, MD, MA

Quantitative Assessment of Glenohumeral Translation in Baseball Players: A Comparison of Pitchers Versus Nonpitching Athletes
Sethi PM, Tibone JE, Lee TQ (Orthopedic and Neurosurgical Associates, Greenwich, Conn; Univ of Southern California, Los Angeles; VA Long Beach Healthcare System, Calif)
Am J Sports Med 32:1711-1715, 2004   5–18

Introduction.—Thorough understanding of adaptations of the throwing shoulder and careful interpretation of the physical examination are equally important in both normal and pathologic shoulders. Of particular interest is how the capsuloligamentous injuries associated with the throwing shoulder relate to pitching mechanisms and to pathomechanics and anatomy of the shoulder. Side-to-side differences in shoulder translation were measured by using cutaneous electromagnetic sensors and range-of-motion (ROM) in division I college baseball players and professional pitchers.

Findings.—Nineteen position players and 37 pitchers were evaluated. Pitchers had a significant increase in external rotation of the dominant arm compared with the nondominant arm ($P = .02$); this difference was not significant among position players ($P = .34$). The mean ROM for the dominant arm in pitchers was 110° external rotation to 68° internal rotation; for position players, it was 100° external rotation to 85° internal rotation ($P = .278$). The mean anteroposterior translation in the dominant and nondominant arm was 33.30 mm and 29.84 mm, respectively ($P = .0001$). This difference was not seen in position players ($P = .88$). One in 19 position players had a side-to-side shoulder translation difference greater than 3 mm compared with 22 of 37 pitchers ($P = .0001$).

Conclusion.—Pitchers have a greater amount of glenohumeral translation in the dominant arm compared with nonpitching players. These differences make the side-to-side comparison less useful in pitchers and should be considered when making therapeutic decisions in these athletes.

▶ This is a prospective cross-sectional study of baseball pitchers to examine whether there are greater differences in side-to-side anteroposterior translation of their throwing shoulders compared with position players. The authors' conclusion was that pitchers have a greater amount of glenohumeral translation in the dominant arm, which was not the case with position players.

R. C. Cantu, MD, MA

Knee Biomechanics of the Support Leg in Soccer Kicks From Three Angles of Approach

Kellis E, Katis A, Gissis I (Aristotle Univ of Thessaloniki, Serres, Greece)
Med Sci Sports Exerc 36:1017-1028, 2004   5–19

Background.—The most important move in soccer is the kick, but the magnitudes of ground reaction forces (GRF) have not been thoroughly studied. An investigation was done of knee joint kinematics, electromyographic (EMG) activity of the vastus medialis (VM), vastus lateralis (VL), biceps femoris (BF), and GRF during maximal instep soccer kicks from 3 different approach angles.

Study Design.—The study included 10 male amateur soccer players. The players performed a series of maximal soccer kicks from 0 radian (K0), 0.81 radian (K45) and 1.62 radian (K90) (0°, 45°, and 90°, respectively) angles of approach on a piezoelectric force platform to record GRF. EMG activity was also recorded. Digital cameras recorded the kicks for motion and ball speed analyses.

Findings.—K90 and K45 were associated with increased medial and posterior GRF and decreased anterior GRF than was the result with K0. K90 and K45 were also associated with significantly increased external rotation displacement, maximum flexion, internal rotation, abduction, and adduction velocity of the tibia relative to the femur of the support leg. BF EMG was also significantly increased for K90 and K45 kicks compared with that of K0.

Conclusions.—Soccer kicks with a high angle of approach have increased medial and posterior GRF, which may have negative implications for performance. These kicks are associated with significant alterations in knee joint kinematics and BF activation strategies. Angled soccer kicks may induce significant loads to the knee joint of the supporting leg.

▶ These authors have studied 10 amateur soccer players, their approach to the soccer ball from an angle, and have looked at the biomechanics associated with this angled kick. They concluded that kicking with a high angle approach increases the medial and posterior GRF, which may have a negative impact on soccer kick performance. In addition, these angled kicks increase loads to knee joint ligaments.

R. C. Cantu, MD, MA

An Acute Bout of Static Stretching: Effects on Force and Jumping Performance
Power K, Behm D, Cahill F, et al (Mem Univ of Newfoundland, St John's, Canada; Univ of Ballarat, Victoria, Australia)
Med Sci Sports Exerc 36:1389-1396, 2004   5–20

Background.—Light aerobic activity followed by stretching is the recommended routine preceding exercise. Stretching has been shown to increase the range of motion (ROM) around joints, decrease muscle soreness, reduce or prevent injury caused by tight muscles, and promote rehabilitation after an injury. More current studies have questioned the capability of stretching to achieve these effects but have focused on more sustained stretching than is normally performed. Static stretching (SS) routines were assessed for their role in decreasing isometric force, activating muscles, and influencing jump power while improving ROM.

Methods.—The 12 men who participated ranged in age from 20 to 44 years and acted as their own control group. Tests were done before and at various points after performing a SS routine of the quadriceps and plantar flexors (PF) or before and after a similar period of no stretching (control). Maximal voluntary force (MVC), evoked contractile properties, surface integrated electromyographic (EMG) activity of the agonist and antagonist muscle groups, and muscle inactivation (interpolated twitch technique [ITT]) were determined. Measurements of vertical jumping included unilateral concentric-only jump height and drop jump (DJ) height and contact time. ROM was determined for seated hip flexion, prone hip extension, and plantar flexion and dorsiflexion.

Results.—A significant 9.5% decline in MVC force of the quadriceps resulted after SS, and significant decreases between 8.4% and 10.4% were noted for the 120-minute duration of testing. Neither the control condition nor PF MVC changed significantly. The ITT revealed a significant overall 5.4% increase in quadriceps inactivation with SS. Quadriceps EMG activity declined 15.1% immediately and 16.5% after 120 minutes. PF EMG activity increased 6.5% immediately and decreased 13.5% after 120 minutes. Immediately after SS, the evoked contractile properties increased 0.5%; they declined 2.1% 120 minutes after the test. The DJ height contact times decreased nonsignificantly from 2.6% to 10.1% within 120 minutes of SS. DJ heights decreased nonsignificantly from 5.1% to 6.5%. Concentric-only jump height declined 2% to 4.5% over 120 minutes. A significant increase in the sit and reach ROM was produced by SS and lasted 120 minutes. Immediately after testing, the ROM increase was 10%; it then declined to 8% at 30 minutes, 7% at 60 minutes, 6% at 90 minutes, and 6% at 120 minutes after SS.

Conclusions.—The SS routine produced significant declines in the MVC and ITT of the quadriceps. MVC force remained significantly decreased for at least 120 minutes. Hip extensor ROM was significantly increased by SS for 120 minutes. Jump performance variables were not changed by SS. Thus, SS may impair isometric force production for as long as 120 minutes. When maximal force output is sought, SS should be avoided for at least 120 minutes before the effort. Jumping activities may proceed after SS with no change in performance.

▶ This study confirms previous studies that showed that an acute bout of stretching decreases force production. Although decreases in jumping height with stretching were not statistically significant, the magnitude of the decrease was similar to that in previous studies. The study further shows that at least part of the mechanism responsible is a decreased ability to activate the muscle and is not just due to local muscle damage.

I. Shrier, MD, PhD

Effect of Acute Static Stretching on Force, Balance, Reaction Time, and Movement Time
Behm DG, Bambury A, Cahill F, et al (Mem Univ of Newfoundland, St John's, Canada)
Med Sci Sports Exerc 36:1397-1402, 2004   5–21

Background.—Stretching increases the range of motion around a joint and theoretically improves an athlete's performance, but no substantial evidence has supported the latter use. Several studies indicate that vigorous and prolonged stretching may decrease force, thereby negatively affecting human performance. The stiffness of the musculotendinous unit can determine how effectively and how quickly internal forces generated by the muscle are transmitted to the skeletal system. If the musculotendinous unit length, stiffness, force output, and muscle activation greatly change, afferent proprioception and efferent muscle activation may be altered. Impairments induced by stretching could affect balance and stability or limb proprioception. The effect on balance, proprioception, reaction time (RT), and movement time (MT) of a vigorous bout of lower limb static stretching was assessed.

Methods.—Static stretching of the quadriceps, hamstrings, and plantar flexors or a control condition lasting the same time was undertaken by 16 participants. The components of the stretching were a 5-minute cycle ergometer warm-up, 3 stretches to the point of discomfort lasting 45 seconds each, and a 15-second rest period for each muscle group. The maximal voluntary isometric contraction force of the leg extensors, static balance as determined on a computerized wobble board, RT and MT time of the dominant lower limb, and the ability to achieve 30% and 50% maximal voluntary isometric contraction forces with or without visual feedback were determined for each research subject.

Results.—Static balance, RT, and MT differed significantly between the control data and those obtained with stretching. The force output and perceived force did not differ between the 2 conditions. The control condition improved balance significantly (17.3%), but the stretch condition resulted in a nonsignificant 2.2% decline in balance scores. The same type of reverse trend was noted for RT and MT. Under control conditions, RT improved 5.8%, and MT improved 5.7%. With stretching, RT was impaired 4.0%, and MT was impaired 1.9%.

Conclusions.—A moderate bout of stretching held to the point of discomfort resulted in impaired balance, RT, and MT compared with control conditions. The use of stretching nullified the beneficial effects of the warm-up and induced a small decrement in performance compared with pretest scores.

▶ As a companion to the article by Power et al (see Abstract 5–20), this study further shows that stretching decreases performance on balance tests and RT. Readers should note that, although force decreases were not significantly different, greater decreases were seen in the stretching group, and the magnitude was similar to previous studies showing statistically significant results.

I. Shrier, MD, PhD

Reliability of a Device Measuring Triceps Surae Muscle Fatigability
Haber M, Golan E, Azoulay L, et al (SMBD-Jewish Gen Hosp, Montreal)
Br J Sports Med 38:163-167, 2004   5–22

Objective.—To examine the test-retest reliability of a protocol using an apparatus designed to standardise the standing heel rise test for the triceps surae muscle (Fig 1).

Subjects.—40 healthy subjects volunteered to test short and medium term test-retest reliability (group SM, median age 24 years), and a convenience sample of 38 subjects with a history of unilateral deep vein thrombosis (DVT) volunteered to test long term test-retest reliability (group L, median age 52 years).

Design.—Subjects carried out 23 heel rises per minute until either the pace or the height could no longer be maintained. Group SM subjects repeated the test 30 minutes later (short term), and again 48 hours later (medium term). Subjects in group L did the test on the unaffected leg, and repeated the test one week later (long term).

Results.—The median number of heel rises achieved per trial in group SM was 34 (range 16 to 120). The intraclass coefficient (ICC) was 0.93 (SEM 2.1) for both 30 minute and 48 hour test-retest reliability. In group L, the median number of heel rises was 27 (range 9 to 97), with ICC 0.88 and SEM 3.4.

Conclusions.—The apparatus is a simple and inexpensive standardised tool that reliably measures triceps surae fatigability in subjects with no current injury. Future research should assess its use in injured patients.

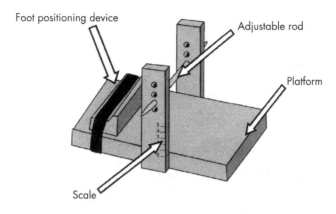

Foot positioning device

Adjustable rod

Platform

Scale

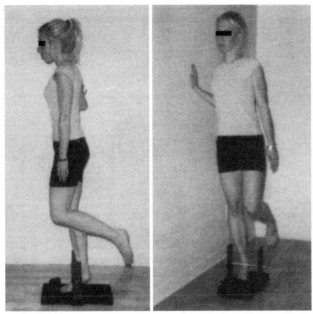

FIGURE 1.—The Haberometer. Before each trial the foot positioning device and rod are adjusted to limit each heel rise to the desired height. The subject stands on the platform barefooted with the knee fully extended and the contralateral leg suspended in air. Following a metronome, the subject does heel rises, touching the rod with the navicular bone each time until either the pace or the height can no longer be maintained, at which time the test is terminated. The pictures of the subject show her foot positioned with the distal end of her toes touching the foot positioning device (lateral view), and the navicular bone touching the rod during the maximum height of the heel lift (anterior view). The subject is allowed to place one hand lightly on a wall to improve balance. (Courtesy of Haber M, Golan E, Azoulay L, et al: Reliability of a device measuring triceps surae muscle fatigability. *Br J Sports Med* 38:163-167, 2004. Reprinted with permission from the BMJ Publishing Group.)

▶ Muscle fatigue and weakness is an important risk factor for injury during sports activities. The standing heel raise test is often used to test the fatigability of the calf muscles, but the test requires refinement to determine the criteria for fatigue. The reliability of a testing device for the heel raise exercise was tested. The device determines when fatigue has occurred due to inability to raise the foot to a certain level in the device. This is evaluated by contact of the navicular with a specific point of contact on the device. This device, the Haberometer, was found to have good reliability, low cost, and simplicity of use in measuring triceps surae fatigability in normal subjects. Reliability of the device with subjects with muscle strain injuries to the calf muscles, Achilles tendonitis, or osteoarthritis has not yet been established.

M. J. L. Alexander, PhD

Fatigability of the Elbow Flexor Muscle for a Sustained Submaximal Contraction Is Similar in Men and Women Matched for Strength
Hunter SK, Critchlow A, Shin I-S, et al (Univ of Colorado, Boulder; Marquette Univ, Milwaukee, Wisconsin; Seoul Natl Univ, Korea)
J Appl Physiol 96:195-202, 2004   5–23

Introduction.—The time to task failure for an isometric contraction sustained at a submaximal intensity is greater for women than for men. No trials have directly examined the contribution of absolute strength and the associated pressor response to the sex differences in time to task failure for a sustained contraction of a large muscle group in which the intramuscular pressures are likely to be great. The time to task failure for a submaximal fatiguing contraction sustained with the elbow flexor muscles by men and women who were matched for strength was compared.

Methods.—Ten men and 10 women, aged 18-35 years, were matched for strength based on the torque exerted at the wrist during a maximal voluntary contraction (MVC). The pressor response (mean arterial pressure and heart rate) and the electromyogram (EMG) activity of multiple muscles were measured. The pressor response revealed the cardiovascular adjustments during the task. The electromyogram EMG activity (average rectified EMG and bursting activity) was documented for comparison with previously observed gender differences between men who were stronger than women.

Results.—The maximal torque exerted at the wrist was similar for men and women (64.5 ± 8.7 [standard deviation] vs 64.5 ± 8.3 N/m; $P < .05$), meaning that the average torque exerted during the fatiguing contraction (20% of MVC) was similar for both sexes. Time to failure was similar in strength-matched men and women (819 ± 306 vs 864 ± 391 seconds; $P < .05$). The mean arterial pressure was similar at the start of the contraction for men (97 ± 12 mm Hg) and women (96 ± 15 mm Hg; $P > .05$) and at task failure (134 ± 18 vs 126 ± 26 mm Hg; $P > .05$, respectively) (Fig 3).

The increases in heart rate, torque fluctuations, and rating of perceived exertion during the fatigue contraction were similar in men and women. The EMG activity was different for men and women; the rate of increase in the average of the rectified EMG (percentage peak MVC) for all elbow flexor muscles was less for women than for men ($P < .05$). The bursts of EMG activity for the elbow flexor muscles increased toward exhaustion for all participants, yet at a greater rate for women than for men ($P < .05$).

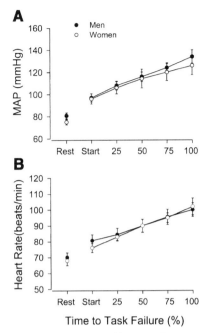

FIGURE 3.—Mean arterial pressure (*MAP*) (**A**) and heart rate (**B**) at rest and during the fatiguing contraction for men and women who were matched for strength. Values are means ± SE of 15-second intervals at 25% increments of the time to task failure. The increase in MAP and heart rate was similar for the men and women ($P < .05$). (Courtesy of Hunter SK, Critchlow A, Shin I-S, et al: Fatigability of the elbow flexor muscle for a sustained submaximal contraction is similar in men and women matched for strength. *J Appl Physiol* 96:195-202, 2004. Copyright The American Physiological Society.)

Conclusion.—Strength-matched men and women had similar levels of muscle fatigue and cardiovascular adjustments during a sustained low-force isometric contraction despite differences in EMG activity.

▶ Gender differences in epidemiology and physiology are a hot topic today. On the molecular and histologic level, muscle is muscle. Since muscle strength is directly linked to the number of active cross-bridges, I always found it difficult to understand how there could be gender differences. The interpretation that women fatigue less than men was based on fatigue times at the same relative strength. However, this type of comparison is only valid if the relationship is linear throughout the strength range.

This study suggests it is not and further shows that when men and women of equal strength are compared, there are no gender differences in time to exhaustion or heart rate/blood pressure responses. Considering the potential for unknown confounding, I am never surprised when basic physiologic principles hold true over epidemiologic observations and always surprised by the contrary. As an epidemiologist, I still have to point out that many questions cannot be answered by basic science because we need to know how systems interact within the complex milieu of the entire body.

I. Shrier, MD, PhD

Effect of Lower-extremity Muscle Fatigue on Postural Control

Gribble PA, Hertel J (Pennsylvania State Univ, University Park)
Arch Phys Med Rehabil 85:589-592, 2004   5–24

Objective.—To examine the effects of fatigue of the lower extremity on postural control during single-leg stance.

Design.—Pretest-posttest.

Setting.—University research laboratory.

Participants.—Fourteen healthy volunteers (age, 21 ± 2y) with no history of lower-extremity injury or neurologic deficits.

Interventions.—Testing consisted of isokinetically fatiguing the sagittal plane movers of the ankle, knee, or hip with measures of static postural control. Postural control was assessed with three 30-second trials during unilateral stance with eyes open.

Main Outcome Measures.—Center of pressure excursion velocity (COPV) in the frontal and sagittal planes.

Results.—Fatigue at the knee and hip led to postural control impairment in the frontal plane, whereas fatigue at the ankle did not (Fig 1). In the sagittal plane, fatigue at all 3 joints contributed to postural control impairment.

Conclusions.—Our results suggest that there is an effect of localized fatigue of the sagittal plane movers of the lower extremity on COPV. It appears that fatigue about the hip and knee had a greater adverse affect on COPV.

▶ Postural control is usually measured as COPV on a force plate. The subjects were fatigued by flexion-extension movements to exhaustion on the Biodex machine. Fatigue of the knee flexors and extensors caused substantial postural control impairments in both the sagittal and frontal planes. Fatigue of the ankle plantarflexors and dorsiflexors caused only slight postural impairments in the sagittal plane. Slowed conduction of the afferent signal from the fatigued muscle may lead to slower efferent signals to help maintain posture. Fatigue will place the individual at a greater risk for musculoskeletal injury, so rehabilitation procedures should avoid muscle fatigue exercises.

M. J. L. Alexander, PhD

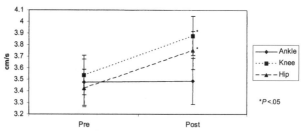

FIGURE 1.—Frontal plane COPV (COP$_{frontal}$). A significant condition by joint interaction (F$_{2,26}$ = 3.18, P = .05) demonstrated that fatigue to the hip and knee musculature led to greater impairments in mediolateral postural sway. (Reprinted from Gribble PA, Hertel J: Effect of lower-extremity muscle fatigue on postural control. *Arch Phys Med Rehabil* 85:589-592, 2004. Copyright 2004 with permission from The American Congress of Rehabilitation Medicine and the American Academy of Physical Medicine and Rehabilitation.)

Sports Massage After Eccentric Exercise

Jönhagen S, Ackermann P, Eriksson T, et al (Institutionen Södersjukhuset, Stockholm; Karolinska Inst, Stockholm)

Am J Sports Med 32:1499-1503, 2004   5–25

Background.—The use of sports massage is very common in the athletic community. However, only a few studies have shown any therapeutic effect of massage.

Hypothesis.—Sports massage can improve the recovery after eccentric exercise.

Study Design.—Prospective randomized clinical trial.

Methods.—Sixteen subjects performed 300 maximal eccentric contractions of the quadriceps muscle bilaterally. Massage was given to 1 leg, whereas the other leg served as a control (Fig 1). Subjects were treated once daily for 3 days. Maximal strength was tested on a Kin-Com dynamometer, and functional tests were based on 1-leg long jumps. Pain was evaluated using a visual analog scale.

Results.—There was a marked loss of strength and function of the quadriceps directly after exercise and on the third day after exercise. The massage treatment did not affect the level or duration of pain or the loss of strength or function following exercise.

Conclusion.—Sports massage could not improve the recovery after eccentric exercise.

▶ Massage therapy has become a popular modality for competitive athletes in many sports, primarily to increase the speed of recovery for the next exercise bout. Massage is believed to reduce the risk of delayed-onset muscle

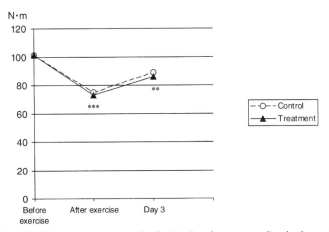

FIGURE 1.—Quadriceps strength measured with a Kin-Com dynamometer directly after, and 3 days after a training session including 300 maximal eccentric contractions. Sports massage was given once daily to 1 leg (treatment); the other leg was not treated. No difference between the groups was found ($P < .05$, $N = 16$). The strength was reduced directly after exercise (***$P < .001$) and at day 3 (**$P < .01$). (Courtesy of Jönhagen S, Ackermann P, Eriksson T, et al: Sports massage after eccentric exercise. *Am J Sports Med* 32:1499-1503, 2004.)

soreness and possibly decrease strength losses. However, few studies have actually proven the effectiveness of sport massage in maintaining muscle function after intense exercise. This study exercised both legs using strenuous eccentric exercise, and massage therapy was applied on 1 leg following the exercise. No difference was found in pain between the massage-treated leg and the control leg, and massage did not shorten the duration of the soreness of the legs. Although sport massage showed no positive effects on muscle strength and soreness in this study, it is possible that some positive effects were not measured by the current protocol. These could include an improved psychological state of the athlete, or improved afferent flow from the muscle.

M. J. L. Alexander, PhD

Effects of Massage on Limb and Skin Blood Flow After Quadriceps Exercise

Hinds T, McEwan I, Perkes J, et al (Manchester Metropolitan Univ, Alsager, England; Aberdeen Univ, Scotland; Liverpool John Moores Univ, England)
Med Sci Sports Exerc 36:1308-1313, 2004   5–26

Background.—Athletes and therapists use massage in the belief that it enhances muscle recovery and reduces soreness after intense physical activity. The proposed mechanism is enhanced muscle blood flow, which increases oxygen delivery to the tissue, enhances healing, promotes metabolite removal, and prompts a return to homeostasis. To evaluate the phenomenon, Doppler US has been used to measure muscle and skin blood flow (SKBF), but the results have not consistently found therapeutic value for massage after exercise. Doppler US and laser Doppler flowmetry were used to integrate femoral artery blood flow (FABF) and SKBF, and skin and muscle temperatures (SKT and MT, respectively) were determined to provide more insight into the effects of massage physiologically and metabolically.

Methods.—Measurements were obtained in 13 men (mean age, 21.0 years) who engaged in dynamic quadriceps exercise. Each volunteer performed three 2-minute bouts of concentric quadriceps exercises and then two 6-minute sets of deep effleurage and pétrissage massage or a rest period (control) lasting the same time. At baseline, immediately after exercise, and midway through and at the end of the massage or rest period, FABF, SKBF, SKT, MT, the blood lactate concentration, heart rate (HR), and blood pressure were determined.

Results.—Work completed and mean total work completed were similar for the trials for all 3 exercise bouts and between trials. Increased FABF was noted between rest and after exercise in both trials; FABF then returned to baseline values. SKBF increased significantly with exercise and was further elevated in the massage trial but returned to normal in the control trial. SKT increased with exercise and continued to increase when massage was performed but remained stable under control conditions. Time and treatment variables interacted significantly, which suggests a variant response in skin temperature between trials with increasing time. MT increased with exercise and declined in both the massage and control conditions, although it did not return to baseline levels. The blood lactate concentration increased significantly with exercise and remained significantly elevated over baseline values with massage and under control conditions. HR increased significantly with exercise. Both HR and blood pressure returned toward baseline values at the end of the trials.

Conclusions.—Massage produced no effect on FABF in the various trials. Thus, limb blood flow is not increased by postexercise massage, but massage produced significant increases in SKBF and ST. With no increase in FABF, some muscle blood flow may be diverted to the cutaneous circulation, but the blood flow diversion is strictly limited. Postexercise massage does not seem to have any effect on the recovery process as far as physiologic variables are concerned.

▶ Because of the popularity of massage and other forms of manual therapy among athletes, studies on their effects are very important. This study adds to our knowledge about potential mechanisms through which massage may or may not act. However, the suggestion that recovery might be impaired because blood flow might be diverted from muscles is overstated. Blood flow to muscles is under tight autoregulation. For instance, if skin vasodilation caused a fall in femoral arterial pressure because of the decrease in resistance, a muscle that required more blood flow would vasodilate to offset the reduced perfusion pressure. Future studies should directly assess recovery through measures of force and both central fatigue (which includes psychological effects) and peripheral fatigue (which includes only direct effects on the muscle).

I. Shrier, MD, PhD

Effects of Leg Massage on Recovery From High Intensity Cycling Exercise
Robertson A, Watt JM, Galloway SDR (Univ of Stirling, Scotland)
Br J Sports Med 38:173-176, 2004   5–27

Background.—Massage research has not produced evidence of clear benefit. This well-controlled study investigated the effects of leg massage on lactate clearance, muscle power output, and fatigue after high-intensity cycling exercise.

Study Design.—The study group consisted of 9 healthy male team sports players aged 20 to 22 years. These volunteers rested for 15 minutes, then had a baseline blood sample drawn. They then performed a standardized warm-up, a short stretch and then 6 × 30–second high-intensity cycling bouts with 30 seconds of active recovery between each bout. This was followed by 5 minutes of active recovery and a 20-minute intervention.

Participants were randomly assigned to either 20 minutes of passive supine rest or 20 minutes of leg massage. The intervention period was followed by a standardized warm-up and stretch and then a 30-second highest-intensity exercise bout (Wingate test). The heart rate was recorded throughout and blood samples collected for lactate analysis after the initial exercise, during intervention, and after the Wingate test. Wingate test variables included peak power, mean power, and fatigue index.

Findings.—There was no significant effect of massage compared to rest on blood lactate levels, maximum power, or mean power during the subsequent Wingate test. However, there was a significantly lower fatigue index after massage.

Conclusion.—Massage did not appear to affect blood lactate levels after exercise, but there was an effect on fatigue index that should be investigated further.

▶ Many rehabilitation techniques lack evidence from scientific studies, and massage is only one example. This study suggests that it has no effect on recovery. However, stretching was incorporated as part of the pretest warm-up, and stretching immediately before a test of performance has been shown to impair performance. This study is a good first step in assessing the true value of massage therapy for performance enhancement, and we should encourage more research into this area, using different types of warm-ups and different types of fatiguing protocols.

I. Shrier, MD, PhD

Influence of Therapeutic Ultrasound on Skeletal Muscle Regeneration Following Blunt Contusion
Wilkin LD, Merrick MA, Kirby TE, et al (Ohio State Univ, Columbus)
Int J Sports Med 25:73-77, 2004   5–28

Introduction.—Therapeutic US is one of the most commonly used treatment modalities for various athletic injuries. Yet in spite of more than 60 years of clinical use, the effectiveness of US in the treatment of pain, musculoskeletal injuries, and soft tissue lesions remains controversial. Most US research has focused on noncontractile tissue, even though about 90% of all sports-associated injuries are skeletal muscle contusions and strains.

Eighty male Wistar rats were evaluated to compare contusion injury to the gastrocnemius (GTN) muscles in animals treated and not treated by US. Measurements were made of muscle mass, total protein concentration, and fiber cross-sectional area; the number of nuclei per fiber in US-treated and nontreated GTN were compared; and comparisons were made of myonuclear density from the contusion-injured US-treated and nontreated GTN muscles.

Methods.—After anesthetic administration, each rat received a bilateral contusion to the GTN muscle. Pulsed US treatment was initiated 6 hours after contusion injury unilaterally on the right GTN muscle once daily for 7 days. The left (non–US-treated) and right (US-treated) GTN muscles of 10 rats/group were excised at 1, 3, 5, 7, 14, 21, 28, and 40 days after contusion injury.

Results.—No differences were observed in muscle mass, total protein concentration, or fiber cross-sectional area (Fig 3) between the right and left

Fiber Cross-sectional Area (micrometers^2)

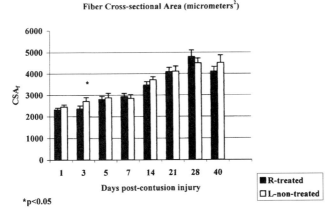

*p<0.05

FIGURE 3.—Absolute fiber cross-sectional area (CSA_f) of the gastrocnemius (GTN) muscles for 8 different time points. The right GTN was treated with US and the left GTN received no treatment. (Courtesy of Wilkin LD, Merrick MA, Kirby TE, et al: Influence of therapeutic ultrasound on skeletal muscle regeneration following blunt contusion. *Int J Sports Med* 25:73-77, 2004. Georg Thieme Verlag.)

GTN muscles at any post-injury time point evaluated. When fiber cross-sectional area was normalized to muscle mass, no differences were observed. There were no significant between-group differences in myonuclear number or cross-sectional area per myonuclei between the right and left GTN muscles.

Conclusion.—The use of US, as administered in this rat model of blunt contusion of skeletal muscle, does not hasten or improve the regeneration of skeletal muscle following contusion injury.

▶ Most of the research on US has examined superficial noncontractile tissue. Clinical experiments on injured patients have not shown much benefit, but some have suggested this is because of nonuniform types of pathology. In this animal study, US again had no effect, even though the muscle contusion was produced using standardized methods. Believers in US will likely remark that this study used 3 MHz, and it may be likely that other settings could provide benefit. However, given the current evidence, the burden of proof should now fall on the shoulders of the proponents of US to demonstrate some clinical effectiveness, under at least some conditions.

I. Shrier, MD, PhD

Core Stability Exercises On and Off a Swiss Ball
Marshall PW, Murphy BA (Univ of Auckland, New Zealand)
Arch Phys Med Rehabil 86:242-249, 2005   5–29

Objectives.—To assess lumbopelvic muscle activity during different core stability exercises on and off a Swiss ball.

Design.—Prospective comparison study.

Setting.—Research laboratory.

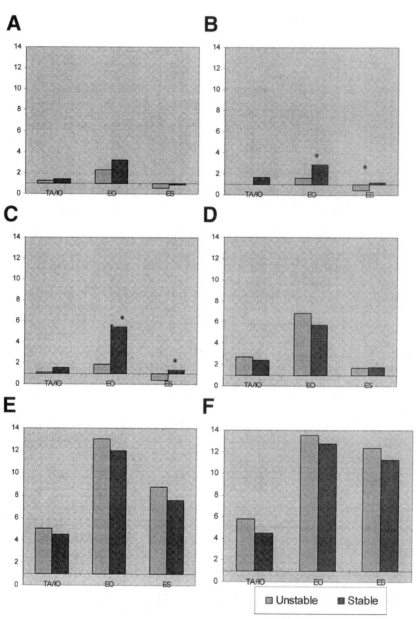

FIGURE 3.—Mean ratio of muscle activity: the rectus abdominis for each exercise, comparing the relationship between test surfaces for each task: (A) roll outs, B single leg hold, C press-up top position, D press-up bottom position, E quadruped with right arm and left leg, and F quadruped with left arm and right leg. *$P < .05$. The ratio of 1:1 indicates equal relative activity of the comparison muscle: rectus abdominus. (Reprinted from Marshall PW, Murphy BA: Core stability exercises on and off a Swiss ball. *Arch Phys Med Rehabil* 86:242-249, 2005. Copyright 2005 with permission from The American Congress of Rehabilitation Medicine and the American Academy of Physical Medicine and Rehabilitation.)

Participants.—Eight healthy volunteers from a university population.

Intervention.—Subjects performed 4 exercises on and off a Swiss ball: inclined press-up, upper body roll-out, single-leg hold, and quadruped exercise.

Main Outcome Measures.—Surface electromyography from selected lumbopelvic muscles, normalized to maximum voluntary isometric contraction, and median frequency analysis of electromyography power spectrum. Visual analog scale for perception of task difficulty.

Results.—There was a significant increase in the activation of the rectus abdominus with performance of the single-leg hold and at the top of the press-up on the Swiss ball (Fig 3). This led to changes in the relation between the activation levels of the lumbopelvic muscles measured.

Conclusions.—Although there was evidence to suggest that the Swiss ball provides a training stimulus for the rectus abdominus, the relevance of this change to core stability training requires further research because the focus of stabilization training is on minimizing rectus abdominus activity. Further support has also been provided about the quality of the quadruped exercise for core stability.

▶ Swiss ball has received a lot of attention by the public and fitness trainers. There are many claims being made, and I look forward to further research that helps me decide which likely myths are likely truths.

I. Shrier, MD, PhD

Interaction of the Human Body and Surfaces of Different Stiffness During Drop Jumps
Arampatzis A, Stafilidis S, Morey-Klapsing G, et al (German Sport Univ of Cologne, Germany)
Med Sci Sports Exerc 36:451-459, 2004   5–30

Introduction.—The means by which humans adjust their behavior to surfaces with different stiffness during activities in which the goal is to maximize take off velocity has yet to be reported in the literature. Ten female varsity gymnasts were evaluated to determine whether the stiffness of a surface influences the leg stiffness of the individual during drop jumps and to ascertain whether drop jump performance (jumping height and energy rates of the individual's center of mass during the contact phase) increases when reducing surface stiffness due to the greater energy storage capacity of the surface at a given force.

Methods.—Participants performed a series of drop jumps from 0.4-m height onto 2 sprung surfaces with different stiffness. Every trial of every research subject displaying the maximal mechanical power during the upward phase was examined. Ground reaction forces were determined by means of a force plate. Sagittal kinematics of the participant's body positions and the deformation of the surface were documented with 2 high-speed video cameras.

Results.—On the soft surface, the jumping height and the energy rates of participants during the contact phase were greater, compared with the hard surface. The energy delivered by the participants during the upward phase, leg and joint stiffness, and the range of motion remained unchanged for both surfaces The mechanical work performed by participants during the downward phase was greater for the hard surface.

Conclusion.—The absolute energy loss is lower for the hard surface; jumping performance is greater for the soft surface. This is due to a higher ratio of positive to negative mechanical work performed by participants during the contact phase. The adjustment of participants to different surfaces depends on both the stiffness of the surface and the intensity of the movement.

▶ This study highlights the complex interaction between body, surface, and type of exercise with respect to performance. The optimal combination is likely to be different for different athletes.

I. Shrier, MD, PhD

Effect of Positioning and Bracing on Passive Position Sense of Shoulder Joint
Ulkar B, Kunduracioglu B, Çetin C, et al (Ankara Univ, Turkey; Suleyman Demirel Univ, Isparta, Turkey)
Br J Sports Med 38:549-552, 2004   5–31

Objective.—To examine the effects of positioning and sleeve type bracing on passive position sense of shoulder joints of healthy untrained subjects.

Method.—A cross over study was carried out on 26 subjects (13 male, 13 female) with a proprioception measurement device. The selected method of testing was passive reproduction of a target angle. Both shoulder joints of all the subjects were evaluated with and without a compressive neoprene sleeve type of brace at two different start positions (45° internal rotation, 75° external rotation) with an angular rotational movement at a constant speed of 0.5°/s (Fig 1). The angular displacements from the target angles at the end of the reproduction tests were recorded as position sense deficit scores.

Results.—The overall mean (SD) deficit score (0.99 [0.06]) was significantly ($P < 0.001$) lower with the brace than without, and the overall mean deficit score was significantly ($P < 0.001$) higher at the 45° internal rotation start position than at the 75° external rotation start position. However, there was no significant ($P < 0.05$) interaction between brace application and start position.

Conclusion.—Terminal limits of range of motion facilitate the position sense of shoulder joints. Compressive brace application improves the passive positioning sense possibly by stimulating cutaneous mechanoreceptors.

▶ Bracing of the ankle and knee joints is common practice and has been found to have positive effects on the neuromuscular function of these joints. No

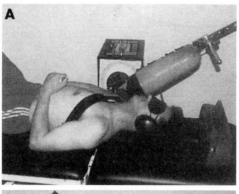

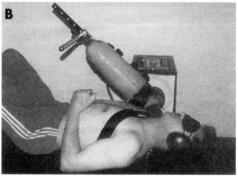

FIGURE 1.—Proprioception measuring device. Passive position matching tests were performed with and without neoprene sleeve type braces at two different start positions: 45° internal rotation and 75° external rotation. The subjects were asked to stop the motion with the hand held disengage switch when they thought the arm had reached the target angle. The deficit scores were recorded from the display present at the top of the machine. (Courtesy of Ulkar B, Kunduracioglu B, Çetin C, et al: Effect of positioning and bracing on passive position sense of shoulder joint. *Br J Sports Med* 38:549-552, 2004. Reprinted with permission from the BMJ Publishing Group.)

studies have been performed to examine the effects of compressive brace application on the proprioception of the shoulder joint. This study examined the ability of the subjects to reproduce target angles in the shoulder joint with and without a compressive sleeve. They determined that proprioceptive ability of the shoulder joint is improved significantly by the application of a neoprene compressive brace. In addition, the application of an external brace appears to promote the sensation of stability in the subject. Although compressive braces do not provide much mechanical support, they may help patients by enhancing neuromuscular performance and proprioceptive ability by stimulating cutaneous receptors.

M. J. L. Alexander, PhD

Measures of Accuracy for Active Shoulder Movements at 3 Different Speeds With Kinesthetic and Visual Feedback

Brindle TJ, Nitz AJ, Uhl TL, et al (NIH, Bethesda, Md; Univ of Kentucky, Lexington)

J Orthop Sports Phys Ther 34:468-478, 2004   5–32

Study Design.—Repeated-measures experiment.

Objective.—To compare measures of end point accuracy (EPA) for 2 feedback conditions: (1) visual and kinesthetic feedback and (2) kinesthetic feedback alone, during shoulder movements, at 3 different speeds.

Background.—Shoulder joint kinesthesia is typically reported with EPA measures, such as constant error. Reporting multiple measures of EPA, such as variable error and absolute error, could provide a more detailed description of performance.

Methods and Measures.—Subjects were seated with the shoulder abducted 90 degrees in the scapular plane and externally rotated 75°, with the forearm placed in a custom shoulder wheel (Fig 1). Subjects internally rotated the shoulder 27° to a target position at 48° of shoulder external rotation for both conditions. Motion analysis was used to determine peak angular velocity and 3 EPA measures for shoulder movements. Each EPA measure was compared between the 2 feedback conditions and among the 3 speeds with a separate 2-way analysis of variance.

Results.—Movements performed with kinesthetic feedback alone, measured by constant error ($P < .01$), variable error ($P < .01$), and absolute error ($P < .01$), were less accurate than movements performed with visual and kinesthetic feedback. Faster movements were less accurate when measured by constant error ($P = .01$) and absolute error ($P < .01$) than slower movements. Subjects tended to overshoot the target in the absence of visual feedback; however, movement speed played minimal role in the overshooting.

Conclusions.—Multiple measures of EPA, such as constant, variable, and absolute error during simple restricted shoulder movements may provide additional information regarding the evaluation of a motor performance or identify different central nervous system control mechanisms for joint kinesthesia.

▶ Shoulder kinesthetic feedback by reproducing joint positions in shoulder rotation movements was measured by use of a custom-made shoulder wheel. As expected, movements performed with only kinesthetic feedback were less

FIGURE 1.—(A) The glenohumeral joint is maintained at 90° abduction in the scapular plane (ie, 30° anterior to the frontal plane). (B) Subject positioned in shoulder wheel. Direct visualization of shoulder wheel and arm is prevented by the subject wearing goggles and shield (†). Retroflective markers used to measure shoulder angular position and velocity are located at the axis of rotation (1) on the stationary arm (2) and the movable arm (3) of the shoulder wheel. A thumb switch is located near the right hand. C The starting position was 75° of external rotation in the scapular plane; the glenohumeral joint was internally rotated (27° to the target position of 48° of external rotation. (Reprinted from Brindle TJ, Nitz AJ, Uhl TL, et al: Measures of accuracy for active shoulder movements at 3 different speeds with kinesthetic and visual feedback. *J Orthop Sports Phys Ther* 34:468-478, 2004, with permission of the Orthopaedic and Sports Sections of the American Physical Therapy Association.)

FIGURE 1

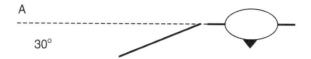

A

30°

B

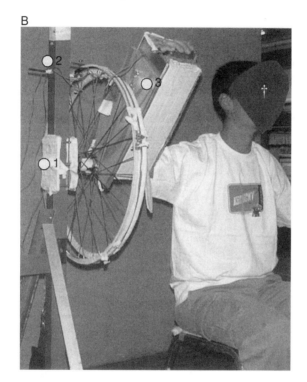

C
90° external rotation

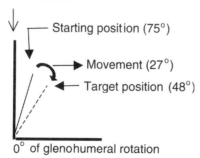

Starting position (75°)

Movement (27°)

Target position (48°)

0° of glenohumeral rotation

accurate than those with kinesthetic and visual feedback. Faster movements were less accurate than slower movements. Collection of data on shoulder position sense in healthy subjects enables comparison with motor performance of subjects with shoulder pathology that have impaired kinesthetic feedback. Identification of shoulder impairment as well as tracking of progress in rehabilitation are important outcomes of kinesthetic testing.

M. J. L. Alexander, PhD

Functional Fatigue Decreases 3-Dimensional Multijoint Position Reproduction Acuity in the Overhead-Throwing Athlete
Tripp BL, Boswell L, Gansnerder BM, et al (Univ of Kentucky, Lexington; Naval Service Training Command, Great Lakes, Ill; Univ of Virginia, Charlottesville; et al)
J Athl Train 39:316-320, 2004   5–33

Objective.—To determine the effects of functional fatigue on active multijoint position reproduction in overhead-throwing athletes.

Design and Setting.—A standard, repeated-measures, randomized-ordered, counterbalanced, 2-period (crossover) design was used. During the first test session, we randomly assigned subjects to either the nonfatigue or fatigue condition. Subjects underwent pretest measurements and then either a functional fatigue protocol or rest period, followed by posttest measurements. After a recovery period, subjects crossed over to the opposing condition for the second testing session.

Subjects.—Thirteen overhead-throwing athletes competing in National Collegiate Athletic Association Division I or club baseball, with no history

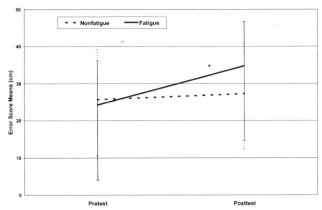

FIGURE 3.—Pretest and posttest mean error scores (cm) for the nonfatigue and fatigue conditions. *Significantly different from nonfatigue condition. (Reprinted from Tripp BL, Boswell L, Gansnerder BM, et al: Functional fatigue decreases 3-dimensional multijoint position reproduction acuity in the overhead-throwing athlete. *J Athl Train* 39:316-320, 2004. Copyright 2004, with permission from The National Athletic Trainers' Association.)

of upper extremity or central nervous system disorders, volunteered for this study.

Measurements.—We measured active multijoint position reproduction accuracy in 3 dimensions using an electromagnetic tracking device. We noted each subject's ability to reproduce 3 positions corresponding with distinct moments of his throwing motion. A variable error score was calculated to compare the locations of the reproduced points with reference to the target point.

Results.—A significant difference occurred between the pretest and posttest error scores in the fatigue condition. Comparisons between positions indicated that more errors were seen in the arm-cocked position than in the follow-through position under both fatigue and nonfatigue conditions (Fig 3).

Conclusions.—Functional fatigue decreased joint position sense acuity in overhead-throwing athletes. Our findings using this novel testing measurement method are in agreement with past research, with one exception. The trend toward higher error scores in the arm-cocked position would appear to contradict findings that sensorimotor system acuity increases toward end ranges of motion.

▶ Fatigue has long been considered a risk factor for injury. This study suggests that one possible mechanism is a fatigue-induced decrease in proprioception. If true, one would expect increased gleno-humeral movement due to lack of appropriate muscle control, and increased stress to various periarticular structures. Although the results of the study support this theory, it remains unclear whether strength, endurance, or proprioceptive training is most likely to minimize the fatigue-induced effects.

I. Shrier, MD, PhD

Contributions of Selected Fundamental Factors to Wheelchair Basketball Performance
Wang YT, Chen S, Limroongreungrat W, et al (Georgia State Univ, Atlanta; Hong Kong Inst of Education)
Med Sci Sports Exerc 37:130-137, 2005   5–34

Purpose.—The purpose of this study was to determine the contributions of selected fundamental factors, such as arm length, sitting height, simple vision reaction time (SVRT), choice vision reaction time (CVRT), muscle strength, and range of motion (ROM) at the shoulder, elbow, and wrist joints to wheelchair basketball (WCB) performance as measured by season statistics and coaches' evaluation.

Methods.—Thirty-seven Paralympic WCB players from seven countries participated in this study. A computerized reaction time system was used to test the SVRT and CVRT. The ROM and muscle strengths of the shoulder, elbow, and wrist joints were measured using a goniometer and MP DA100B BioPac force measurement system, respectively. Stepwise regression analysis was used to identify the contributions of these fundamental factors and "dimensional variables" (DV) derived from the selected factors fundamental to WCB performance. A DV represented a dimension or category of the factor, for example, the wrist flexion/extension DV represented the ROM of the wrist in flexion and extension, and the WCB performance DV represented average points, rebounds, assists, blocks, and steals per game.

Results.—The results of this study demonstrated that elbow extension and wrist extension had significant contributions to average points. Sitting height, shoulder internal rotation, and elbow flexion had significant contributions to the average rebounds. Arm length had a significant contribution to average assists, and SVRT had a significant contribution to the average blocks. Wrist flexion/extension ROM DV and wrist flexion/extension strength DV had significant contributions to the WCB performance DV.

Conclusion.—Shoulder internal rotation, elbow extension, and wrist flexion/extension ROM, CVRT, and wrist flexion/extension muscle strength are important to WCB performance and should be addressed in WCB training.

▶ WCB is one of the most popular team sports in the Paralympics. This sport is characterized by intermittent high-intensity activity for wheelchair maneuvers and ball handling. Sports science is now providing the level of support that able-bodied athletes already experience and as a result, determination of biomechanical factors influencing success has become a priority. This study demonstrates that elbow and wrist extension are important in relation to point scoring, whereas sitting height, shoulder internal rotation, and elbow flexion are more important for rebounding. It also found that arm length is related to assists and visual reaction time to blocking. All of these factors should be addressed either in talent identification programs or in training methods.

P. McCrory, MBBS, PhD

Relation Between Median and Ulnar Nerve Function and Wrist Kinematics During Wheelchair Propulsion

Boninger ML, Impink BG, Cooper RA, et al (Univ of Pittsburgh, Pa)
Arch Phys Med Rehabil 85:1141-1145, 2004   5–35

Background.—Carpal tunnel syndrome and ulnar nerve injury are common diagnoses among manual wheelchair users. These upper limb injuries have significant consequences for these individuals, who rely on their arms for mobility, transfers, and most activities of daily living. A link has already been established between wheelchair propulsion and carpal tunnel syndrome. An investigation was undertaken to determine whether wrist motion during wheelchair propulsion is related to median and ulnar nerve functioning. Two hypotheses were formulated: (1) that greater peak flexion, extension, and radial and ulnar deviation would occur with decreased median and ulnar nerve functioning and (2) that an increased absolute range of motion (ROM) would produce worse median and ulnar nerve functioning.

Methods.—The investigation took place in the biomechanics laboratory at a veterans' health administration facility and in an electrodiagnostic laboratory at a university hospital. Participants were 35 individuals with spinal cord injuries who used manual wheelchairs; they ranged in age from 18 to 65 years (average age, 38.9 years). These individuals propelled their own wheelchairs on a dynamometer at speeds of 0.9 and 1.8 m/s. Force and moment sensing pushrims and a kinematic system obtained bilateral biomechanical data. Participants also underwent bilateral median and ulnar nerve conduction studies. Measurements included wrist flexion and extension, radial and ulnar deviation peaks, and ROM with respect to median and ulnar motor and sensory amplitudes, as well as peak pushrim forces and moments and stroke frequency.

Results.—Several significant relationships were noted between physical characteristics (eg, age, height, and body mass) and median sensory amplitude, latency, ulnar sensory amplitude, ulnar motor latency, and median motor latency. A nearly significant difference was noted between mean peak wrist flexion and less motion at faster speeds. Significant negative correlations were noted between wrist flexion and extension ROM, age, and body mass. A significant positive correlation held for wrist flexion and extension ROM and median motor amplitude and ulnar motor amplitude. Higher ranges of wrist motion were related to increased median and ulnar motor amplitudes. Wrist ROM and median and ulnar nerve amplitude were positively correlated, not negatively correlated as had been hypothesized. Significant negative correlations were found between wrist flexion and extension ROM and stroke frequency and resultant force.

Conclusions.—Greater wrist ROM translated to larger amplitudes in median and ulnar motor nerve responses. With the larger wrist ROM, lower forces, moments, and cadence were found during the propulsive stroke. Therefore, study participants who used a greater ROM during propulsion had better nerve functioning than did those who used a smaller ROM. The larger ROM required fewer strokes and less force, which produced less strain on the ulnar and median nerves. Thus, manual wheelchair users may reduce injury by using long smooth strokes to propel themselves.

▶ Sport medicine physicians are often presented with patients who have pain performing their sport. Rather than suggesting that patients discontinue the activity, physicians generally find it preferable to suggest modifications that decrease the stress of the affected area. This study yields important insights into the mechanics of wheelchair propulsion, and the findings may help clinicians advise their patients on how to modify techniques so that they can continue to participate in their sport.

I. Shrier, MD, PhD

Effect of Lateral Ankle Ligament Anesthesia on Single-Leg Stance Stability

Riemann BL, Myers JB, Stone DA, et al (Univ of Pittsburgh, Pa; Georgia Southern Univ, Statesboro)
Med Sci Sports Exerc 36:388-396, 2004   5–36

Introduction.—There is a lack of understanding concerning the significance of articular mechanoreceptor information to postural control, as well as numerous reports of orthopedic injury adversely impacting both the sensory and motor components of the body. However, the orthopedic community has largely considered postural control from only an afferent perspective. Few trials have focused only on the function of ankle articular receptors in postural control. The contribution of lateral ankle ligament mechanoreceptors to postural stability during single leg static (eyes open, eyes closed) and landing tasks was examined in 14 recreationally active healthy research subjects.

Methods.—Nine male and 5 female research subjects underwent 2 different treatment conditions (control, anesthesia) in a counterbalanced order at 48-hour intervals. During the anesthetic experiment, lidocaine was injected into the regions of the anterior talofibular and calcaneofibular ligament (1.5 mL each). Postural stability was determined by means of forceplate and kinematic variables. The average of each variable across multiple trials under each treatment for the 3 tasks was evaluated.

Results.—The results of none of the statistical analyses showed significant alterations ($P > .05$) in postural control attributable to the treatment condition.

Conclusion.—Lateral ankle ligament mechanoreceptors do not make a significant contribution to single leg stance stability; do not have a unique, irreplaceable role; or have a role too subtle to be observed, given the measurement techniques used. The theory that single leg stability is changed after ankle joint injury due to proprioceptive disruption was not supported. Postural control alterations after repetitive ankle injury more likely occur due to alterations in mechanical stability, motor components, or central motor programming.

▶ Epidemiologic studies have suggested that proprioception training reduces the likelihood of recurrent ankle sprains. However, whether most of the proprioceptive information is provided mainly by the ligaments or by the muscles remains controversial. The current study used balance platforms to study 2 tests of static stability and 1 test of dynamic stability, and the results suggested that ligaments are not the major source of information under these conditions. Although muscle proprioception would be the likely source, the authors also suggest central programming might be the source.

I. Shrier, MD, PhD

Electromyographic Analysis of the Rotator Cuff and Deltoid Musculature During Common Shoulder External Rotation Exercises
Reinold MM, Wilk KE, Fleisig GS, et al (American Sports Medicine Inst, Birmingham, Ala; Univ of Florida, Gainesville; Univ of Vermont, Burlington)
J Orthop Sports Phys Ther 34:385-394, 2004   5-37

Study Design.—Prospective single-group repeated-measures design.

Objectives.—To quantify electromyographic (EMG) muscle activity of the infraspinatus, teres minor, supraspinatus, posterior deltoid, and middle deltoid during exercises commonly used to strengthen the shoulder external rotators.

Background.—Exercises to strengthen the external rotators are commonly prescribed in rehabilitation, but the amount of EMG activity of the infraspinatus, teres minor, supraspinatus, and deltoid during these exercises has not been thoroughly studied to determine which exercises would be most effective to achieve strength gains.

Methods and Measures.—EMG measured using intramuscular electrodes were analyzed in 10 healthy subjects during 7 shoulder exercises: prone horizontal abduction at 100° of abduction and full external rotation (ER), prone ER at 90° of abduction, standing ER at 90° of abduction, standing ER in the scapular plane (45° abduction, 30° horizontal adduction), standing ER at 0° of abduction, standing ER at 0° of abduction with a towel roll, and sidelying ER at 0° of abduction. The peak percentage of maximal voluntary isometric contraction (MVIC) for each muscle was compared among exercises using a 1-way repeated-measures analysis of variance ($P < .05$).

Results.—EMG activity varied significantly among the 7 exercises. Sidelying ER produced the greatest amount of EMG activity for the infraspinatus (62% MVIC) and teres minor (67% MVIC). The greatest amount of activity of the supraspinatus (82% MVIC), middle deltoid (87% MVIC), and posterior deltoid (88% MVIC) was observed during prone horizontal abduction at 100° with full ER.

Conclusions.—Results from this study provide initial information to develop rehabilitation programs. It also provides information helpful for the design and conduct of future studies.

▶ Rotator cuff injuries are common in throwing athletes, usually caused by the rapid deceleration of shoulder medial rotation and horizontal adduction following release of the ball. The muscle regions most often injured are the midsupraspinatus to the midinfraspinatus, so these muscles are often emphasized in rehabilitation programs for the shoulder. This study used intramuscular electrodes to measure EMG activity in the 4 ERs during 7 shoulder exercises used to strengthen these muscles. They determined that the largest amount of ER activity occurred in sidelying external rotation and prone horizontal abduction. This study provides a useful contribution for rehabilitation professionals regarding the most effective exercises for rehabilitation of ERs.

M. J. L. Alexander, PhD

Comparing the Function of the Upper and Lower Parts of the Serratus Anterior Muscle Using Surface Electromyography

Ekstrom RA, Bifulco KM, Lopau CJ, et al (Univ of South Dakota, Vermillion; North Platte Physical Therapy, Sundance, Wyo; VA Black Hills Healthcare System, Fort Meade, SD; et al)

J Orthop Sports Phys Ther 34:235-243, 2004   5–38

Study Design.—Prospective single-group repeated-measures design.

Objective.—To use electromyographic (EMG) analysis during muscle testing to determine if there is a difference in function of the upper and lower parts of the serratus anterior (SA) muscle.

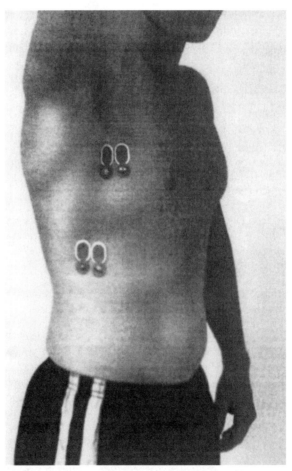

FIGURE 2.—Electrode placement over the third rib for recording from the upper serratus anterior and placement over the seventh rib for recording from the lower serratus anterior. (Reprinted from Ekstrom RA, Bifulco KM, Lopau CJ, et al: Comparing the function of the upper and lower parts of the serratus anterior muscle using surface electromyography. *J Orthop Sports Phys Ther* 34:235-243, 2004, with permission of the Orthopaedic and Sports Sections of the American Physical Therapy Association.)

Background.—The SA muscle is a very important scapular protractor and upward rotator. Authors have anatomically described the muscle as being divided into 2 or 3 parts, and have suggested that the upper part is more suited for protraction and the lower part for upward rotation of the scapula.

Methods and Measures.—Surface electrodes recorded EMG activity of the upper and lower parts of the SA muscle during 9 different muscle tests in 29 healthy subjects (Fig 2).

Results.—Three muscle tests demonstrated significantly greater ($P < .05$) EMG activity in the lower part of the SA as compared to the upper part. There was no significant difference in the EMG activity of the upper and lower parts of the SA when the other 6 muscle tests were analyzed.

Conclusion.—When upward rotation was the primary position of the scapula during the muscle tests, the lower part of the SA was activated to a greater degree than the upper part. Muscle tests with maximum scapular protraction with varying degrees of upward rotation produced EMG activity with no significant difference when comparing the upper and lower parts of the SA. This information may be helpful for clinicians when muscle testing and developing exercise programs for the SA muscle.

▶ The SA muscle has been described as an abductor (protractor) and upward rotator of the scapula, with different parts of the muscle differing in their actions. The muscle can be divided into 3 structural components as follows: the lower part produces upward rotation and protraction of the scapula, while the upper portions are arranged to abduct or protract the scapula. The very lowest 2 or 3 digitations may also assist in depression of the scapula. This EMG study of SA during a number of resisted shoulder movements verified these as primary actions. Resisted upward rotation of the scapula produced greater EMG in the lower part of SA. Protraction of the scapula was seen to elicit greater activity in the upper part of SA. These findings suggest that training SA may require several upper-limb exercises, using different shoulder joint movements for each part of the muscle.

M. J. L. Alexander, PhD

Combining Isometric Knee Extension Exercises With Hip Adduction or Abduction Does Not Increase Quadriceps EMG Activity

Hertel J, Earl JE, Tsang KKW, et al (Penn State Univ, University Park; Univ of Wisconsin-Milwaukee; Michigan State Univ, East Lansing)
Br J Sports Med 38:210-213, 2004   5–39

Objective.—To determine if the combined isometric contractions of knee extension/hip adduction and knee extension/hip abduction will elicit a different quadriceps and gluteus medius electromyographic (EMG) pattern as compared to isometric contraction of a uniplanar knee extension exercise.

Methods.—Eight healthy young adult volunteers without history of knee or quadriceps injury participated. Surface EMG data were collected from the vastus medialis oblique (VMO), vastus lateralis (VL), and gluteus me-

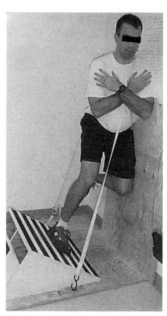

FIGURE 3.—Knee extension/hip abduction exercise. (Courtesy of Hertel J, Earl JE, Tsang KKW, et al: Combining isometric knee extension exercises with hip adduction or abduction does not increase quadriceps EMG activity. *Br J Sports Med* 38:210-213, 2004. Reprinted with permission from the BMJ Publishing Group.)

dius (Gmed) muscles of the dominant leg of each subject during three single leg, weight bearing, isometric exercises (uniplanar knee extension, knee extension/hip adduction, knee extension/hip abduction) (Fig 3). All exercises were performed at a position of 60° knee flexion. Three trials lasting 5 s each were performed for each of the three exercises. EMG data from each muscle were integrated and the maximum root mean square activity over a 0.5 s window for each trial was averaged. Analyses of variance were performed with exercise (straight extension, extension/adduction, extension/abduction) as the independent variable and VMO, VL, and Gmed activity and VMO:VL ratio as dependent variables.

Results.—A significant main effect for exercise was found for the VMO ($P = 0.006$) and VL ($P = 0.02$), but not the Gmed ($P = 0.25$) or the VMO:VL ratio ($P = 0.13$). For the VMO and VL, the uniplanar knee extension task produced significantly more EMG activity than the extension/adduction or extension/abduction tasks.

Conclusions.—Uniplanar knee extension exercises may be more appropriate than combining isometric knee extension exercises with hip adduction or abduction when eliciting maximal VMO and VL contractions.

▶ Quadriceps function is important in prevention and control of patellofemoral pain syndrome, especially the activation of the vastus medialis muscle. Because the fibers of the vastus medialis (VM) attach to the adductor magnus muscle, activation of VM may be enhanced by combining knee extension with hip adduction. The EMG findings revealed that uniplanar knee extension tasks produced the greatest quadriceps activity and that the activity decreased when hip adduction or hip abduction was combined with knee extension.

M. J. L. Alexander, PhD

Reliability of Biomechanical Variables of Sprint Running
Hunter JP, Marshall RN, McNair P (Univ of Auckland, New Zealand; Eastern Inst of Technology, Hawkes Bay, New Zealand; Auckland Univ of Technology, New Zealand)
Med Sci Sports Exerc 36:850-861, 2004   5–40

Purpose.—The purpose of this paper was to report the reliability of variables used in the biomechanical assessment of sprint running and to document how these reliability measures are likely to improve when using the average score of multiple trials.

Methods.—Twenty-eight male athletes performed maximal-effort sprints. Video and ground reaction force data were collected at the 16-m mark. The reliability (systematic bias, random error, and retest correlation) for a single score was calculated for 26 kinematic and 7 kinetic variables. In addition, the reliability (random error and retest correlation) for the average score of 2, 3, 4, and 5 trials was predicted from the reliability of a single score.

Results.—For all variables, there was no evidence of systematic bias. The measures of random error and retest correlation differed widely among the variables. Variables describing horizontal velocity of the body's center of mass were the most reliable, whereas variables based on vertical displacement of the body's center of mass or braking ground reaction force were the least reliable. For all variables, reliability improved notably when the average score of multiple trials was the measurement of interest.

Conclusion.—Although it is up to the researcher to judge whether a measurement is reliable enough for its intended use, some of the lower-reliability variables were possibly too unreliable to monitor small changes in an athlete's performance. Nonetheless, there was a consistent trend for reliability to improve notably when the average score of multiple trials was the measurement of interest. Subsequently, if resources permit, researchers and applied sports-scientists may like to consider using the average score of multiple trials to gain the advantages that improved reliability offers.

▶ A high level of reliability in skill technique measurement is important to the biomechanist to detect changes in performance that are due to an intervention or increased training regimes. Even with highly sophisticated measuring methods, errors in biomechanical measurements will usually occur because of equipment limitations and biological variation of the subject. The measures of random error and retest correlation varied widely among the variables. Variables such as horizontal velocity of the center of mass were the most reliable, and variables that were based on vertical displacement of the body's center of mass were the least reliable. Average scores of multiple trials were found to improve reliability on all variables. However, in skills, such as sprinting, the number of valid trials is limited because of fatigue in the subjects.

M. J. L. Alexander, PhD

Effect of Swim Suit Design on Passive Drag
Mollendorf JC, Termin AC II, Oppenheim E, et al (Univ of Buffalo, NY)
Med Sci Sports Exerc 36:1029-1035, 2004   5–41

Introduction.—The drag (D) of seven (7) male swimmers wearing five (5) swimsuits was investigated.

Methods.—The drag was measured during passive surface tows at speeds from 0.2 up to 2.2 m/s and during starts and push-offs. The swimsuits varied in body coverage from shoulder-to-ankle (SA), shoulder-to-knee (SK), waist-to-ankle (WA) and waist-to-knee (WK) and briefs (CS).

Results.—Differences in total drag among the suits were small, but significant. In terms of least drag at 2.2 m/s, the swimsuits ranked: SK, SA, WA, WK and CS. The drag was decomposed into its pressure drag (DP), skin friction drag (DSF) and wave drag (DW) components using nonlinear regression and classical formulations for each drag component. The transition-to-turbulence Reynolds number and decreasing frontal area with speed were taken into account. The transition-to-turbulence Reynolds number location was found to be very close to the swimmers' "leading edge," i.e. the head. Flow was neither completely laminar, nor completely turbulent; but rather, it was transitional over most of the body. The DP contributed the most to drag at low speeds (<1.0 m/s) and DW the least at all speeds. DSF contributed the most at higher speeds for SA and SK suits, whereas DP and DW were reduced compared with the other suits.

Conclusion.—The decomposition of swimmer drag into DSF, DP and DW suggests that increasing DSF on the upper-body of a swimmer reduces DP and DW by tripping the boundary layer and attaching the flow to the body from the shoulder to the knees. It is possible that body suits that cover the torso and legs may reduce drag and improve performance of swimmers.

▶ Modern competitive swimmers often wear lycra body suits while racing, because of the decreased drag forces produced by these suits. This study examined 5 different styles of lycra swim suits, to determine which style decreased drag forces the most. The styles included SA, SK, WA, WK, and CS. The most efficient suit was found to be the SK suit, and the least efficient in drag forces was the CS. The body suit was found to alter the flow around the body during swimming by attaching the flow closer to the suit. Suits that cover from the shoulder may improve performance at velocities above 1.5 m/s, but not below this critical speed.

M. J. L. Alexander, PhD

In Professional Road Cyclists, Low Pedaling Cadences Are Less Efficient
Lucia A, San Juan AF, Montilla M, et al (European Univ of Madrid; Univ Alphonse X, Madrid; Cooper Inst, Dallas)
Med Sci Sports Exerc 36:1048-1053, 2004   5–42

Purpose.—To determine the effects of changes in pedaling frequency on the gross efficiency (GE) and other physiological variables (oxygen uptake (VO_2), HR, lactate, pH, ventilation, motor unit recruitment estimated by EMG) of professional cyclists while generating high power outputs(PO).

Methods.—Following a counterbalanced, cross-over design, eight professional cyclists (age (mean ± SD): 26 ± 2 y, VO_{2max}: 74.0 ± 5.7 mL/kg/min) performed three 6-min bouts at a fixed PO (mean of 366 ± 37 W) and at a cadence of 60, 80, and 100 rpm.

Results.—Values of GE averaged 22.4 ± 1.7, 23.6 ± 1.8 and 24.2 ± 2.0% at 60, 80, and 100 rpm, respectively. Mean GE at 100 rpm was significantly higher than at 60 rpm ($P < 0.05$). Similarly, mean values of VO_2, HR, rates of perceived exertion (RPE), lactate and normalized root-mean square EMG (rms-EMG) in both vastus lateralis and gluteus maximum muscles decreased at increasing cadences.

Conclusions.—In professional road cyclists riding at high PO, GE/economy improves at increasing pedaling cadences.

▶ Top road cyclists are more efficient during their races by using higher pedaling cadences. The highest oxygen uptake (4700 mL/min) occurred at a pedaling rate of 60 rpm, while a lower uptake of 4400 mL/min occurred at 100 rpm. This may be due to several reasons, 1 of which is the lower recruitment of type II muscle fibres that have more anaerobic metabolism. Also, the cardiac output increases with cadence and produces a more efficient return of venous blood to the heart. This may produce a more efficient function of the heart in pumping blood to the leg muscles. At lower cadences (95 rpm), both lactate levels and the individual's perception of fatigue are increased.

M. J. L. Alexander, PhD

Effect of Ski Binding Parameters on Knee Biomechanics: A Three-Dimensional Computational Study
St-Onge N, Chevalier Y, Hagemeister N, et al (Univ of Montreal; Univ of Quebec, Montreal)
Med Sci Sports Exerc 36:1218-1225, 2004   5–43

Introduction.—Downhill skiing is a relatively safe sport, but many potentially avoidable injuries do occur. Whereas tibia and ankle injuries have been declining, severe knee sprains usually involving the anterior cruciate ligament (ACL) have increased from the 1970s to the 1990s. The goal of the present study was to evaluate the effect of the position of the binding pivot point and binding release characteristics on ACL strain during a phantom-foot fall.

Methods.—We computed ACL strain using a biomechanical computer knee model to simulate the phantom-foot ACL-injury mechanism. This mechanism, which is one of the most common mechanisms of ACL injury in downhill skiing, occurs when the weight of the skier is on the inner edge of the ski during a backward fall, resulting in a sharp uncontrolled inward turn of the ski.

Results.—The model predicts, that under simulated phantom-foot conditions, a binding with fast-release characteristics with a pivot positioned in front of the center of the boot produces less strain on the ACL. Current bindings have their pivot point approximately at the center of the heel radius. A pivot positioned at the back of the binding is more effective for sensing loads that occur at the tip of the ski. However, it is less effective for sensing loads that occur at the tail of the ski and, therefore, offers less protection during a phantom-foot fall.

Conclusion.—A binding with two pivot points, one positioned in front and the other at the back, could sense twist loads applied to the ski both at the front and at the back, and might, therefore, be a solution to reduce the occurrence of ACL injuries.

▶ This study reported that there has been a 60% reduction of lower-extremity injuries in downhill skiing during the past 20 years. Although there has been a dramatic decrease in tibia and ankle injuries, there has been a dramatic increase in ACL sprains and ruptures. These ACL sprains may be related to the design of modern downhill skis, which are designed to turn more easily when weight is put on the edge. If too much weight is placed on the inner edge during a fall, a sharp inward turn of the ski occurs, producing ACL sprains or ruptures. This is called the phantom-foot injury mechanism and, in this study, it was modeled using a biomechanical computer knee model to determine the pivot point on the ski during ACL strain. The model determined that a binding with fast release and the pivot point positioned in front of the center of the boot produces less strain on the ACL than a binding with the pivot point located further back on the boot. They recommended a binding designed with 2 pivot points that could sense twist on both the front and back of the boot that may reduce the occurrence of ACL strains.

M. J. L. Alexander, PhD

Altered Quadriceps Control in People With Anterior Cruciate Ligament Deficiency
Williams GN, Barrance PJ, Snyder-Mackler L, et al (Univ of Delaware, Newark)
Med Sci Sports Exerc 36:1089-1097, 2004   5–44

Purpose.—The purpose of this study was to determine whether similar patterns of quadriceps dysfunction are observed when people with anterior cruciate ligament (ACL) deficiency perform static and dynamic tasks.

Methods.—EMG data were collected from 15 subjects with an ACL deficient knee and 15 uninjured subjects as they performed static and dynamic tasks that were isolated to the knee and presented no threat to joint stability. The dynamic task was cyclic flexion and extension in the terminal 30° of knee extension; the static task was an established isometric target-matching protocol. The muscle activity patterns observed during the tasks were evaluated and compared.

Results.—The subjects with ACL deficiency exhibited quadriceps muscle control strategies that were significantly different from those of the uninjured subjects. This was true in both the dynamic and the static tasks. The findings were most noteworthy in the vastus lateralis muscle. Good agreement ($r = -0.73$ to -0.75) was observed in subjects' static and dynamic VL results; more moderate agreement was observed in results of the other quadriceps muscles.

Conclusion.—Diminished quadriceps control was observed when people with ACL deficiency performed static and dynamic tasks. The most striking feature of this impaired control was failure to turn the quadriceps "off" when performing flexion tasks in which the knee extensors are usually "silent." Our findings suggest that quadriceps dyskinesia after ACL injury is relatively global. Changes in neural function and muscle physiology after ACL injury are put forth as the most likely source of the observed dyskinesia.

▶ It has been previously reported that there is decreased proprioception and kinesthetic sense from the knee ligaments after an ACL injury. It is not clear if patients who have sustained an ACL injury will always have altered voluntary muscle control. Electromyographic (EMG) data collected during static and dynamic knee movement tests indicated that the muscle control strategies in the ACL-deficient subjects differed significantly from those of normal controls. Injured subjects tended to fire their quadriceps first in response to sudden loads, while uninjured subjects responded with a hamstrings-first response. Since the quadriceps pull increases the load on the injured ACL by placing an anterior shear on the tibia, this increases the stress on an already compromised structure. The hamstrings act as an agonist to the ACL, as it helps to pull the tibia posteriorly and decrease the stress on the ACL. This neuromuscular deficit after ACL injury may be related to the injury to the sensory nerves in the ACL that can no longer provide normal feedback.

M. J. L. Alexander, PhD

Effects of 20 Days of Bed Rest on the Viscoelastic Properties of Tendon Structures in Lower Limb Muscles

Kubo K, Akima H, Ushiyama J, et al (Univ of Tokyo; Nagoya Univ, Aichi, Japan; Natl Inst of Health and Nutrition, Shinjuku, Tokyo; et al)
Br J Sports Med 38:324-330, 2004   5–45

Objectives.—The purpose of this study was to investigate the effects of 20 days' bed rest on the viscoelastic properties of human tendon structures in knee extensor and plantar flexor muscles in vivo.

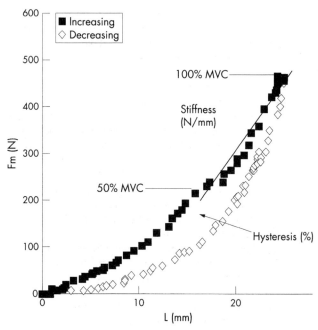

FIGURE 2.—Typical example of estimated muscle force (Fm)-tendon elongation (L) relationship in medial gastrocnemius muscle. (Courtesy of Kubo K, Akima H, Ushiyama J, et al: Effects of 20 days of bed rest on the viscoelastic properties of tendon structures in lower limb muscles. *Br J Sports Med* 38:324-330, 2004. Reprinted with permission from the BMJ Publishing Group.)

Methods.—Eight healthy men (age: 24±4 years, height: 172±9 m, body mass: 69±13 kg) carried out a 6° head-down bed rest for 20 days. Before and after bed rest, elongation (L) of the tendon and aponeurosis of vastus lateralis (VL) and medial gastrocnemius muscles (MG) during isometric knee extension and plantar flexion, respectively, were determined using real-time ultrasonic apparatus, while the subjects performed ramp isometric contraction up to the voluntary maximum, followed by ramp relaxation. The relationship between estimated muscle force (Fm) and tendon elongation (L) was fitted to a linear regression, the slope of which was defined as stiffness (Fig 2). The hysteresis was calculated as the ratio of the area within the Fm-L loop to the area beneath the load portion of the curve.

Results.—L values above 100 N were significantly greater after bed rest for VL, while there were no significant differences in L values between before and after for MG. The stiffness decreased after bed rest for VL (70.3±27.4 vs 50.1±24.8 N/mm, before and after bed rest, respectively; $P = 0.003$) and MG (29.4±7.5 vs 25.6±7.8 N/mm, before and after bed rest, respectively; $P = 0.054$). In addition, hysteresis increased after bed rest for VL (16.5±7.1% vs 28.2±12.9%, before and after bed rest, respectively; $P = 0.017$), but not for MG (17.4±4.4% vs 17.7±6.1%, before and after bed rest, respectively; $P = 0.925$).

Conclusions.—These results suggested that bed rest decreased the stiffness of human tendon structures and increased their hysteresis, and that these changes were found in knee extensors, but not the plantar flexors.

▶ It is well known that skeletal muscle function deteriorates following bed rest or space flight, usually with significant strength losses. Other outcomes of immobilization include a decrease in stiffness, times to peak torque and half relaxation, and maximum rate of tension development. This study reported that 20 days of bed rest produced a significant decrease in stiffness of tendon structures in knee extensors. This decreased stiffness would lead to longer transmission of tension from muscle fibers to bone, decreasing the effectiveness of muscle contraction. The hysteresis curve for tendon structures also increased significantly after bed rest, which suggests an increase in the viscosity of the tendon. The decrease in stiffness was less in plantar flexors than in knee extensors, suggesting differences in the plasticity of the tissues caused by differences in the levels of daily activity between these muscle groups.

M. J. L. Alexander, PhD

6 Physical Activity and Cardiorespiratory Diseases

Recall of Physical Activity in Distant Past: The 32-Year Follow-up of the Prospective Population Study of Women in Göteborg, Sweden
Lissner L, Potischman N, Troiano R, et al (Göteborg Univ, Sweden)
Am J Epidemiol 159:304-307, 2004   6–1

Background.—The accuracy with which elderly persons can recall their physical activity patterns in the distant past is important to research on chronic disease epidemiology. This was 1 question explored in the Prospective Population Study of Women in Göteborg, Sweden, a 32-year follow-up study.

Methods.—Four hundred thirty-three participants, currently aged 70 to 92 years, were asked to recall their leisure-time physical activity at the initial examination in 1968, when they were 38 to 60 years of age. Using a 4-point scale, participants reported leisure-time activity in the preceding 12 months. Identical questionnaires were completed in 2000 about 1968 and current levels of such activity.

Findings.—Participants were more likely to overestimate than underestimate their previous activity levels. Only 7.4% underestimated their previous activity levels, whereas 48.7% overestimated them. Classifications at the 2 examinations were consistent for 43.9% (Table 1). The use of current activity as a proxy for recalled levels did not improve the moderate agreement with activity reported initially in 1968. The mean magnitude of the recall bias was 0.5 unit on the 4-point scale. It did not correlate significantly with age or body mass index.

Conclusions.—Systematic errors were documented in remote recalls of physical activity by elderly women. In general, the participants recalled being more active 32 years earlier than they had reported originally. Physical activity recall questionnaires to determine levels in the distant past should be used cautiously.

TABLE 1.—Cross-classification of Response Frequencies for Original Activity Levels, Recalled Levels, and Current Levels in 2000,* Göteborg, Sweden

	Recalled Level†							
	Inactive		Moderately Active		Active		Very Active	
	No.	%	No.	%	No.	%	No.	%
Original level in 1968†								
Inactive	5	1.15	38	8.78	15	3.46	2	0.46
Moderately active	15	3.46	147	33.95	150	34.64	4	0.92
Active	0		17	3.93	38	8.78	2	0.46
Very active	0		0		0		0	

	Recalled Level†							
	Inactive		Moderately Active		Active		Very Active	
	No.	%	No.	%	No.	%	No.	%
Current level in 2000†								
Inactive	10	2.31	33	7.62	10	4.62	1	0.23
Moderately active	8	1.85	146	33.72	95	21.94	3	0.69
Active	2	0.46	21	4.85	88	20.32	3	0.69
Very active	0		2	0.46	0		1	0.23

	Original level in 1968†							
	Inactive		Moderately Active		Active		Very Active‡	
	No.	%	No.	%	No.	%	No.	%
Current level in 2000†								
Inactive	15	3.46	45	10.39	4	0.92	0	
Moderately active	33	7.62	191	44.11	28	6.47	0	
Active	11	2.54	79	18.24	24	5.54	0	
Very active	1	0.23	1	0.23	1	0.23	0	

*Cell percentages given relative to total per 4 × 4 table.
† Group mean for "recalled": 2.46 (standard deviation, 0.62); "current": 2.12 (standard deviation, 0.65); "original": 1.99 (standard deviation, 0.52).
‡No subject in the follow-up sample classified herself as very active in 1968.
(Courtesy of Lissner L, Potischman N, Troiano R, et al: Recall of physical activity in distant past: The 32-year follow-up of the prospective population study of women in Göteborg, Sweden. Am J Epidemiol 159:304-307, 2004. Reprinted by permission of Oxford University Press.)

▶ Many of the questions that exercise epidemiologists would like to pose concern the long-term health benefits of physical activity, and, because of the expense and logistic problems associated with longitudinal studies, subjects are often asked to recall their levels of physical activity in the distant past. The present report suggests that distance adds beauty to the view, with many elderly women overreporting their level of physical activity 32 years previously. The average error was 0.5 unit on a 4-unit physical activity scale. At first inspection, this does not seem too large a problem. In fact, however, about half of the sample who initially had stated that they were only "moderately active" reported being "active" when questioning was repeated 32 years later—a large enough error to confound many potential epidemiologic studies. A further problem is that the time-related change in reporting of physical activity is inconsistent. An earlier study of similar duration found that physical activity was underreported after 30 years had elapsed.[1]

R. J. Shephard, MD, PhD, DPE

Reference

1. Falkner KL, McCann SE, Trevisan M: Participant characteristics and quality of recall of physical activity in the distant past. *Am J Epidemiol* 154:865-872, 2001.

Body Mass Index, Physical Activity, and the Risk of Decline in Overall Health and Physical Functioning in Late Middle Age
He XZ, Baker DW (Northwestern Univ, Chicago)
Am J Public Health 94:1567-1573, 2004
6–2

Introduction.—Few large longitudinal trials have evaluated the association between body mass index (BMI), physical activity, and the risk of a decline in overall health and physical functioning. Data from the Health and Retirement Study was used to assess the correlation between BMI, physical activity, and the risk of a decline in self-reported overall health and physical functioning during a 4-year period among a national sample of US adults 51 to 61 years of age in 1992.

Methods.—Self-reported overall health, physical activity level, and physical difficulties were evaluated in 7887 participants. BMI was calculated with the use of self-reported body mass and height. Adjusted relative risks (ARRs) were ascertained by logistic regression.

Results.—Overweight and obesity were independently correlated with a health decline (ARRs, 1.29 and 1.36, respectively) and the development of a new physical difficulty (ARR, 1.27 and 1.45, respectively). Regular exercise significantly decreased the risk of a health decline and the development of a new physical difficulty, even among obese individuals (Table 2).

Conclusion.—Maintaining one's ideal body mass is important in preventing a decline in overall health and physical functioning. Regular exercise can diminish the risk of a decline, even among individuals who cannot achieve their ideal mass.

▶ For a number of years, I have argued that an enhanced quality of life during retirement may be one of the more important reasons for maintaining a physically active lifestyle.[1] A number of recent authors have taken up this theme. The article by He and associates notes relationships between physical activity, 2 potential indicators of inactivity (ie, overweight and obesity), and declines in health and the development of physical difficulty over a 4-year period. The study participants were relatively young at the outset (51-61 years), and the follow-up period was quite short. Larger effects might have been seen with an older age of initial contact and a longer follow-up. Another limitation of the study is that physical activity, height, and weight were all self-reported. Finally, no steps were taken to ensure that those initially inactive were not in poorer health than those who were active even at the start of the investigation. Surprisingly, in the light of some epidemiologic studies,[2] many of the sample reported that their occupation required much physical effort, but this had no im-

TABLE 2.—Risk of Major Decline in Self-Reported Overall Health and Development of a New Mobility Difficulty, by Average Body Mass Index

Variable	Average Body Mass Index				
	Normal	Overweight	Obesity	Extreme Obesity
No. of participants eligible for analysis	2625	3213	1704	235
Decline in overall health				
Major decline, n (%)	222 (7.5)	363 (10.4)***	228 (12.4)***	34 (14.2)***
Relative risk of decline (95% CI)				
Crude	Reference	1.39 (1.15, 1.67)**	1.64 (1.37, 1.97)**	1.89 (1.37, 2.57)**
Adjusted[a]	Reference	1.29 (1.02, 1.62)*	1.36 (1.06, 1.72)*	1.45 (0.98, 2.10)
New mobility difficulty				
Mobility difficulty, n (%)	397 (14.7)	575 (17.3)***	418 (23.5)***	68 (28.4)***
Relative risk of mobility difficulty (95% CI)				
Crude	Reference	1.18 (1.03, 1.35)*	1.60 (1.42, 1.80)**	1.93 (1.53, 2.40)**
Adjusted[a]	Reference	1.27 (1.11, 1.45)**	1.75 (1.55, 1.96)**	2.43 (1.94, 2.96)**

Note: Data were adjusted for the complex design of the survey and for the person-level analytic weights. *P* values are for the comparison with normal-weight participants (the reference category).

[a]Relative risks have been adjusted for age, sex, race or ethnic group, income, educational level, marital status, smoking and drinking behaviors, self-reported overall health, mobility status, insurance status, and frequency of light exercise, vigorous exercise or household chores, and work-related physical activity.

*P < .05; **P < .01; ***P < .001.

(Courtesy of He XZ, Baker DW: Body mass index, physical activity, and the risk of decline in overall health and physical functioning in late middle age. *Am J Public Health* 94:1567-1573, 2004. Copyright 2004, American Public Health Association.)

pact on the prognosis. Possibly, the occupational tasks involved lifting rather than sustained aerobic energy expenditures.

R. J. Shephard, MD, PhD, DPE

References

1. Shephard RJ: *Aging, Physical Activity and Health.* Champaign, Ill, Human Kinetics Publishers, 1997.
2. King GA, Fitzhugh EC, Bassett DR, et al: Relationship of leisure-time physical activity and occupational activity to the prevalence of obesity. *Int J Obesity* 25:606-612, 2001.

Consistency of the Talk Test for Exercise Prescription
Persinger R, Foster C, Gibson M, et al (Univ of Wisconsin-La Crosse)
Med Sci Sports Exerc 36:1632-1636, 2004   6–3

Introduction.—The Talk Test, well correlated with the ventilatory threshold, accepted guidelines for exercise prescription, and the ischemic threshold, seems to be a valuable yet simple method of exercise prescription. The consistency of the Talk Test was evaluated by comparing responses during various modes of exercise.

Methods.—Sixteen healthy volunteers performed incremental exercise on a treadmill and on a cycle ergometer. Trials were conducted while respiratory gas exchange measurements were made and while performing the Talk Test. The last positive response, an equivocal response, and the first negative response on the Talk Test were then correlated with the ventilatory threshold.

Results.—The $\%\dot{V}O_{2peak}$, $\%\dot{V}O_2$ reserve, the percentage of peak heart rate ($\%HR_{peak}$), and $\%HR$ reserve at the ventilatory threshold on a treadmill versus a cycle ergometer (77%, 75%, 89%, and 84% vs 67%, 64%, 82%, and 74%) were not significantly different compared with the equivocal stage of the Talk Test (83%, 82%, 86%, and 80% vs 73%, 70%, 87%, and 81%). The $\dot{V}O_2$ at the ventilatory threshold was well correlated with the $\dot{V}O_2$ at the last positive, equivocal, and negative stages of the Talk Test during treadmill and cycle ergometry exercise.

Conclusion.—The Talk Test approximates the ventilatory threshold on both treadmill and cycle testing. At the time speech first became difficult, the exercise intensity was nearly exactly equivalent to the ventilatory threshold. When speech was not comfortable, the exercise intensity was consistently above the ventilatory threshold. The talk test may be a highly consistent approach to exercise prescription.

▶ The Talk Test has the merit of offering an approximate measure of the intensity of a patient's exercise without the need for a lot of complicated laboratory testing, and the approach is simple enough that it should be understood by most of the general population. One limitation with regard to its theoretical basis is that much of the research on the use of the test has been published by 1 laboratory.[1,2] The present article is based on findings in a small sample of fit young men and women. On average, the oxygen consumption at which talking becomes difficult corresponds quite closely with the individually determined ventilatory threshold (V-slope method) during both treadmill running and cycle ergometry. Coefficients of correlation between the 2 data sets also look quite close; nevertheless, individual subjects show substantial discrepancies (eg, in 1 person, an oxygen consumption of 2.2 L/min is reached on the basis of the talk test, when it is intended to prescribe a value of 1.6 L/min). What is needed is a determination of the 95% CIs of departures from the intended oxygen consumption in a large group of naive subjects using the talk test. However, for the present, it seems that, like other methods of exercise prescription, such as HRs and ratings of perceived exertion, the talk test has unacceptable margins of error in some patients.

R. J. Shephard, MD, PhD, DPE

References

1. Dehart-Beverley M, Foster C, Porcari JP, et al: Relationship between the talk test and the ventilatory threshold. *Clin Exerc Physiol* 2:34-38, 2000.
2. Voleker SA, Foster C, Skemp-Arlt M, et al: Relationship between the talk test and ventilatory threshold in cardiac patients. *Clin Exerc Physiol* 4:120-123, 2002.

Validation of the Adult OMNI Scale of Perceived Exertion for Walking/ Running Exercise
Utter AC, Robertson RJ, Green JM, et al (Appalachian State Univ, Boone, NC; Univ of Pittsburgh, Pa; Univ of Alabama, Tuscaloosa; et al)
Med Sci Sports Exerc 36:1776-1780, 2004   6–4

Purpose.—Concurrent and construct validity of the OMNI-Walk/Run Scale of Perceived Exertion was examined using young adult women and men (18-36 yr).

Methods.—Concurrent validity was established by correlating OMNI-Walk/Run Scale ratings of perceived exertion (RPE-OMNI) with oxygen uptake ($\dot{V}O_2$), relative maximal oxygen uptake (%$\dot{V}O_{2max}$), ventilation ($\dot{V}_E$), respiratory rate (RR), respiratory exchange ratio (RER), and heart rate (HR) to a graded exercise test on a treadmill. Construct validity was established by correlating RPE-OMNI with RPE from the Borg (6-20) Scale (RPE-BORG). Measurements were made every min throughout the test.

Results.—The range of exercise responses across the incremental walking/ running test for the female and male groups were: $\dot{V}O_2$ = 0.99-3.9 L/min, HR = 98-190 beats/min and RPE-OMNI = 1.3-9.4. Correlation/regression analyses indicated that RPE-OMNI distributed as a positive linear function for all criterion measures; r = 0.67 to 0.88 ($P < 0.05$). RPE-OMNI was positively and linearly related to the RPE-BORG; r = 0.96 ($P < 0.01$) for both the female and male groups.

Conclusions.—Concurrent and construct evidence supports use of the OMNI-Walk/Run Scale by adult women and men to estimate RPE during graded exercise test on a treadmill.

▶ This study showed that the new OMNI-Walk/Run Scale of Perceived Exertion is a valid instrument for use with men and women during graded treadmill tests. The OMNI-Walk/Run scale is easy to use (0 to 10 scale, with 0 = extremely easy, and 10 = extremely hard) and uses a pictorial format to reinforce the number-descriptor relationships. In using the OMNI scale, subjects are asked to use both the pictures and words to help select a number.

D. C. Nieman, DrPH

Individual Interdependence Between Nocturnal ANS Activity and Performance in Swimmers
Garet M, Tournaire N, Roche F, et al (Univ Jean Monnet, France; Univ Blaise Pascal Clermont-Ferrand II, France; Cusset Swimming Team, France; et al)
Med Sci Sports Exerc 36:2112-2118, 2004   6–5

Background.—Physical training is usually accomplished with cycles of intensive training followed by a recovery period, which is needed for supercompensation, which is related to better performances. The goal of current physical training regimens is to optimize the load during the intensive physical training period as well as the duration of training and the recovery period at an individual level. The activity of the autonomic nervous system (ANS) is decreased for up to 2 days after a single bout of exercise. Activity in the ANS increases during recovery, eventually presenting a rebound with higher values than those measured before the exercise session. The associations between training load and ANS activity and between performance and ANS activity seem highly individual. However, variations in ANS and variations in performances have been shown to be correlated at the group level in swimmers. The strength of that relationship at the individual level was investigated.

Methods.—Seven regional-level swimmers (4 male) with a mean age of 16.6 ± 0.5 years and a mean of 6.4 ± 0.9 years of practice were included in the study. The swimmers performed maximal aerobic performance on a 400-m freestyle race before and after a 3-week period of intensive training and after a 2-week tapering period. ANS activity was assessed through heart rate variability (HRV) indices measured the night before each race and twice weekly along the protocol.

Results.—There were alterations in all HRV indices, with global and parasympathetic indices decreasing from week 1 to week 3 in the whole group. The indices increased to week 5 in 5 swimmers and continually decreased in the other 2 swimmers. The best performances for each swimmer were realized when global and parasympathetic indices of HRV were highest. The relationship between the changes in performance and the changes in HRV indices was strong.

Conclusions.—Athletic performance in swimmers is correlated with nocturnal activity of the ANS at an individual level. The decrease in ANS activity during intensive training is correlated with a loss in performance, and the rebound in ANS activity during tapering is correlated with the gain in performance. However, the speed of the rebound during the tapering period was quite different between swimmers. The measurement of ANS activity may be useful in the design and control of individual training periods and in optimizing the duration of tapering.

▶ HRV continues to show promise as a marker for a variety of conditions. This study extends population-based data and suggests that HRV is also useful in following an individual over time. The next few years will likely lead to studies designed to work out mechanisms, causal pathways, and potential confounders/effect modifiers.

I. Shrier, MD, PhD

Longitudinal Changes in Cardiorespiratory Fitness: Measurement Error or True Change?
Jackson AS, Kampert JB, Barlow CE, et al (Univ of Houston; The Cooper Inst, Dallas; Univ of North Texas, Denton)
Med Sci Sports Exerc 36:1175-1180, 2004   6–6

Background.—The beneficial effects of aerobic exercise and fitness on health have been well-documented. This link has been based on prospective observations that show that physical activity measured by self-reported physical activity (SR-PA) and maximum treadmill performance is related to the risk of all-cause and cardiovascular disease mortality. It has been proposed by the Aerobics Center Longitudinal Study (ACLS) that men with a low state of fitness could reduce their risk of mortality by improving their aerobic fitness. However, the validity of this observation has been questioned by Williams, who proposed that the change in fitness and health risk reported in the ACLS cohort was a statistical artifact resulting from a measurement error. Whether the longitudinal changes in cardiorespiratory fitness reported in the ACLS study were reflective of true changes or a measurement error was determined.

Methods.—The results of 3 serial maximal treadmill tests (T1, T2, and T3) were used to evaluate the serial changes in cardiorespiratory fitness of 4675 men. The mean durations between the 3 serial tests were 1.9 years for T2 to T1, 6.1 years for T3 to T2, and 8 years for T3 to T1. The maximum and resting heart rate, body mass index (BMI), SR-PA, and maximum Balke treadmill duration were measured on each occasion.

Results.—General linear analysis indicated that the change in treadmill time performance was a function of independent changes in SR-PA, BMI, and resting heart rate when the change in maximum heart rate was statistically controlled; these variables accounted for significant proportions (7%, 9%, and 12%) of the change in treadmill time variance.

Conclusions.—The findings of this study were supportive of the results of the ACLS. The variations in serial ACLS treadmill tests were not the result of a measurement error alone but were also associated with a systematic variation linked with changes in lifestyle.

▶ Given the large test–retest errors inherent in most physiologic measurements, it is a dangerous business to assume that a change in the fitness score from one visit to another reflects a change in lifestyle.[1-3] This is particularly true if a clinician chooses to assess aerobic fitness by the simple expedient of measuring treadmill endurance time. Various formal statistical techniques exist to distinguish a true change of lifestyle from an artifact due to measurement errors.[2,3] Faced by a challenge to their previously published conclusions, Jackson and associates have elected the alternative, empirical approach of testing correlations between any change in treadmill time and parallel changes in such independent indices of lifestyle as SR-PA, BMI, and resting heart rate. The 3 independent indices account for small but statistically significant percentages (7%-12%) of the variance in an individual's treadmill time. Thus, although a change in treadmill time provides only a crude measure of an increase or decrease in aerobic fitness, it seems that the numbers do contain a small nub of fitness information that can be used for prognostic purposes.

R. J. Shephard, MD, PhD, DPE

References

1. Williams PT: The illusion of improved fitness and reduced mortality. *Med Sci Sports Exerc* 35:736-740, 2003.
2. Shephard RJ: Regression to the mean: A threat to exercise science? *Sports Med* 33:575-584, 2003.
3. Shephard RJ, Rankinen T, Bouchard C: Test-retest errors and the apparent heterogeneity of training response. *Eur J Appl Physiol* 91:199-203, 2004.

Global Risk Scores and Exercise Testing for Predicting All-Cause Mortality in a Preventive Medicine Program
Aktas MK, Ozduran V, Pothier CE, et al (Cleveland Clinic Found, Ohio)
JAMA 292:1462-1468, 2004
6–7

Background.—Exercise testing has been shown to be of limited usefulness in the detection of coronary artery disease in asymptomatic stress testing. However, recent guidelines have suggested that coronary artery disease screening with exercise testing may be valuable in persons with at least an intermediate risk for adverse events. The goals were to determine the validity for prediction of all-cause mortality of the Framingham Risk Score and of a recently described European global scoring system Systematic Coronary Risk Evaluation (SCORE) for cardiovascular mortality among asymptomatic individuals evaluated in a clinical setting and to determine the potential prognostic value of exercise stress testing once these baseline risks are known.

Methods.—A prospective cohort study was conducted of 3554 asymptomatic adults between the ages of 50 and 75 years who underwent exercise stress testing as part of an executive health program between October 1990 and December 2002. The study participants were monitored for a mean of 8 years. The main outcome measures were global risk based on the Framingham Risk Score and the European SCORE. Exercise stress test result abnormalities, including impaired physical fitness, abnormal heart rate recovery, ventricular ectopy, and ST-segment abnormalities, were prospectively recorded. The primary end point was all-cause mortality.

Results.—There were 114 deaths. The c-index, which corresponds to receiver operating characteristic curve values and the Akaike Information Criteria indicated that the European SCORE was superior to the Framingham Risk Score in estimation of global mortality risk. A multivariable model showed that independent predictors of death were a higher SCORE, impaired functional capacity, and an abnormal heart rate recovery. ST-segment depression was not predictive of mortality. Among patients in the highest tertile from the SCORE, an abnormal exercise stress test (defined as either impaired functional capacity or an abnormal heart rate recovery) were indicative of a mortality risk of more than 1% per year.

Conclusions.—Exercise testing in combination with the European global risk SCORE may facilitate the stratification of risk in asymptomatic persons in a comprehensive executive health screening program.

▶ The key to effective exercise stress testing of asymptomatic patients is to increase the prevalence of disease among the population that is exercised through some form of preliminary triage.[1] This reduces the number of false-positive tests. Although the patients for this study were drawn from the Cleveland Clinic, the instrument developed by the European College of Cardiology in 2003 (SCORE)[2] proved a better method of triage than the Framingham risk factor assessment,[3] at least in terms of predicting the likelihood of all-cause deaths. However, the increase in likelihood of death for each 1% increase in risk score was not large, the respective mean values and 95% confidence limits for the 2 tests being 1.09 (1.07-1.11) and 1.07 (0.92-1.23). The main difference between the European and Framingham scores was the greater scatter of values for the Framingham index. The European SCORE assessment takes account of age, sex, total cholesterol, systolic blood pressure, smoking status, and region of the world (high or low risk). The Framingham score is somewhat similar, being based on age, sex, smoking status, total and high-density lipoprotein cholesterol, and diabetes; it may have worked less well in the present trial because it was designed to predict coronary events rather than all-cause deaths. The question remains that if exercise testing is made diagnostically effective by a preliminary SCORE triage, does this information alter patient management or outcome significantly?

R. J. Shephard, MD, PhD, DPE

References

1. Greenland P, Smith SC, Grundy SM: Improving coronary heart disease risk assessment in asymptomatic people: Role of traditional risk factors and non-invasive cardiovascular tests. *Circulation* 104:1863-1867, 2001.
2. Conroy RM, Pyorala K, Fitzgerald AP, et al: Estimation of ten-year risk of fatal cardiovascular disease in Europe: The SCORE project. *Eur Heart J* 24:987-1003, 2003.
3. D'Agostino RB, Grundy S, Sullivan ML, et al: Validation of the Framingham coronary heart disease prediction scores: Results of a multiple ethnic groups investigation. *JAMA* 286:180-187, 2001.

Nitric Oxide Is Released Into Circulation With Whole-Body, Periodic Acceleration

Sackner MA, Gummels E, Adams JA (Mount Sinai Med Ctr, Miami Beach, Fla; Non-Invasive Monitoring Systems, Inc, North Bay Village, Fla)
Chest 127:30-39, 2005   6–8

Study Objective.—To determine if comfortably applied, whole-body, periodic acceleration releases significant amounts of nitric oxide (NO) into the circulation of healthy subjects and patients with inflammatory diseases.

Materials.—Fourteen healthy adults and 40 adult patients with inflammatory diseases underwent single 45-min trials of whole-body, periodic acceleration with a new "passive exercise" device, while an ECG and a digital pulse wave were obtained with a photoelectric-plethysmograph sensor.

Methods.—The position of the dicrotic notch from the pulse waveform was computed from the amplitude of the pulse divided by the height of the dicrotic notch above the end-diastolic level (a/b ratio). Increase of the a/b ratio reflects the vasodilator action of NO that causes downward movement of the dicrotic notch in the diastolic limb of the digital pulse, thereby elevating the a/b ratio.

Results.—Application of whole-body, periodic acceleration was well tolerated in all participants, and all completed the 45-min treatment. The peak value of the a/b ratio markedly rose during periodic acceleration and returned to baseline during a 5-min recovery period in all healthy subjects and patients with inflammatory diseases.

Conclusions.—Whole-body, periodic acceleration increased pulsatile shear stress to the endothelium leading to vasodilatation and a fall in the dicrotic notch, consistent with increased NO bioactivity in every healthy adult and adult patient with inflammatory disease so treated. Therefore, passive exercise using whole-body, periodic acceleration produces an important benefit that occurs with active exercise.

▶ When a subject exercises, NO is released into the circulation. This agent has direct vasodilator and antiatherosclerotic properties as well as indirect anti-inflammatory and antitumorigenic actions. In short, this is one of the most important metabolic effects of exercise. The authors tested a passive exercise machine that gave a whole-body, periodic acceleration and noted that this form of exercise had a beneficial effect on NO synthesis. The authors did declare their conflict of interest as officers and stakeholders in the company manufacturing this passive exercise system.

P. McCrory, MBBS, PhD

Altered Cardiac Function and Minimal Cardiac Damage During Prolonged Exercise

Shave R, Dawson E, Whyte G, et al (Brunel Univ, Uxbridge, England; Rigshospitalet, Copenhagen; Olympic Med Inst, London; et al)
Med Sci Sports Exerc 36:1098-1103, 2004   6–9

Background.—Recent studies in ultra-endurance exercise (>10 hours) have reported evidence of exercise-induced cardiac fatigue. This fatigue has been characterized by a decrease in both systolic and diastolic functioning. In contrast, a number of studies of shorter duration endurance exercise (<4 hours) have demonstrated no significant decrease in cardiac functioning after exercise. There are limited data on the effects of endurance lasting 4 to 10 hours; thus, the duration of endurance exercise required to trigger exercise-induced cardiac fatigue has not been determined. Markers of cardiac functioning and damage during a simulated half-ironman triathalon were examined in highly trained athletes.

Methods.—The study group was composed of 9 highly trained male triathletes with a mean ± SD age of 33 ± 3 years and a mean ± SD body mass of 77.7 ± 3.2 kg. All study subjects completed a half-ironman triathalon under controlled conditions, including a 1.9-km swim in an indoor pool, a laboratory-based 90-km cycle, and a 21.1-km run. Venous blood samples were drawn, and echocardiographic assessments were performed before the start of exercise, immediately after each stage, and 24 hours after exercise. Serum was analyzed for total creatine kinase activity (CK), creatine kinase isoenzyme MB_{mass} (CK-MB_{mass}), and the cardiac troponin (cTnT) level. Left ventricular systolic and diastolic measurements were obtained from the echocardiographic assessment.

Results.—The mean time for completion of the half-ironman triathalon was 301 ± 28 minutes. Left ventricular contractility was significantly reduced after the half-ironman triathalon. A significant reduction in the ratio of early to late ventricular filling was observed after the run segment of the triathalon. Significant increases in CK and CK-MB_{mass} were observed during and after the triathalon, and cTnT levels were elevated in 4 study subjects over the course of the triathalon.

Conclusions.—The physiologic demand of the half-ironman triathalon resulted in a reduced left ventricular contractility and altered diastolic filling but minimal cardiac damage in this group of highly trained male triathletes. However, the mechanisms of this altered cardiac functioning and cardiac damage after prolonged exercise have not been determined.

▶ Early articles on cardiac damage after triathlon participation[1,2] were somewhat suspect because of the lack of specificity in the assays of cTnT. However, a highly specific test is now available; this shows no cross-reactivity with muscle damage.[3] As the present article shows, the new technology confirms that participation in sustained-endurance exercise such as a triathlon can cause minor cardiac damage. In general, it seems that normal cardiac functioning is restored within a day or so, but there remains a need to examine whether cumulative effects result from repeated exposure of the heart to exercise of this duration.

R. J. Shephard, MD, PhD, DPE

References

1. Whyte G, George K, Sharma S, et al: Cardiac fatigue following prolonged endurance exercise of differing distances. *Med Sci Sports Exerc* 32:1067-1072, 2000.
2. Neumayr G, Pfister R, Mitterbauer G, et al: Effect of the "Race across the Alps" on plasma cardiac troponins I and T. *Am J Cardiol* 89:484-486, 2002.
3. Shave R, Dawson E, Whyte G, et al: The cardiospecificity of the third generation cTnT assay after exercise-induced muscle damage. *Med Sci Sports Exerc* 34:651-654, 2002.

Postexercise Left Ventricular Function and cTnT in Recreational Marathon Runners
George K, Whyte G, Stephenson C, et al (Liverpool John Moores Univ, England; Northwick Park Hosp, Harrow, Middlesex, England; Manchester Metropolitan Univ, Alsager, England; et al)
Med Sci Sports Exerc 36:1709-1715, 2004   6–10

Background.—Evidence is accumulating to suggest that prolonged exercise may induce a transient reduction in left ventricular (LV) function (fatigue) and promote the appearance of cardiac-specific troponins (cTnT and cTnI), which are normally indicative of myocyte necrosis. Currently, most of the available literature has studied young, well-trained athletes from ultra-endurance events, such as the Ironman Triathlon, or exercise of even longer duration. Few data are available on prolonged exercise in a broader range of ages and training levels. As more recreational athletes participate in physical activities, such as marathon running, and in light of the uncertain clinical significance of depressed LV function and cTnT appearance, it is important to investigate postexercise LV function in these athletes. The effect of prolonged exercise on LV function and the appearance of cTnT in older and recreational athletes were assessed.

Methods.—The study included 35 participants (ages 22-57 years) with a finishing time of 157 to 341 minutes for the marathon. Heart rate (HR), blood pressures, and cTnT were recorded prerace and postrace. Echocardiograms were used to assess stroke volume (SV), ejection fraction (EF), sBP/LV end-systolic volume (sBP/ESV), diastolic filling (E:A) ratio as well as preload (LV internal dimension at end-diastole [LVIDd]) and afterload (LV wall stress). HR and core temperature were recorded in-event. Changes in LV function were analyzed by repeated measures t-test. Delta scores for LV function and cTnT data were correlated with each other, age, finishing time, alterations in loading, and in-event data.

Results.—A significant decrease was noted in the mean SV postrace (109 mL vs 85 mL), which was likely the result of a significant decrease in LVIDd. LV wall stress and sBP/ESV were virtually unchanged postrace and were not related to age or finishing time. E:A ratio was significantly reduced after the race, and this reduction could not be explained by an increased HR, a reduced LVIDd, age, finishing time, or in-event data. After the race, 26 of 33 subjects had cTnT values in the range of 0.024 to 0.080 µg/L that were not related to changes in LV function, loading, age, finishing time, or in-event data.

Conclusions.—No evidence was noted of load-independent depression in LV systolic function postrace in marathon runners. Changes in cTnT and E:A were not related, and their cause is uncertain.

▶ Discussion of possible cardiac damage from participation in ultra-endurance events has so far been limited mainly to observations on young and well-trained competitors.[1,2] One might hypothesize that the dangers of cardiac damage would be greater if older and less-fit individuals undertook similar physical activities, but data from the London marathon do not offer much support to this view. The subjects in the sample of George and associates covered a wide range of ages (36 ± 9 years), and the finishing times (256 ± 46 min) also indicate that most of the group had only moderate fitness levels. The SVs of participants were decreased by more than 20% at the end of the event, but on average, EFs were unchanged. Postrace, the concentrations of cardio-specific troponins in 26 out of 33 subjects were in the zone suggestive of minor cardiac injury (0.02-0.08 µg/L),[3] but there was no obvious relationship between changes in cardiac function and cardiac troponin concentration. Thus, the significance of the increase in cardiac troponins remains unclear. The relatively minor cardiac changes seen in this group of subjects probably reflects the fact that older competitors match their running velocity to their physical abilities. It would be worth collecting further data on even older individuals, including, if possible, those who have maintained a high level of performance.

R. J. Shephard, MD, PhD, DPE

References

1. Dawson E, George K, Shave R, et al: Does the heart fatigue subsequent to prolonged exercise in humans? *Sports Med* 33:365-380, 2003.
2. McGavock JM, Warburton DER, Taylor D, et al: The effects of prolonged strenuous exercise on left ventricular function: A brief review. *Heart Lung* 31:279-292, 2002.
3. Collinson PO, Boa FG, Gaze DC: Measurement of cardiac troponins. *Ann Clin Biochem* 38:423-449, 2001.

Effects of Prolonged Strenuous Exercise (Marathon Running) on Biochemical and Haematological Markers Used in the Investigation of Patients in the Emergency Department

Smith JE, Garbutt G, Lopes P, et al (Royal London Hosp; Univ of East London; Homerton Hosp, London)
Br J Sports Med 38:292-294, 2004   6–11

Introduction.—Exercise may affect the results of biochemical and hematologic measurements in asymptomatic healthy research subjects, especially if the exercise is prolonged or strenuous. Many trials addressing this issue have been performed in the laboratory. The effects of strenuous exercise on commonly used biochemical and hematologic variables were assessed in participants of the 2002 Flora London marathon.

Methods.—Blood samples were obtained in 34 healthy volunteers (7 female, 27 male) before the race at registration and after completion of the marathon to measure concentrations of urea and electrolytes, creatine kinase (CK), CK-MB isoenzyme, myoglobin, troponin I, and D-dimers. A full blood count, a clotting screen, and liver function tests were also performed.

Results.—Significant increases were observed in CK, CK-MB, aspartate aminotransferase, lactate dehydrogenase, and myoglobulin levels after the marathon. No significant change was seen in the level of troponin I. After the marathon, activation of the coagulation and fibrinolytic cascades was evidenced by a decrease in the activated partial thromboplastin time, a decrease in the fibrinogen level, and an increase in the D-dimer level (Table 2).

TABLE 2.—Summary of the Results Before and After Exercise, Giving Normal Ranges

Variable (Units)	Normal Range	Mean (SD) Pre-Exercise	Mean (SD) Post-Exercise	Change and *P* Value
Sodium (mmol/l)	135 to 147	140.3 (1.6)	140.0 (3.3)	NS
Potassium (mmol/l)	3.4 to 4.9	4.4 (0.2)	4.5 (0.5)	NS
Urea (mmol/l)	2.0 to 6.6	5.3 (1.0)	6.1 (1.0)	Increase (p<0.001)
Creatinine (µmol/l)	55 to 110	98.1 (9.5)	118.9 (18.6)	Increase (p<0.001)
AST (U/l)	5 to 35	31.6 (12.8)	47.6 (16.1)	Increase (p<0.001)
LDH (U/l)	230 to 460	429.2 (64.5)	824.5 (220.9)	Increase (p<0.001)
CK (U/l)	<165	195.0 (125.8)	707.8 (376.7)	Increase (p<0.001)
CK-MB (U/l)	0.0 to 4.3	3.6 (2.2)	13.5 (9.6)	Increase (p<0.001)
Myoglobin (ng/ml)	0 to 107	74.8 (6.2)	>500	Increase
Troponin I (ng/ml^{-1})	0.0 to 1.0	0.03 (0.06)	0.01 (0.05)	NS
Haemoglobin (g/dl)	11.5 to 18	14.8 (1.3)	14.7 (1.5)	NS
PCV (%)	40 to 54	44.2 (0.3)	43.2 (0.4)	Decrease (p<0.05)
WBC (10^9/l)	4.0 to 11.0	6.4 (1.4)	17.4 (3.6)	Increase (p<0.001)
Platelet count (10^9/l)	150 to 400	244.2 (50.5)	267.9 (54.9)	Increase (p<0.001)
PT (s)	9.0 to 11.0	11.3 (0.6)	11.9 (0.7)	Increase (p<0.001)
APTT (s)	25.0 to 33.0	26.3 (1.9)	22.6 (1.4)	Decrease (p<0.001)
Fibrinogen (g/dl)	1.5 to 4.5	2.51 (0.47)	2.34 (0.41)	Decrease (p<0.001)
D-dimers (ng/ml)	<250	234.0 (130.6)	553.7 (378.6)	Increase (p<0.001)

Abbreviations: APTT, Activated partial thromboplastin time; *AST,* aspartate aminotransferase; *CK,* creatine kinase; *CK-MB,* creatine kinase MB isoenzyme; *LDH,* lactate dehydrogenase; *PCV,* packed cell volume; *PT,* prothrombin time; *WBC,* white blood cell.

(Courtesy of Smith JE, Garbutt G, Lopes P, et al: Effects of prolonged strenuous exercise (marathon running) on biochemical and haematological markers used in the investigation of patients in the emergency department. *Br J Sports Med* 38:292-294, 2004. Reprinted with permission from the BMJ Publishing Group.)

Conclusion.—These findings are similar to those of prior trials on marathon running and hematologic testing that is routinely performed in the hospital. Several laboratory tests evaluated were affected by prolonged exercise; "abnormal" results may be normal after prolonged exercise and, therefore, not diagnostic of a disease process. Thus, results in patients who have been exercising should be interpreted with caution.

▶ The use of autoanalyzers has made it very easy for the physician to obtain values for a wide range of biochemical variables. However, it is important not to overinterpret deviations from published norms, particularly when evaluating individuals who have just engaged in a prolonged bout of endurance exercise. The data of Smith and associates were obtained from 34 healthy individuals who had just completed a marathon. Many showed elevations of traditional markers of cardiac injury (although the results for a third-generation assay of troponin I remained within normal limits). D-dimer levels were also increased, which could be misinterpreted as evidence of a thromboembolic disorder, and neutrophilia was present, which might be thought indicative of an infection. Plainly, it is important to base treatment on clinical findings rather than to simply react to abnormal test results.

R. J. Shephard, MD, PhD, DPE

The "Weekend Warrior" and Risk of Mortality

Lee I-M, Sesso HD, Oguma Y, et al (Harvard School of Public Health, Boston; Harvard Med School, Boston)
Am J Epidemiol 160:636-641, 2004   6–12

Introduction.—The health benefits of physical activity are well known. Daily exercise is currently recommended. Little is understood concerning any health benefits associated with the "weekend warrior" exercise bouts that infrequently generate the recommended energy expenditure. Whether health benefits are associated with infrequent bouts of exercise (1-2 episodes per week) and can affect all-cause mortality rates was determined in a prospective cohort investigation of 8421 men with no major chronic diseases in the Harvard Health Study.

Methods.—Participants (mean age, 66 years) provided information regarding physical activity on mailed surveys in 1988 and 1993. Participants were classified as sedentary (expending <2100 kJ/wk), insufficiently active (2100-4200 kJ/wk), weekend warriors (>4200 kJ/wk from sports/recreation 1-2 times per week), or regularly active (all others expending ≥4200 kJ/wk).

Results.—There were 1234 deaths between 1988 and 1997. The multivariate relative risks [RRs] of mortality for sedentary, insufficiently active, weekend warrior, and regularly active participants were 1.00 (referent), 0.75 (95% CI, 0.62-0.91), 0.85 (95% CI, 0.65-1.11), and 0.64 (95% CI, 0.55-0.73), respectively. In stratified analysis, among participants without major risk factors, weekend warriors were at a lower risk of dying than were sedentary participants (RR, 0.41; 95% CI, 0.21-0.81). This was not ob-

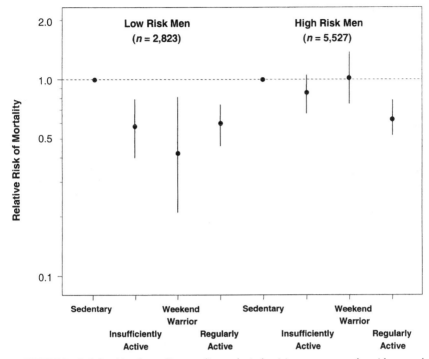

FIGURE 1.—Relative risks of mortality according to physical activity pattern among low-risk men and high-risk men. Harvard Alumni Health Study, 1988-1997. *Lines* represent 95% CIs. Relative risks are adjusted for age, cigarette smoking (never, past, or current), alcohol consumption (never, 1-3 drinks/wk, 4-6 drinks/wk, or daily), red meat intake (<3 servings/month, 1-2 servings/wk, or ≥3 servings/wk), vegetable intake (<1 serving/d, 1-2 servings/d, or ≥3 servings/d), vitamin/mineral supplements, and early parental mortality (both no or yes). "Physical activity pattern" is defined as follows: "sedentary" (men expending <2100 kJ/wk in walking, climbing stairs, and sports/recreation); "insufficiently active" (men expending 2100-4200 kJ/wk in these same activities); "weekend warrior" (men expending ≥4200 kJ/wk by participation in sports/recreation 1-2 times/wk); and "regularly active" (all other men expending ≥4200 kJ/wk in walking, climbing stairs, and sports/recreation). Both weekend warrior and regularly active groups meet the Centers for Disease Control and Prevention/American College of Sports Medicine physical activity recommendation with respect to energy expenditure, that is, at least 4200 kJ/wk. Low-risk men had none of the following risk factors at baseline, but high-risk men had at least one: cigarette smoking, overweight (body mass index, ≥25 kg/m²), history of hypertension, and hypercholesterolemia. (Courtesy of Lee I-M, Sesso HD, Oguma Y, et al: The "weekend warrior" and risk of mortality. *Am J Epidemiol* 160:636-641, 2004. Reprinted by permission of Oxford University Press.)

served among men with at least 1 major risk factor (corresponding RR, 1.02; 95% CI, 0.75-1.38) (Fig 1).

Conclusion.—Regular physical activity generating 4200 kJ/wk or more is recommended for lowering mortality rates in men. In men with no major risk factors, even 1 to 2 episodes of exercise per week generating 4200 kJ/wk or more can postpone mortality.

▶ It is commonly thought that unfit individuals are at greater risk of cardiac catastrophes when they must exercise, and there have been concerns that weekend warriors would worsen rather than improve their prognosis by infrequent but vigorous bouts of exercise. The analysis of Lee and associates suggests that weekend warriors who are free of cardiac risk factors have a substantially lower risk of "all-cause" death than do their sedentary peers, but for those who show cardiac risk factors, their prognosis is on a par with that of their sedentary peers. One weakness in this argument is that those classified as weekend warriors include individuals who engage in vigorous physical activity as often as twice per week; this frequency of activity may be enough to maintain a semblance of physical condition, and it seems quite probable that a different perspective on their prognosis would have been observed if *weekend warriors* had been defined as those who were physically active only once or twice per month. The major impact of cardiac risk factors in this population seems to be a strong argument for including a cardiac risk assessment in the preliminary screening of amateur athletes, as suggested by the American College of Sports Medicine.[1] Possibly, the usefulness of such predictions might be enhanced even further if information on smoking were to be more detailed than a simple yes or no answer.

R. J. Shephard, MD, PhD, DPE

Reference

1. American College of Sports Medicine: *ACSM's Guidelines for Exercise Testing and Prescription*, ed 6. Philadelphia, Lippincott Williams and Wilkins, 2000.

Anginal Threshold Between Stress Tests: Exercise Versus Dobutamine Stress Echocardiography
Arsenault M, Bergeron S, Dumesnil J-G, et al (Quebec Heart and Lung Inst, Ste-Foy)
Med Sci Sports Exerc 37:18-23, 2005   6–13

Background.—Ischemia is usually assessed by exercise stress testing or with pharmacological testing such as dobutamine echocardiography, dipyridamole echocardiography, or nuclear perfusion imaging. Whenever possible, exercise stress testing is preferred because it is also possible to determine the threshold at which angina occurs. This information can be useful in determining clinical management. Dobutamine stress echocardiography is also designed to induce ischemia by increasing cardiac workload, so the monitoring of heart rate (HR) and blood pressure (BP) during this test could offer the same advantage as exercise stress testing, although such information is not currently being used on a routine basis. The purpose of this study was to compare the ischemic threshold between treadmill exercise testing (EX) and dobutamine (DOB).

Methods.—A group of 20 white men with typical chronic stable angina underwent DOB and EX echocardiography in a random order after being weaned from their cardiac medications. Electrocardiography, HR, and systolic BP were recorded every minute. Ischemic threshold was defined as the precise time at which clinical angina occurred.

Results.—Anginal threshold appeared consistently at a higher level for DOB than for EX, as was shown by the higher rate-pressure product (RPP) values, HR, and percent maximal predicted HR. Of the 20 patients tested, 32% presented an ischemic HR above 85% of maximal predicted HR, and 60% had a higher ischemic HR during DOB than during EX.

Conclusions.—Estimation of anginal threshold during DOB stress echocardiography is feasible and is slightly higher (approximately 10%) than during exercise stress testing. The extrapolation of a cut-off target HR from an exercise modality to a pharmaceutical modality may not be valid.

▶ Some authors have chosen to test for myocardial ischemia using pharmacological means, such as dobutamine (DOB), rather than a standardized exercise (EX) test.[1] If the intent is to measure a patient's exercise tolerance and/or offer advice on exercise prescription, it seems logical to undertake an EX test under controlled conditions in the laboratory, rather than provoke ischemia by administration of some synthetic chemical agent. The present study demonstrates that if the ischemia threshold is defined in terms of the rate-pressure product, tolerated values are about 10% higher with DOB than with an EX test. If the DOB test had been carried to 85% of the age-predicted maximal heart rates, as many as 32% of patients would wrongly have been assessed as "normal." The difference in outcome between the 2 types of test reflects differences in cardiac preload and afterload, differences in overall hormonal secretion, and resultant changes in myocardial contractility.[2,3] Plainly, results from DOB and EX tests cannot be considered as interchangeable. Possible weaknesses in the present study include a relatively small sample, and reliance on clinical rather than electrocardiographic evidence for the onset of myocardial ischemia.

R. J. Shephard, MD, PhD, DPE

References

1. Cheitlin MD, Alpert JS, Armstrong WF, et al: Guidelines for the clinical application of echocardiography: A report of the American College of Cardiology/American Heart Association Task Force on Practical Guidelines (Committee on Clinical Application of Echocardiography). Developed in collaboration with the American Society of Echocardiography. *Circulation* 95:1686-1744, 1997.
2. Beleslin BD, Ostojic M, Stepanovic J, et al: Stress echocardiography in the detection of myocardial ischemia. Head to head comparison of exercise, dobutamine, and dipyrimadole tests. *Circulation* 90:1168-1174, 1994.
3. Cohen JL, Ottenweller JE, George AK, et al: Comparison of dobutamine and exercise electrocardiography for detecting coronary artery disease. *Am J Cardiol* 72:1226-1231, 1993.

Effect of Pharmacological Wash-out in Patients Undergoing Exercise Testing After Acute Myocardial Infarction

Bigi R, Verzoni A, Cortigiani L, et al (Clinical Physiology Inst, Milan, Italy; S Paolo Academic Hosp, Milan, Italy; Campo di Marte Hosp, Lucca, Italy; et al)
Int J Cardiol 97:277-281, 2004   6–14

Background.—It is suggested in international guidelines that an exercise electrocardiographic (ECG) test should be the modality for first-line risk stratification in low-risk patients recovering from acute myocardial infarction (MI). The test is generally performed on therapy, even though the advisability of discontinuing drugs is still debated. The effect of pharmacologic therapy on the prognostic value of stress testing was assessed.

Methods.—The study included 362 patients with MI who underwent ECG Holter recording before and after withdrawing β-blockers, calcium antagonists and nitrates. QRS (QRS/h) and ventricular premature beat (VPB/h) counts per hour, repetitive ventricular arrhythmias, ST-segment changes, and patient complaints were evaluated for reproducibility using kappa statistics and the Bland-Altman method.

Results.—No major complications occurred. Of the 362 MI patients, 43 (12%) complained of more than 1 symptom on therapy, and 37 (10%) patients complained of more than 1 symptom off therapy. A mean heart-rate (HR) increase of 8 beats/min was noted in addition to a 5-fold increase in VPB/h after withdrawal of therapy (Fig 2). Repetitive ventricular arrhythmias and ST changes were also more frequent off therapy, but intrapatient reproducibility was poor.

Conclusion.—Early withdrawal of therapy is well tolerated in patients with uncomplicated MI, but a generic risk (not individual) of ventricular arrhythmias and/or transient myocardial ischemia must be considered.

▶ After MI, a large proportion of patients receive drugs, such as β-blockers, that modify their cardiac responses to exercise. The question then arises whether exercise testing should be performed with or without the prescribed treatment. If the objective is to make an appropriate exercise prescription, it seems logical to make observations while the patient is receiving the customary therapeutic regimen; the HR may then change little in response to exercise, and it becomes necessary to rely on other indicators of the intensity of effort, such as the Rating of Perceived Exertion. But if the intent of the exercise test is to determine prognosis, some investigators have argued that more valuable information is obtained when a stress test is performed after withdrawal of medication.[1,2] The sudden withdrawal of cardiac drugs carries its own risks, although in the present sample of patients (all seen soon after MI) no major increases in ischemic episodes or abnormalities of cardiac rhythm were observed after the elimination of prescribed drugs was complete.

R. J. Shephard, MD, PhD, DPE

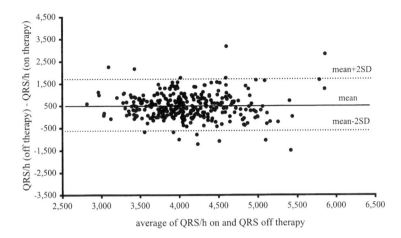

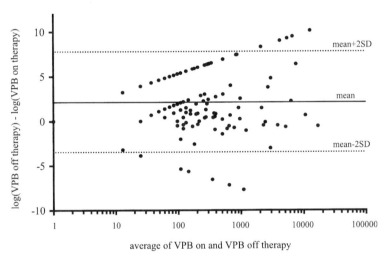

FIGURE 2.—Plots of difference between QRS count and, respectively, logarithm of VPB count on and off therapy against the average of counts on and off therapy. The central, continuous line indicates the mean differences, whereas the upper and lower dotted lines correspond to mean (2 SD). The outliers were not excluded from the calculation of the coefficient of repeatability. (Reprinted by permission of the publisher from Bigi R, Verzoni A, Cortigiani L, et al: Effect of pharmacological wash-out in patients undergoing exercise testing after acute myocardial infarction. *Int J Cardiol* 97:277-281, 2004. Copyright 2004 by Elsevier Science Inc.)

References

1. Ades PA, Thomas JD, Hanson JS et al: Effect of metoprolol on the submaximal stress test performed early after myocardial infarction. *Am J Cardiol* 60:963-966, 1987.
2. Lim R, Dymond DS: Should antianginal medication be stopped for exercise testing? *Lancet* 340:161-162, 1992.

Exercise in Heart Failure: Should Aqua Therapy and Swimming Be Allowed?

Meyer K, Bücking J (Univ of Bern, Switzerland: Caspar Heinrich Clinic, Bad Driburg, Germany)
Med Sci Sports Exerc 36:2017-2023, 2004   6–15

Background.—Aqua exercise and swimming have long been recommended for low-risk cardiac patients. However, there are reservations among some physicians regarding these exercises in patients with severe myocardial infarction (MI) and compensated severe congestive heart failure (CHF). One reason for this concern is the lack of information regarding central hemodynamic volume and pressure responses during immersion in these patients. The purpose of the present study was to investigate the hypothesis that there is a critical point in patients with severe MI and/or severe CHF during graded immersion and swimming during which central hemodynamic alterations change into abnormal cardiac responses.

Methods.—The study was performed in 6 groups: a moderate MI group (group A), a severe MI group (group B), a moderate CHF group (group C), a compensated severe CHF group (group D), and 2 groups of healthy volunteers (groups E and F). Measurements were performed with Swan-Ganz catheterization of the right side of the heart, subxiphoidal echocardiography, and Doppler-echocardiography.

Results.—There were indicators of an increase in preload in patients with moderate and severe MI. In both patient groups, upright immersion to the neck and supine body position at rest in the water resulted in abnormal mean pulmonary artery pressure (PAm) and mean pulmonary capillary pressures (PCPm), respectively. During low-speed swimming (defined as 20-25 m·min^{-1}), the PAm and/or PCPm were higher than during supine cycle ergometry at a power output of 100 W. Left ventricular overload and decrease and/or no change in stroke volume occurred in patients with severe CHF who were immersed to the neck. The well-being of the patients was maintained despite their hemodynamic deterioration.

Conclusions.—The acute responses seen in patients with congestive heart failure and myocardial infarction in this study suggest the need for additional studies on long-term changes in cardiac dimensions and central hemodynamics in these patients who undergo a swimming program compared with nonswimming patients with heart failure who have similar etiology and severity of disease.

▶ The value of progressive exercise programs based on activities such as cycle ergometry is now well established in stable chronic heart failure.[1,2] Given that many of the patients concerned are elderly, with age-related joint problems, the options of aqua therapy and swimming at first seem attractive. Nevertheless, there are theoretical anxieties about the increase of central blood volume induced by hydrostatic compression of the lower half of the body. When a person is immersed to the neck, the central blood volume may be augmented by as much as 700 mL.[3] The data of Meyer and Bücking suggest that those treating patients with congestive heart failure should be cautious until more data are available. It is disturbing to see that patient well-being was maintained despite hemodynamic deterioration. If aqua exercises are practiced by such individuals, these should be limited to shallow water.

R. J. Shephard, MD, PhD, DPE

References

1. Shephard RJ, Kavanagh T, Mertens DJ: On the prediction of physiological responses to aerobic training in patients with stable congestive heart failure. *J Cardiopulm Rehabil* 18:45-51, 1998.
2. Shephard RJ: Exercise for patients with congestive heart failure. *Sports Med* 23:75-92, 1997.
3. Risch WD, Koubenec HJ, Beckmann U, et al: The effect of graded immersion on heart volume, central venous pressure, pulmonary blood distribution and heart rate in man. *Pflügers Arch* 374:115-118, 1978.

Outcome of Exercise Training on the Long-term Burden of Hospitalisation in Patients With Chronic Heart Failure. A Retrospective Study
Hagerman I, Tyni-Lenné R, Gordon A (Huddinge Univ, Stockholm)
Int J Cardiol 98:487-491, 2005   6–16

Aims.—Heart failure is a major cause of hospitalisation, particularly in patients more than 65 years of age in the western world. A common endpoint in studies designed to evaluate treatment effects in heart failure is mortality and morbidity, often reported as an event of hospitalisation. It has recently been reported that this endpoint is misleading with respect to the burden of the disease with regard to the patient, the health service and costs. Furthermore, it can be hypothesized that different treatment effects are bet-

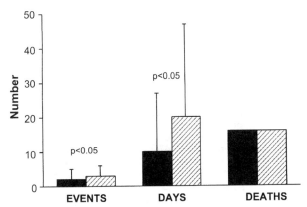

FIGURE 1.—Outcome of exercise training in cardiac hospitalization events and days. *Solid bars* = training group. *Stretched bars* = controls (nontrained). (Reprinted by permission of the publisher from Hagerman I, Tyni-Lenné R, Gordon A: Outcome of exercise training on the long-term burden of hospitalisation in patients with chronic heart failure. A retrospective study. *Int J Cardiol* 98:487-491, 2005. Copyright 2005 by Elsevier Science Inc.)

ter evaluated using more sensitive parameters than those traditionally used in clinical studies. Short-term beneficial effects of exercise training in heart failure patients have previously been showed. Therefore, the aim of this study was to evaluate the long-term effects of exercise training in heart failure patients with regard to different outcome parameters.

Method and Study Group.—Patients with chronic heart failure, stabilised on pharmacological treatment, who had participated in a physical training program for 8 weeks, were analysed retrospectively after 5 years. The study group was compared to a matched control group which received conventional treatment and was diagnosed during the same period but not participating in a training program.

Results.—Exercise training in heart failure patients resulted in significantly less hospitalisation events (2 ± 3 vs. 3 ± 3, $p < 0.05$) and hospitalisation days (10 ± 17 vs. 20 ± 27, $p < 0.05$) due to cardiac problems at 5 years after follow-up (Fig 1). Exercise training did not effect mortality.

Conclusion.—Long-term effects of exercise training on burden of disease in chronic heart failure patients is associated with significantly less events and days of hospitalisation due to worsening of cardiac disease.

▶ From the viewpoint of the patient, one of the most important indices of an effective treatment is its impact upon the health-related quality of life (QOL). Gains in QOL are a welcome consequence of exercise in the treatment of chronic heart failure.[1,2] However, from the viewpoint of the community, the relative impact of various treatments upon health care costs is also an important issue. The 2 questions are not entirely unrelated. Indeed, the present observations showing that hospital usage is reduced, but mortality remains unaffected could well be explained by an exercise-induced enhancement of mood state. This study suggests that the benefits from an 8-week training program persisted as long as 5 years. However, there were some baseline differences between exercise and control groups, and it is unfortunate that there were no final assessments of physical activity patterns to confirm the supposition that exercise levels remained greater in the experimental group. Further work using a prospective randomized controlled design seems warranted.

R. J. Shephard, MD, PhD, DPE

References

1. Kavanagh T, Myers MG, Baigrie RS, et al: Quality of life and cardiorespiratory function in chronic heart failure: Effects of 12 months' aerobic training. *Heart* 76:42-49, 1996.
2. Tynni-Lenné R, Gordon A, Jensen-Urstad M, et al: Exercise-based rehabilitation improves skeletal muscle capacity, exercise intolerance, and quality of life in women as well as men with congestive heart failure. *J Card Fail* 4:9-17, 1998.

Extensive Venous Thrombosis in a Runner: Progression of Symptoms Key to Diagnosis

Fleming A, Frey D (Creighton Univ, Omaha, Neb)
Physician Sportsmed 33(1):34-36, 2005   6–17

Background.—Deep venous thrombosis (DVT) is usually thought of as a disease of sedentary persons. The accepted risk factors for DVT include a sedentary lifestyle, smoking, obesity, and prolonged periods of inactivity. DVT is sometimes found in persons who engage in competitive running, but the diagnosis may not be considered in runners who report pain and swelling in a lower leg because they do not manifest the accepted risk factors for DVT. A failure to promptly diagnose DVT can result in significant morbidity from postphlebitic syndrome or death from pulmonary embolism. A case of DVT occurring in a runner after a race is described.

Case Report.—Man, 40, presented with progressive left lower leg swelling and pain 1 month after completion of a 10-km run. The patient had run regularly for 20 years. He reported having ankle and heel pain and discomfort in the lower leg after finishing the run. He continued to run for another 2 weeks, although the pain and ankle swelling continued. A week off of training provided some improvement, but symptoms returned after a 3-mile run. The development of calf pain and swelling and pain in the medial aspect of the anterior thigh prompted the patient to see his physician. Physical examination showed tenderness to palpation in the left calf, which was swollen. No warmth or erythema of the calf was noted. DVT was thought to be an unlikely diagnosis. However, US and Doppler flow studies showed thrombosis of the left posterior tibial, popliteal, and superficial femoral veins. The patient was admitted to hospital and started on IV heparin and oral warfarin sodium. He returned to work 2 weeks after discharge and continued oral warfarin therapy. Running resumed in the third month after thrombosis, and eventually the patient was able to return to distance running with improved racing times. After the death of his mother from a pulmonary embolus, the patient was rescreened and found to be homozygous for the thermolabile type of methylenetetrahydrofolate reductase deficiency (MTHFR C677T).

Conclusions.—DVT is usually considered a condition of sedentary patients and is not considered when a runner presents with leg discomfort and swelling. As this case demonstrates, it is important to consider DVT in the differential diagnosis of leg pain in runners.

▶ This case report highlights the high degree of clinical suspicion that clinicians must have when faced by an athlete reporting a swollen leg after exercise and where radiologic studies revealed a DVT. It is rare in younger athletes, but in this era of increasing activity in older age groups—and with airline travel being commonplace—this phenomenon will likely be increasingly recognized.

P. McCrory, MBBS, PhD

Severe Acute Respiratory Syndrome and Sport: Facts and Fallacies
So RCH, Ko J, Yuan YWY, et al (Hong Kong Sports Inst; Pamela Youde Nethersole Eastern Hosp, Hong Kong; Centre for Orthopaedic Surgery, Hong Kong; et al)
Sports Med 34:1023-1033, 2004   6–18

Introduction.—Severe Acute Respiratory Syndrome (SARS) not only paralysed economic activities in SARS-affected cities, it also affected sporting activities. SARS was identified in Hong Kong in late February 2003 and the WHO issued a global alert on 12 March, 2003. The incubation period of SARS is usually 4-6 days and patients commonly present with high fever (temperature >38°C), dry cough, chills and rigor, dyspnoea and diarrhoea. Although a specific antiviral agent and vaccines for SARS are not available at the time of writing, a standard treatment protocol for SARS has been developed. The average mortality rate is about 16% in Hong Kong.

The coronavirus is a common pathogen for upper respiratory tract infection and is the most probable pathogen for SARS. Transmission methods may, therefore, be similar for both these infections. Transmission is possible when aerosolised viral particles come into contact with the susceptible host's mucous membrane, most commonly the nose, but also the mouth and eyes.

With appropriate preventive measures to avoid contact with virus, the probability of infection is minimal. Isolation of those who have had close contact with confirmed or suspected SARS patients and/or who have persistent fever will be the most effective and practical method of avoiding contact. Maintaining personal hygiene and frequent hand washing can also reduce the risk of infection. Using diluted bleach (1 part bleach in 99 parts water) to cleanse training areas and equipment is also recommended.

With proper event planning to conform with quarantine measures, special travel arrangements, facility sterilisation and use of venues with good ventilation and filtering systems, sport competition can still proceed.

▶ This article is an interesting summary of the recent SARS epidemic and the issues surrounding hygiene, disease prevention, and the public health procedures put in place to enable sporting activity to continue in this setting. It also summarizes the nature of this illness and the usefulness of exercise prescription in the convalescent period. While the SARS epidemic has been contained, the potential for an influenza pandemic caused by a new strain of influenza, or for other viral epidemic-type illnesses means that this knowledge should be a key aspect of the knowledge for all clinicians.

P. McCrory, MBBS, PhD

Triggers of Subarachnoid Hemorrhage: Role of Physical Exertion, Smoking, and Alcohol in the Australasian Cooperative Research on Subarachnoid Hemorrhage Study (ACROSS)

Anderson C, for the Australasian Cooperative Research on Subarachnoid Hemorrhage Study Group (Univ of Auckland, New Zealand; Imperial College of Science, Technology, and Medicine, London; Royal Perth Hosp, Australia)
Stroke 34:1771-1776, 2003   6–19

Background.—Subarachnoid hemorrhaging (SAH) is a serious disease, and most deaths are the result of the initial severe hemorrhage. With the exception of cigarette smoking, predisposing risk factors for SAH are not known. The beneficial health effects of regular exercise are balanced by the hazards associated with strenuous physical exertion, which is associated with a temporary increase in the risk of acute myocardial infarction, particularly among active individuals. The association between physical exertion (including sexual activity) and SAH was quantified, as was the potential for other modifiable risk factors (such as heavy alcohol consumption and cigarette smoking) to act as triggers for SAH.

Methods.—All cases of first-ever SAH were identified among the combined populations of 4 urban centers in Australia and New Zealand (total population, 2.8 million individuals). Structured interviews were used to obtain information on the type, time, and intensity of exposures in the 26 hours before the onset of SAH. A case-crossover technique was used to assess the risk of SAH associated with transient exposures to heavy cigarette smoking, moderate to extreme physical exertion, and binge alcohol consumption.

Results.—A total of 432 first-ever cases of SAH were registered (62% women; mean age, 56.5 years). A definite time of onset of SAH was determined for 393 of 432 patients (91%), and information on the levels of physical activity in the preceding 26 hours was obtained for 338 patients (78%). Of these patients, 19% engaged in moderate to extreme exertion in the 2 hours before SAH, which was associated with a tripling in the risk of SAH. No evidence was found of any association between heavy cigarette smoking or binge drinking and the risk of SAH in the subsequent 2 hours. Habitual exercise did not appear to have any effect on the risk of SAH associated with moderate to extreme exertion.

Conclusions.—The risk of SAH was tripled with moderate to extreme exertion; however, no association was found between transient heavy smoking or binge drinking and the risk of SAH. Thus, heavy physical activity may trigger SAH.

▶ It has been recognized for many years that vigorous exercise is associated with at least a 5-fold increase in the risk of sudden death, primarily due to cardiac events.[1,2] In the case of heart disease, this immediate hazard is more than offset by an improved prognosis during the period between exercise bouts. The increase of catecholamine levels and the rise of blood pressure that precipitate heart attacks are also likely to increase the risk of SAH in those with cerebral aneurysms. It has been estimated that SAH accounts for some 3% of exercise-induced deaths in those younger than 30 years.[3] The present study was based on questioning of a substantial sample of patients who had sustained a first incident of cerebral hemorrhaging; 19% of the sample reported exertion of 5 metabolic equivalents or greater in the 2 hours before their hemorrhages. Comparison with the normal likelihood of such activity in the individuals concerned suggested that vigorous exercise had increased the risk of a cerebral incident almost 3-fold. In essence, the study participants served as their own controls, in contrast to our earlier study,[1] in which we selected the person sitting in an adjacent office as the control. It might be anticipated that the habit of regular exercise would decrease catecholamine secretion and the rise of blood pressure, thus decreasing the dangers of vigorous exercise, but no evidence of such a benefit was seen in this study. Possibly, those who exercised regularly were liable to engage in bouts of more vigorous exercise than were those who were rarely active so that all experienced similar peaks of catecholamine secretion.

R. J. Shephard, MD, PhD, DPE

References

1. Shephard RJ: Sudden death: A significant hazard of exercise. *Br J Sports Med* 8:101-110, 1974.
2. Vuori I: Sudden death and exercise: Effects of age and type of activity. *Sport Sci Rev* 4:46-84, 1995.
3. Chillag S, Bates M, Vottin R: Sudden death: Myocardial infarction in a runner with normal coronary arteries. *Physician Sportsmed* 18:89-94, 1990.

Treadmill Versus Shuttle Walk Tests of Walking Ability in Intermittent Claudication

Zwierska I, Nawaz S, Walker RD, et al (Sheffield Hallam Univ, England; Univ of Sheffield, England)
Med Sci Sports Exerc 36:1835-1840, 2004   6–20

Background.—Intermittent claudication (IC) is associated with limited walking ability. The functional capacity of patients with IC is usually assessed with a standardized treadmill-walking test. An alternative is the shuttle-walk test, in which patients walk back and forth between 2 cones set apart on flat ground, at a pace controlled by audiotape beeps. The ability of the standardized treadmill-walking test was compared with that of shuttle-walk tests for assessing the functional capacity in patients with CI.

Methods.—The study included 55 patients (ages 52-85 years) with stable IC. Each patient performed an incremental shuttle-walk test, a constant-pace shuttle-walk test and a standardized treadmill test at each session for 3 sessions. Claudication distance (CD), maximum walking distance (MWD), heart rate (HR), and blood pressure (BP) were evaluated. Patients also completed a test-preference questionnaire.

Results.—CD and MWD were greater on the shuttle walks than on the treadmill test. The average coefficients of variation were similar for all types of walking tests. Treadmill walking was associated with greater increases in HR and BP. Most patients preferred shuttle-walking tests.

Conclusions.—Shuttle-walking tests have a similar test-retest reliability as the standardized treadmill-walking tests for functional assessment of patients with IC but are associated with lower levels of cardiovascular stress. Patients with IC generally prefer the shuttle-walking tests. Therefore, shuttle-walking tests can be considered an alternative to standardized treadmill-walking tests to evaluate functional capacity in patients with IC.

▶ The exercise status of patients with IC is commonly assessed by means of a standard uphill-walking treadmill test.[1] However, many older people are nervous when first tested on the treadmill, and consequently, they cover a substantially shorter total distance than when tested by the more natural "shuttle walk." In most patients, fears of the treadmill can be overcome by 1 or more habituation sessions, but this is time consuming, and in view of the good reliability of intermittent shuttle runs, physicians who are testing patients with IC may wish to consider this alternative approach.

R. J. Shephard, MD, PhD, DPE

Reference

1. Hiatt WR: Functional assessment of the claudicant. Importance of treatment and follow-up strategies. *Minerva Cardioangiologica* 47:385-386, 1999.

Field Exercise vs Laboratory Eucapnic Voluntary Hyperventilation to Identify Airway Hyperresponsiveness in Elite Cold Weather Athletes
Rundell KW, Anderson SD, Spiering BA, et al (Marywood Univ, Scranton, Pa; United States Olympic Committee, Lake Placid, NY; Royal Prince Alfred Hosp, Camperdown, NSW, Australia)
Chest 125:909-915, 2004   6–21

Background.—Athletes participating in the 2002 Winter Olympic Games who wished to inhale a β_2-agonist were required to submit objective evidence of asthma or exercise-induced bronchoconstriction (EIB) for approval. Eucapnic voluntary hyperventilation (EVH) was recommended as a method for identifying airway hyperresponsiveness (AHR) consistent with EIB. Change in FEV_1 provoked by EVH in the laboratory was compared with that provoked by field exercise in the cold.

Methods.—Thirty-eight athletes, with a median age of 16 years, underwent 2 challenges performed in random order at least 24 hours apart. For EVH, the participants inhaled dry air containing 5% carbon dioxide for 6 minutes at a target ventilation equivalent to 30 times baseline FEV_1. Exercise consisted of cross-country skiing, ice skating, or running for 6 to 8 minutes. Spirometry was assessed before and for 15 minutes after the challenges. Airway hyperresponsiveness was considered consistent with EIB when there was a 10% decline in FEV_1 or greater from baseline after challenge.

TABLE 1.—Anthropometric Measurements in the 38 Athletes Who Performed 6 Minutes of EVH in the Laboratory at 19°C and 6 to 8 Minutes of Field Exercise at 2°C*

Subject No.	Gender	Ht, cm	Wt, kg	Age, yr	$\dot{V}_E/$ FEV_1	FEV_1 % Pred	FVC % Pred	FEV_1/FVC Ratio	FEF_{25-75} % Pred	% Fall on 6 to 8 min Ex†	% Fall on 6-min EVH†
1	M	183	89	26	28.65	112	112	85	96	1.34	5.01
2‡§	M	170	70	18	28.13	91	113	67	52	27.22	10.63
3	M	173	82	17	29.80	137	128	90	152	3.54	0.6
4	F	173	60	16	26.57	105	93	95	128	7.76	5.37
5	F	168	64	18	26.95	138	125	93	145	4.77	10.51
6	F	170	75	17	28.21	121	116	88	120	1.46	0
7	F	157	66	19	26.00	99	103	84	71	4.62	1.01
8	M	173	70	22	30.76	93	98	81	69	4.83	6.36
9	M	185	77	26	30.20	106	105	84	98	2.59	4.98
10	M	169	60	16	29.43	103	105	81	81	19.89	7.95
11	M	180	68	15	28.58	136	130	86	131	11.9	18.47
12	F	173	57	27	29.12	96	86	98	138	6.16	0.88
13	M	180	73	20	31.38	111	109	87	88	9.33	2.37
14	M	168	68	24	29.48	96	97	86	88	7.18	2.61
15	M	183	83	23	NA	107	114	80	87	6.78	3.21
16§	F	170	61	16	26.50	123	109	99	122	18.55	20.3
17	F	165	52	16	23.94	122	114	94	123	16.76	17.86
18	F	168	57	15	27.30	107	102	89	95	4.52	4.22
19	F	165	59	17	34.29	94	105	76	60	0	3.91
20	F	160	57	16	27.76	131	129	87	119	6.15	10.89
21	F	160	59	17	26.60	130	118	94	143	4.24	9.6
22	F	168	52	15	24.66	126	148	74	78	7.65	17.09
23	F	163	52	13	26.41	107	95	100	121	4.25	8.82
24	F	157	52	14	30.97	119	105	100	141	3.86	9
25	F	163	57	17	21.30	116	110	90	106	4.82	11.45
26	F	165	57	15	28.93	125	109	98	158	14.48	7.77
27	F	163	48	16	21.65	114	100	100	163	15.74	14.51
28§‖¶	F	155	50	14	27.35	91	106	73	48	0	26.32
29§	F	157	50	15	21.47	121	115	94	111	38.29	14.24
30	F	157	55	16	NA	115	106	95	99	4.97	10.6
31§¶	F	152	48	15	27.61	123	105	100	158	20.48	10.24
32	F	165	55	16	22.28	113	103	95	103	7.99	12.13
33	F	178	66	16	29.48	105	103	85	86	0	10.47
34	F	178	60	16	27.76	98	85	100	154	14.53	14.53
35	F	157	50	15	29.31	110	106	93	110	25.61	16.61
36	M	173	68	42	30.43	123	117	87	127	6.25	9.83
37	M	178	70	25	29.47	79	76	88	80	2.11	2
38	M	168	64	18	29.76	122	109	93	131	3.9	2.69
Mean		168	62	18	27.74	112.30	108.14	89.18	109.97	9.07	9.08
SD		8.5	10.3	5.4	2.92	14.23	13.31	8.34	31.10	8.54	6.22

*Average ventilation during EVH is expressed as a multiple of baseline FEV_1.

Abbreviations: Ht, Height; *W*, weight; *Pred*, predicted; *NA*, not available; *Ex*, exercise; *VE*, minute ventilation; *M*, male; *F*, female.

†Expressed as a percentage of baseline FEV_1.

‡Regular therapy: fluticasone/salmeterol.

§Regular therapy: albuterol.

‖Regular therapy: montelukast.

¶Regular therapy: fluticasone.

(Courtesy of Rundell KW, Anderson SD, Spiering BA, et al: Field exercise vs laboratory eucapnic voluntary hyperventilation to identify airway hyperresponsiveness in elite cold weather athletes. *Chest* 125: 909-915, 2004.)

Findings.—Eleven athletes were exercise positive, with a 20.5% drop in FEV_1. Seventeen athletes were EVH positive, with a 14.5% decline in FEV_1. Fifty-eight percent of the 19 athletes with AHR were identified by exercise and 89% by EVH. Eucapnic voluntary hyperventilation identified 9 of 11 exercise-positive athletes and 8 athletes with a potential for EIB. The mean ventilation during EVH was 28 times FEV_1 (Table 1).

Conclusions.—In this study, EVH for 6 minutes in the laboratory was associated with a better chance of identifying AHR than 6 to 8 minutes of field exercise in the cold. The EVH test will also be useful for assessing elite summer athletes.

▶ Subjective reports of EIB are unreliable,[1,2] particularly in elite athletes, and objective documentation is a prerequisite to allowing competitors to use bronchodilator medication,[3] Potential provocative tests include field or laboratory exercise, ECH of dry gas, and inhalation of mannitol powder or hypertonic saline. The present findings are based on a small sample of competitors, not all of whom suffered from EIB. The results suggest that EVH may be not only more convenient than a field exercise challenge but also more effective in diagnosing hyperresponsive airways. Nevertheless, neither method provides an infallible test. Two of the subjects seen by Rundell et al had no response to 6 minutes of EVH despite a clear response to 6 to 8 minutes of exercise in the cold, and several of the 17 "positive" responses to EVH were based on marginal changes of pulmonary function (a 10%-11% decrease of 1-second forced expiratory volume). One weakness of the experimental design was the retesting of subjects within 24 to 36 hours of the first challenge; there may thus have been some delayed effects from the first response (although the authors deny that there was such an effect).

R. J. Shephard, MD, PhD, DPE

References

1. Rundell KW, Im J, Mayers LB, ct al: Self-reported symptoms and exercise-induced asthma in the elite athlete. *Med Sci Sports Exerc* 33:208-213, 2001.
2. Holzer K, Anderson SD, Douglass J: Exercise in elite summer athletes: Challenges for diagnosis. *J Allergy Clin Immunol* 110:374-380, 2002.
3. Anderson SD, Fitch K, Perry CP, et al: Responses to bronchial challenge submitted for approval to use inhaled β2 agonists prior to an event at the 2002 Winter Olympics. *J Allergy Clin Immunol* 111:44-49, 2003.

Airway Cell Composition at Rest and After an All-out Test in Competitive Rowers
Morici G, Bonsignore MR, Zangla D, et al (Univ of Palermo, Italy; Italian Natl Research Council (CNR), Palermo, Italy)
Med Sci Sports Exerc 36:1723-1729, 2004   6–22

Background.—Airway cells at rest in well-trained endurance athletes at rest have been found to have evidence of airway inflammation. Increased neutrophils, eosinophils, and lymphocytes have been reported alone or in combination in runners, swimmers, ice hockey players, and skiers. The status of airway cells at rest in competitive rowers to determine whether rowing affects airway cell composition and whether there is a relationship between the degree of ventilation during exercise and airway cells was investigated.

Methods.—Induced sputum samples were obtained at rest and shortly after an all-out rowing test in 9 young, nonasthmatic competitive rowers with a mean (SD) age of 16.2 ± 1.0 years. The rowing test was 1000 m long. Ventilatory and metabolic variables were recorded breath-by-breath.

Results.—At rest, induced sputum showed a prevalence of neutrophils (60%) over macrophages (40%). There was a tendency for total cell and bronchial epithelial cell (BEC) counts to increase after exercise. In the last minute of exercise, mean ventilation (VE) was 158.0 ± 41.5 L·min⁻¹, and VO₂·kg⁻¹ 62 ± 11 mL·min⁻¹. Exercise VE was correlated directly with post-exercise total cell and macrophage counts. A similar trend was observed for exercise VE and changes in BEC counts from baseline to postexercise. Exercise VE was not correlated with airway neutrophil counts at rest or after exercise. Expression of adhesion molecules by airway neutrophils, macrophages, and eosinophils decreased after the all-out test.

Conclusions.—The same as endurance athletes, nonasthmatic competitive rowers showed increased neutrophils in induced sputum compared with values found in sedentary study subjects. The trend toward increased BEC after exercise may be a reflection of the effects of high airflows on airway epithelium. Postexercise airway macrophages were highest in rowers that demonstrated the most intense exercise hyperpnea, which suggested that intense, short-lived exercise may be associated with a blunted response of airway cells in nonasthmatic well-trained rowers.

▶ Cellular damage of the airways is well documented among top-level winter athletes such as skiers and ice hockey players, and this disease apparently accounts for the high incidence of exercise-induced asthma found in such individuals.[1] The underlying cause is thought to be a prolonged exposure to cold, dry air. It is interesting that similar evidence of inflammatory change in the airways can be demonstrated immediately after a brief, all-out rowing test. The observations of Morici and associates were made in a relatively warm laboratory (23°C), and the ambient air had a fair water content (50% relative humidity). Apparently, the only feature in common with the winter athletes was a very large respiratory minute volume (up to 200 L/min during the bout of exercise), and the total cell and macrophage counts in the sputum were significantly correlated with the individual's respiratory minute volume. The observations merit reproduction on a larger sample of subjects, with inclusion of measurements of airway resistance.

R. J. Shephard, MD, PhD, DPE

Reference

1. Shephard RJ: Does cold air damage the lungs of winter athletes. *Curr Sports Med Rep* 6:289-292, 2004.

Effects of Testosterone and Resistance Training in Men With Chronic Obstructive Pulmonary Disease

Casaburi R, Bhasin S, Cosentino L, et al (Drew Univ, Los Angeles; Harbor-Univ of California, Los Angeles)

Am J Respir Crit Care Med 170:870-878, 2004   6–23

Background.—Exercise intolerance is the chief complaint in many patients with chronic obstructive pulmonary disease (COPD). It has become clear in recent years that dysfunction of the muscles of ambulation is a con-

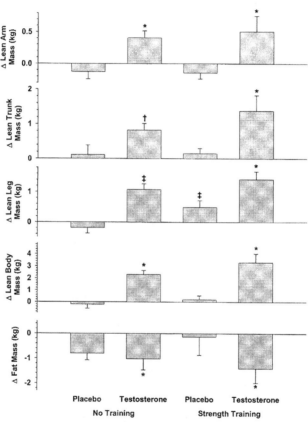

FIGURE 3.—Regional and total body composition changes resulting from the interventions in the four study groups determined by dual-emission X-ray absorptiometry. Study groups are from left to right: placebo + no training, n = 12; testosterone + no training, n = 12; placebo + resistance training, n = 12; testosterone + resistance training, n = 11. The regional (arm, trunk, lean, and total) lean mass increases in the groups receiving testosterone supplementation. In the group undergoing a resistance training program targeting the legs, but not receiving testosterone supplementation, lean mass increases only in the legs. Total fat mass decreases in both groups receiving testosterone. *Response to intervention significantly different from nontestosterone groups. †Response to intervention significantly different from placebo + resistance training group. ‡Response to intervention significantly different from placebo + no training group. (Courtesy of Casaburi R, Bhasin S, Cosentino L, et al: Effects of testosterone and resistance training in men with chronic obstructive pulmonary disease. *Am J Respir Crit Care Med* 170:870-878, 2004. Official Journal of the American Thoracic Society. Copyright, American Lung Association.)

tributor to exercise intolerance in these patients. Rehabilitative programs of exercise tolerance have been shown to significantly increase this important health factor. Both endurance training and resistance training have been found to be effective, and distinct benefits are associated with these 2 training approaches. Endurance training is beneficial in increasing endurance for physical exercises, such as walking and climbing stairs, and resistance training is beneficial in increasing strength for exercises, such as standing from a sitting position and maintaining balance. However, some measures of strength and endurance have shown modest crossover effects. It has also been determined that men with COPD have a high prevalence of low testosterone levels, which may contribute to muscle weakness. Whether testosterone supplementation might have the potential to be an appropriate adjunctive treatment during a program of pulmonary rehabilitation, specifically directed at improving muscle mass and muscle function, was determined.

Methods.—The effects of testosterone supplementation (100 mg injected weekly) on body composition and muscle function, with or without resistance training, were determined in 47 men with COPD. The study participants were randomly assigned to 10 weeks of placebo injections and no training, placebo injections and resistance training, testosterone injections and resistance training, or testosterone injections and no training. The resistance training was performed for 45 minutes 3 times weekly.

Results.—The testosterone injections provided a mean increase of 271 ng/dL in the nadir serum testosterone concentration (to the middle of the normal range for young men) (Fig 3). The average increase in lean body mass, as determined by dual-energy x-ray absorptiometry, was 2.3 kg with testosterone alone and 3.3 kg with combined testosterone and resistance training. The increase in 1-repetition peak leg press force averaged 17.2% with testosterone alone, 17.4% with resistance training alone, and 26.8% with testosterone plus resistance training. The interventions were well tolerated, with no abnormalities in safety measures.

Conclusions.—A need exists for more studies to determine the long-term benefits of adding testosterone supplementation and resistance training to rehabilitative programs for carefully screened men with COPD and low testosterone levels.

▶ It is now widely accepted that weakness of the major muscles contributes substantially to the dyspnea of COPD, [1] and resistance training can increase the exercise tolerance of affected individuals considerably.[2] Given that androgen production is limited in the typical elderly COPD patient, it seems logical to augment the training response by administering substantial doses of testosterone (100 mg/wk). The present data offer convincing evidence of the immediate advantages obtained by this strategy in increases in body mass and leg strength. Longer-term studies are still needed to examine the possible risks of testosterone supplementation—alterations of personality, decreases of HDL cholesterol, liver damage, and a facilitation of the growth of pre-existing prostate tumors.

R. J. Shephard, MD, PhD, DPE

References

1. American Thoracic Society and European Respiratory Society Statement: Skeletal muscle dysfunction in chronic obstructive lung disease. *Am J Respir Crit Care Med* 159:1S-40S, 1999.
2. Ries AL, Carlin BW, Carrieri-Kohlman V, et al: Pulmonary rehabilitation: Evidence-based guidelines. *Chest* 112:1363-1396, 1997.

Inspiratory Muscle Training Improves Lung Function and Exercise Capacity in Adults With Cystic Fibrosis

Enright S, Chatham K, Ionescu AA, et al (Univ of Salford, Manchester, England; Llandough Hosp NHS Trust, Cardiff, Wales; Syracuse Univ, NY)
Chest 126:405-411, 2004   6–24

Introduction.—Increases in exercise capacity have been linked with lower rates of mortality in patients with cystic fibrosis (CF). The effect of controlled inspiratory muscle training (IMT), with no additional form of aerobic training, on exercise performance and psychosocial status in patients with chronic pulmonary disease, has yet to be determined. The effect of an 8-week IMT program with a fixed workload on inspiratory muscle functioning (IMF), diaphragm thickness, lung functioning, physical work capacity (PWC), and psychosocial status was examined in 29 adult patients with CF.

Methods.—Patients were randomly assigned to 3 groups: 2 were required to participate in an 8-week program of IMT in which the training intensity was established at either 80% of maximal effort (group 1; 9 patients) or 20% of maximal effort (group 2; 10 patients). A third patient group did not participate in any training and acted as control subjects (group 3; 10 patients).

Results.—For all participants, baseline and postintervention measures of IMF were ascertained via maximal inspiratory pressure (PImax) and sustained PImax (SPImax); pulmonary functioning, body composition, and physical activity status were also measured. The diaphragm thickness was measured by US at functional residual capacity (FRC) and total lung capacity. The diaphragm thickening ratio [TR] was determined (TR = thickness during PImax at FRC/mean thickness at FRC). Participants also completed an incremental cycle ergometer test to exhaustion and 2 symptom-associated questionnaires, before and after training.

Results.—After training, significant increases in PImax and SPImax ($P < .05$) the diaphragm thickness as measured by US at total lung capacity ($P < .05$), TR ($P < .05$), vital capacity ($P < .05$), total lung capacity ($P < .05$), and PWC ($P < .05$) were detected; reductions in anxiety scores ($P < .05$) and depression scores ($P < .01$) were seen in group 1 patients compared with group 3 patients. Group 2 patients significantly improved PImax and SPImax (both $P < .05$) only in comparison with group 3 patients. No significant differences were seen in group 3 patients (Table 4).

Conclusion.—An 8-week program of high-intensity IMT produced significant benefits for patients with CF, including increased IMF and thickness

TABLE 4.—Pretraining and Posttraining PWC and Psychosocial Status Scores*

Variable	Pretest	Posttest	P Value
PWC, kg/min			
Group 1	328 ± 140	496 ± 159	< 0.05†
Group 2	389 ± 153	371 ± 159	NS
Group 3	343 ± 154	330 ± 165	NS
PWC, min			
Group 1	7.2 ± 2.7	10.3 ± 1.8	< 0.05†
Group 2	7.4 ± 3.0	7.1 ± 3.0	NS
Group 3	6.5 ± 2.7	6.4 ± 2.9	NS
Anxiety			
Group 1	6.0 ± 4.3	3.1 ± 2.7	< 0.05†
Group 2	4.6 ± 3.6	3.7 ± 3.6	NS
Group 3	4.1 ± 3.6	3.7 ± 3.4	NS
Depression			
Group 1	2.8 ± 1.8	0.8 ± 0.7	< 0.01†
Group 2	2.3 ± 1.4	2.0 ± 1.7	NS
Group 3	3.0 ± 2.9	3.3 ± 2.1	NS
CRDQ			
Dyspnea			
Group 1	16.6 ± 4.4	16.2 ± 4.2	NS
Group 2	17.7 ± 4.5	18.4 ± 2.8	NS
Group 3	19.0 ± 2.6	19.6 ± 2.5	NS
Mastery			
Group 1	23.1 ± 1.9	22.1 ± 3.1	NS
Group 2	22.8 ± 4.2	22.5 ± 3.9	NS
Group 3	23.4 ± 3.3	25.1 ± 2.8	NS
Fatigue			
Group 1	15.0 ± 2.3	16.0 ± 3.2	NS
Group 2	20.0 ± 3.4	21.5 ± 2.3	NS
Group 3	20.4 ± 4.4	22.1 ± 2.3	NS
Emotion			
Group 1	32.8 ± 5.0	32.4 ± 8.2	NS
Group 2	37.6 ± 10.5	35.7 ± 9.2	NS
Group 3	36.2 ± 5.9	37.4 ± 5.2	NS

*Values given as mean ± SD, unless otherwise indicated.
†Group 1 had significantly higher PWC values and lower anxiety and depression scores than group 2 and 3 posttraining, although there were no significant differences between groups 2 and 3.
Abbreviations.—PWC, Physical work capacity; CRDQ, chronic respiratory disease questionnaire; NS, not significant.
(Courtesy of Enright S, Chatham K, Ionescu AA, et al: Inspiratory muscle training improves lung function and exercise capacity in adults with cystic fibrosis. *Chest* 126:405-411, 2004.)

of the diaphragm (during contraction), improved lung volumes, increased PWC, and improved psychosocial status.

▶ This is a relatively small study, but it has some unique features, including the introduction of both a control group and a group of patients that received homeopathic IMT. Progressive increases in muscle loading were also included as the muscles became stronger so that the training process could continue. The power output on a cycle ergometer was measured in watts, but the units of physical working capacity used in Table 4 (perhaps kg · m/min?) are unclear. Despite this, the numerical values suggest a very substantial increase of working capacity in the therapeutic group, as contrasted with a small deterioration of performance in the control group and in those receiving homeopathic treatment.

R. J. Shephard, MD, PhD, DPE

7 Visceral and Metabolic Disorders, Other Medical Conditions, and Immune Function

Interindividual Variation in Abdominal Subcutaneous and Visceral Adipose Tissue: Influence of Measurement Site

Lee SJ, Janssen I, Ross R (Queen's Univ, Kingston, Ont, Canada)

J Appl Physiol 97:948-954, 2004   7–1

Introduction.—We evaluated the influence of measurement site on the ranking (low to high) of abdominal subcutaneous (SAT) and visceral (VAT) adipose tissue. We also determined the influence of measurement site on the prediction of abdominal SAT and VAT mass. The subjects included 100 men with computed tomography (CT) measurements at L_4-L_5 and L_3-L_4 levels and 100 men with magnetic resonance imaging (MRI) measurements at L_4-L_5 and 5 cm above L_4-L_5 (L_4-L_5 +5 cm). Corresponding mass values were determined by using multiple-image protocols. For SAT, 90 and 92 of the 100 subjects for CT and MRI, respectively, had a difference in rank position at the two levels. The change in rank position exceeded the error or measurement for approximately 75% of the subjects for both methods. For VAT, 91 and 95 of the 100 subjects for CT and MRI, respectively, had a difference in rank position at the two levels. The change in rank position exceeded the error of measurement for 36% of the subjects for CT and for 8% of the subjects for MRI. For both imaging modalities, the variance explained in SAT and VAT mass (kg) was comparable for L_4-L_5, L_4-L_5 +5 cm, and L_3-L_4 levels. In conclusion, the ranking of subjects for abdominal SAT and VAT quantity is influenced by measurement location. However, the ability to predict SAT and VAT mass by using single images obtained at the L_4-L_5, L_4-L_5 +5 cm, or L_3-L_4 levels is comparable.

▶ Criterion methods for quantifying VAT include imaging techniques such as CT and MRI. For various reasons, including time and cost, most investigators and clinicians use a single image at the L_4-L_5 level to estimate VAT. This approach assumes that the distribution of VAT in the abdomen is similar between individuals. This study showed that although measurement location influenced the visceral adipose ranking across subjects, the effect was small, and that the ability to predict VAT by using the L_4-L_5 level was precise enough to support using the single-image approach.

D. C. Nieman, DrPH

Three-Compartment Model: Critical Evaluation Based on Neutron Activation Analysis
Silva AM, Shen W, Wang Z, et al (Technical Univ of Lisbon, Portugal; Columbia Univ, New York; Winthrop Univ, Mineola, NY; et al)
Am J Physiol Endocrinol Metab 287:E962-E969, 2004   7–2

Introduction.—There is renewed interest in Siri's classic three-compartment (3C) body composition model, requiring body volume (BV) and total body water (TBW) estimates, because dual-energy X-ray absorptiometry (DEXA) and in vivo neutron activation (IVNA) systems cannot accommodate subjects with severe obesity. However, the 3C model assumption of a constant ratio (α) of mineral (M) to total body protein (TBPro) and related residual mass density (D_{RES}) based on cadaver analyses might not be valid across groups differing in sex, race, age, and weight. The aim of this study was to derive new 3C model coefficients in vivo and to compare these estimates to those derived by Siri. Healthy adults (n = 323) were evaluated with IVNA and DEXA and the measured components used to derive α and D_{RES}. For all subjects combined, values of α and D_{RES} (means ± SD, 0.351 ± 0.043; 1.565 ± 0.023 kg/l) were similar to Siri's proposed values of 0.35 and 1.565 kg/l, respectively. However, α and D_{RES} varied significantly as a function of sex, race, weight, and age. Expected errors in percent body fat arising by application of Siri's model were illustrated in a second group of 264 adults, including some whose size exceeded DEXA limits but whose BV and TBW had been measured by hydrodensitometry and ^2H_2O dilution, respectively. Extrapolation of predictions by newly developed models to very high weights allows percent fat error estimation when Siri's model is applied in morbidly obese subjects. The present study results provide a critical evaluation of potential errors in the classic 3C model and present new formulas for use in selected populations.

▶ Most DEXA systems cannot accommodate subjects with severe or morbid obesity. To measure body composition in these individuals, the authors recommend measurement of BV through underwater weighing and TBW through deuterium dilution (^{2}H$_2$O), with these variables passed through an adapted form of the Siri 3C equation: Fat mass = 2.122 × BV (L) − 0.779 × TBW (kg) − 1.356 × body mass (kg).

D. C. Nieman, DrPH

Lifestyle Behaviors Associated With Lower Risk of Having the Metabolic Syndrome
Zhu S, St-Onge M-P, Heshka S, et al (Med College of Wisconsin, Milwaukee; Columbia Univ, New York)
Metabolism 53:1503-1511, 2004   7–3

Introduction.—The metabolic syndrome is a cluster of risk factors that predisposes individuals to cardiovascular disease (CVD) and diabetes and is present in almost one fourth of adult Americans. Risk factors involved with the metabolic syndrome can be altered via modifiable lifestyle factors, such as diet, physical activity, and smoking and drinking habits. The objective of this study was to examine the extent to which these modifiable lifestyle behaviors are associated with the risk of having the metabolic syndrome. Data from the Third National Health and Nutrition Examination Survey (NHANES III), conducted between 1988 and 1994, were used to measure the risk of having the metabolic syndrome in healthy adult Americans who follow certain lifestyle behaviors, such as dietary practices, levels of physical activity, smoking and drinking habits. Low physical activity level, high carbohydrate (CHO) intake, and current smoking habits were all significantly associated with an increased risk of having the metabolic syndrome, even after adjusting for other related covariates. Relative to physically inactive subjects, being physically active was associated with lower odds ratio (OR) (0.36, confidence interval [CI] 0.21 to 0.68, $P < .01$) in overweight men and in normal weight (0.36, CI 0.18 to 0.70, $P < .01$) and overweight (0.61, CI 0.38 to 0.97, $P < .05$) women. Although the type of CHO could not be distinguished, relative to a high CHO diet, men having a low or moderate CHO intake had a lower risk of having the metabolic syndrome with respective ORs of 0.41 (CI 0.24 to 0.67, $P < .01$) and 0.44 (CI 0.25 to 0.77, $P < .01$); no effect of dietary CHO was observed in women. Moderate alcohol consumption was not significantly related to the risk of having the metabolic syndrome in men, but was associated with a lower OR in women (0.76, CI 0.61 to 0.95, $P < .05$) (Fig 1). Regression models indicate a reduced risk of having the metabolic syndrome when selected low-risk lifestyle factors are present in combination, particularly in subjects with body mass index (BMI) < 30 kg/m^2). According to our cross-sectional logistic models, the risk of having the metabolic syndrome is substantially lower in individuals who are physically active, nonsmoking, have a relatively low CHO intake and moderate alcohol consumption, and who maintain a BMI in the non-obese range. These observations have potentially important value for public health recommendations.

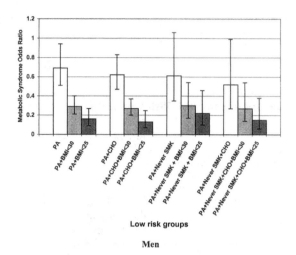

Men

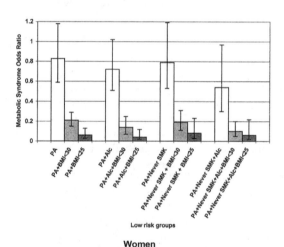

Women

FIGURE 1.—Odds ratios of having the metabolic syndrome with low-risk behaviors or lifestyle. Factors: physically active, low and moderate CHO intake (for men), light-to-moderate alcohol consumption (for women), and nonsmoking, overall (*white bar*) and with additional conditions of normal weight (BMI < 25 kg/m², *black bar*) and overweight (BMI < 30 kg/m², *gray bar*). In each case, the reference group for the comparison is with subjects who do not qualify for that low-risk behavior or lifestyle category. *Abbreviations: PA,* Physically active; *CHO,* low and moderate carbohydrate intakes; *Alc,* light to moderate alcohol consumption; *SMK,* smoking. (Courtesy of Zhu S, St-Onge M-P, Heshka S, et al: Lifestyle behaviors associated with lower risk of having the metabolic syndrome. *Metabolism* 53:1503-1511, 2004.)

▶ About 1 in 4 adults have the metabolic syndrome. This large cross-sectional study showed that the majority of Americans would not be diagnosed with the metabolic syndrome if they had appropriate lifestyle behaviors, such as being physically active, having a low carbohydrate intake for men or light to moderate alcohol-drinking habits for women, not smoking, and having a BMI less than 30 kg/m² (see Fig 1). Of these lifestyle factors, physical activity was most strongly associated with a lower risk of having the metabolic syndrome. It should be noted that this analysis did not discriminate between simple and complex carbohydrates.

D. C. Nieman, DrPH

Associations of Fitness and Fatness With Mortality in Russian and American Men in the Lipids Research Clinics Study
Steven J, Evenson KR, Thomas O, et al (Univ of North Carolina, Chapel Hill)
Int J Obes 28:1463-1470, 2004   7–4

Objective.—To examine the relative size of the effects of fitness and fatness on mortality in Russian men, and to make comparison to US men.

Design.—Prospective closed cohort.

Subjects.—1359 Russian men and 1716 US men aged 40-59 y at baseline (1972-1977) who were enrolled in the Lipids Research Clinics (LRC) Study.

Measurements.—Fitness was assessed using a treadmill test and fatness was assessed as body mass index (BMI) calculated from measured height and weight. Hazard ratios were calculated using proportional hazard models that included covariates for age, education, smoking, alcohol intake and dietary keys score. All-cause and cardiovascular disease (CVD) mortality were assessed through 1995.

Results.—In Russian men, fitness was associated with all-cause and CVD mortality, but fatness was not. For mortality from all causes, compared to the fit-not fat, the adjusted hazard ratios were 0.87 (95% CI: 0.55, 1.37) among the fit-fat, 1.86 (95% CI: 1.31, 2.62) among the unfit-not fat and 1.68 (95% CI: 1.06, 2.68) among the unfit-fat. Among US men, the same hazard ratios were 1.40 (95% CI: 1.07, 1.83), 1.41 (95% CI: 1.12, 1.77) and 1.54 (95% CI: 1.24, 2.06), respectively (Fig 1). There were no statistically significant interactions between fitness and fatness in either group of men for all-cause or CVD mortality.

Conclusion.—The effects of fitness on mortality may be more robust across populations than are the effects of fatness.

▶ A heated debate exists in regard to the "fit and fat" data advanced by the Aerobics Center Longitudinal Study. These studies indicate that fitness is a more potent risk factor for mortality than is fatness.[1] On the other hand, other studies indicate that fit men and women are not protected from the increased disease risk associated with fatness.[2] These data on Russian and American men from the Lipids Research Clinics Study indicate that across populations, cardiorespiratory fitness (ie, duration of the treadmill exercise test in minutes) was a better predictor of all-cause and cardiovascular disease mortality than BMI (Fig 1). For US men, however, being "fit and fat" was less desirable in mortality than being "fit and not fat." Thus, the debate continues.

D. C. Nieman, DrPH

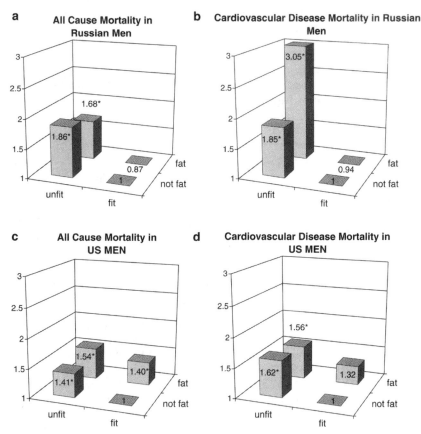

FIGURE 1.—Relative hazard in LRC participants categorized by fitness level (quintile 1 vs 2-5) and BMI (quintiles 1-4 vs 5) adjusted for age, education, smoking, alcohol, and Keys score. * = $P < 0.05$. Hazard ratios were calculated using the fit-not fat group as the reference. Estimates and 95% confidence intervals (CI) for the fit-fat, the unfit-not fat, and the unfit-fat were: all-cause mortality in Russian men, 0.87 (0.55, 1.37), 1.86 (1.31, 2.62), 1.68 (1.06, 2.68); CVD mortality in Russian men, 0.94 (0.49, 1.81), 1.85 (1.09, 3.15), 3.05 (1.74, 5.34); all-cause mortality in US men, 1.40 (1.07, 1.83), 1.41 (1.12, 1.77), 1.54 (1.24, 2.06); CVD mortality in US men, 1.32 (0.85, 2.06), 1.62 (1.01, 2.58), 1.56 (1.08, 2.24). (Courtesy of Steven J, Evenson KR, Thomas O, et al: Associations of fitness and fatness with mortality in Russian and American men in the Lipids Research Clinics study. *Int J Obes* 28:1463-1470, 2004. Copyright 2004 Nature Publishing Group.)

References

1. Lee C, Jackson A, Blair S: US weight guidelines: Is it also important to consider cardiorespiratory fitness? *Int J Obes Relat Metab Disord* 22:2S-7S, 1998.
2. Stevens J, Cai J, Evenson K, et al: Fitness and fatness as predictors of mortality from all causes and from cardiovascular disease in men and women in the Lipid Research Clinics Study. *Am J Epidemiol* 156:832-841, 2002.

Severe Obesity Associated With Cardiovascular Deconditioning, High Prevalence of Cardiovascular Risk Factors, Diabetes Mellitus/Hyperinsulinemia, and Respiratory Compromise

Gidding SS, Nehgme R, Heise C, et al (AI duPont Hosp for Children, Wilmington, Del; Thomas Jefferson Univ, Philadelphia)
J Pediatr 144:766-769, 2004   7–5

Objective.—To determine the extent and severity of obesity-related cardiorespiratory morbidity in children with body mass index (BMI) $\geq$ 40 kg/m^2

Study Design.—Cross-sectional analysis of a cohort comprised of 48 boys and girls aged 8 to 17 years with BMI $\geq$ 40 kg/m^2. Cardiorespiratory fitness (graded cycle exercise test), left ventricular (LV) mass (echocardiography), blood pressure, fasting lipid profile, fasting insulin, fasting glucose, HbA1c, and pulmonary function (spirometry and sleep studies) were measured.

Results.—The cohort averaged 14.2 ± 2 years of age with mean BMI of 45.5 kg/m^2. Only 2 patients had normal fitness; 37 of 48 had peak oxygen consumption < 20 mL O$_2$/minute. Hypertension was present in 10 of 48 patients. Mean lipid values were: triglycerides 103 ± 48 mg/dL, HDL cholesterol 41 ± 10 mg/dL, and LDL cholesterol 108 ± 26 mg/dL. Type II diabetes mellitus was diagnosed in 6 patients. Mean fasting insulin was 31 ± 19 µU/mL. Asthma treatment, small airways disease by pulmonary function testing, or both were present in 35 of 48 patients; upper airway obstruction was present in 7 patients. LV hypertrophy was present in 8 patients, with a mean LV mass of 43 ± 11 g/m$^{2.7}$

Conclusions.—Children and adolescents with BMI $\geq$ 40 kg/m^2 have substantial cardiorespiratory morbidity including severe physical deconditioning.

▶ This is an interesting cross-sectional study of an emerging cohort-severely obese youth. In this group of 48 children and adolescents with an average BMI of 45.5 kg/m^2, cardiorespiratory fitness was extremely low, and dyslipidemia, hyperinsulinemia, elevated blood pressure, and respiratory abnormalities were present in the majority of patients. The authors urge that youth with BMI levels of 40 kg/m^{2}and higher "require a complete cardiac, respiratory, and metabolic workup to identify treatable comorbidities and to initiate individualized treatment programs that include regular exercise and physical activity."

D. C. Nieman, DrPH

Effect of Training Status on Regional Disposal of Circulating Free Fatty Acids in the Liver and Skeletal Muscle During Physiological Hyperinsulinemia

Iozzo P, Takala T, Oikonen V, et al (Univ of Turku, Finland; PET Centre, Pisa, Italy; Univ of Pisa, Italy)
Diabetes Care 27:2172-2177, 2004   7–6

Objective.—Fat metabolism is increasingly implicated in the pathogenesis of type 2 diabetes. Endurance training has been shown to prevent hepatic steatosis and to alter skeletal muscle fat metabolism, and regional free fatty acid (FFA) uptake adaptations were suggested as a mechanism. Thus, we tested whether endurance training modifies the uptake of plasma FFAs occurring in the liver and in skeletal muscle during anabolic, i.e., hyperinsulinemic, conditions.

Research Design and Methods.—Trained and untrained healthy male subjects underwent positron emission tomography scanning of the liver and thigh regions, with the FFA analog $14(R,S)$-$[^{18}F]$fluoro-6-thia-heptadecanoic acid, during euglycemic hyperinsulinemia. Tracer influx rate constants in skeletal muscle (MK_i) and liver (LK_i) were multiplied by plasma FFA levels to obtain FFA uptake for skeletal muscle (MFU) and liver (LFU), respectively.

Results.—Athletes showed increased VO_{2max} ($P < 0.0001$), insulin-mediated glucose disposal (M value, 61 ± 4 vs. 46 ± 3 μmol·min^{-1}·kg^{-1}, $P = 0.01$), and plasma lactate levels during the clamp and lower percentage of body fat mass ($P = 0.002$). MK_i was 25% higher in athletes than in sedentary men ($P = 0.03$). In all subjects, MK_i and MFU were positively correlated with the M value ($r = 0.56$, $P = 0.02$, and $r = 0.51$, $P = 0.03$, respectively) and with plasma lactate levels ($r = 0.63$, $P = 0.006$, and $r = 0.63$, $P = 0.005$, respectively). LK_i was significantly reduced by 20% in the athletes ($P = 0.04$). By multiple regression, LFU was inversely correlated with the two fitness categories ($P = 0.008$), and it was lower in athletes. Linear fitting of liver data showed time consistency, indicating no release of FFAs as a mechanism for the reduced liver retention in athletes.

Conclusions.—We conclude that endurance training promotes insulin-mediated glucose and FFA disposal in skeletal muscle, while lowering hepatic FFA uptake. Such changes may result in a divergent pattern of fat accumulation in the two organs.

▶ Impaired tissue uptake of plasma FFAs is a common finding in patients with impaired glucose tolerance. Other metabolic changes in these patients include raised circulating FFA levels and fat accumulation in nonadipose tissues such as liver and skeletal muscle. It is this latter phenomenon that has been proposed as the key step in the genesis or progression to insulin resistance and type 2 diabetes. This study clearly demonstrates that endurance exercise training (the nature of which was not specified in the report) promotes FFA uptake in skeletal muscle while lowering FFA uptake in the liver. The clinical implications of this suggest that exercise may have an important role in reducing hepatic fat accumulation while improving overall metabolic function in those with or at risk of diabetes.

P. McCrory, MBBS, PhD

Determinants of Fat Oxidation During Exercise in Healthy Men and Women: A Cross-sectional study
Venables MC, Achten J, Jeukendrup AE (Univ of Birmingham, Edgbaston, England)
J Appl Physiol 98:160-167, 2005   7–7

Introduction.—The aim of the present study was to establish fat oxidation rates over a range of exercise intensities in a large group of healthy men and women. It was hypothesised that exercise intensity is of primary importance to the regulation of fat oxidation and that gender, body composition, physical activity level, and training status are secondary and can explain part of the observed interindividual variation. For this purpose, 300 healthy men and women (157 men and 143 women) performed an incremental exercise test to exhaustion on a treadmill [adapted from a previous protocol (Achten J, Venables MC, and Jeukendrup AE. Metabolism 52: 747-752, 2003)]. Substrate oxidation was determined using indirect calorimetry. For each individual, maximal fat oxidation (MFO) and the intensity at which MFO occurred (Fat$_{max}$) were determined. On average, MFO was 7.8 ± 0.13 mg/kg fat-free mass (FFM)/min and occurred at 48.3 ± 0.9% maximal oxygen uptake ($\dot{V}O_{2max}$), equivalent to 61.5 ± 0.6% maximal heart rate. MFO (7.4 ± 0.2 vs. 8.3 ± 0.2 mg·kg/FFM/min; $P < 0.01$) and Fat$_{max}$ (45 ± 1 vs. 52 ± 1% $\dot{V}O_{2max}$; $P < 0.01$) were significantly lower in men compared with women. When corrected for FFM, MFO was predicted by physical activity (self-reported physical activity level), $\dot{V}O_{2max}$, and gender ($R^2 = 0.12$) but not with fat mass. Men compared with women had lower rates of fat oxidation and an earlier shift to using carbohydrate as the dominant fuel. Physical activity, $\dot{V}O_{2max}$, and gender explained only 12% of the interindividual variation in MFO during exercise, whereas body fatness was not a predictor. The interindividual variation in fat oxidation remains largely unexplained.

▶ Fat oxidation during exercise varies widely at set exercise workloads. In this large study of 300 men and women, self-reported physical activity, aerobic fitness ($\dot{V}O_{2max}$), and gender, but not fat mass, explained only 12% of the variation in maximal fat oxidation (0.18-1.01 g/min) during exercise. Thus, this study, along with others, failed to determine what factors explain the large variation in fat oxidation during exercise between individuals. This quest, explained the authors, "is important for the development of interventions allowing effective treatment of conditions in which fat oxidation is disturbed."

D. C. Nieman, DrPH

Validation of the BodyGem™ Hand-held Calorimeter

Melanson EL, Coelho LB, Tran ZV, et al (Univ of Colorado, Denver; HealtheTech Inc, Golden, Colo)
Int J Obes 28:1479-1484, 2004   7–8

Objective.—To assess the validity and reliability of a hand-held indirect calorimeter.

Design.—Resting metabolic rate (RMR) was measured on two separate mornings.

Subjects.—A heterogeneous sample of 41 healthy adults.

Measurements.—RMR using both a metabolic cart (Sensormedics 2900, SM-2900) and a hand-held indirect calorimeter (BodyGem, BG).

Results.—There were no trial-to-trial differences in RMR measured by the BG (6756 ± 163 vs 6697 ± 163 kJ/day) or the SM-2900 (6400 ± 163 vs 6396 ± 167 kJ/day). RMR measured by the BG was significantly higher than that measured by the SM-2900 during both trials. In a sample of 10 subjects, the energy cost of holding the BG in position was determined to be (0.17 ± 0.04 kJ/min, or 255 ± 84 kJ/day). After applying this adjustment, the differences between systems were no longer significant during trial 1 (mean difference = 101 ± 67 kJ/day) or trial 2 (46 ± 75 kJ/day). In overweight and obese individuals, RMR measured by the BodyGem was more accurate than that estimated by the Harris-Benedict equations.

Conclusion.—The BodyGem provides valid and reliable measurements of RMR. The BodyGem produces significantly higher values than the Sensor Medics 2900 indirect calorimeter, with the increase largely due to an increased energy demand required to hold the BG in position.

▶ Several validation studies now show that the BodyGem handheld calorimeter is a valid and precise instrument for measuring RMR in both children and adults.[1,2] The advanced sensor technology in this device has made the measurement of RMR much easier and less costly relative to metabolic carts and Douglas bag systems.

D. C. Nieman, DrPH

References

1. Nieman DC, Trone GA, Austin MD: A new handheld device for measuring resting metabolic rate and oxygen consumption. *J Am Diet Assoc* 103:588-593, 2003.
2. Nieman DC, Austin MD, Chilcote SM, et al: Validation of a new handheld device for measuring resting metabolic rate and oxygen consumption in children. *Int J Sport Nutr Exerc Metab* 14:208-216, 2005.

High Energy Flux Mediates the Tonically Augmented β-Adrenergic Support of Resting Metabolic Rate in Habitually Exercising Older Adults

Bell C, Day DS, Jones PP, et al (Univ of Colorado, Boulder; Colorado State Univ, Fort Collins; Univ of Colorado, Denver)
J Clin Endocrinol Metab 89:3573-3578, 2004   7–9

Background.—As the largest contributing factor in daily energy expenditure, resting metabolic rate (RMR) is an important regulatory factor in energy balance. Low RMR is an independent predictor of future weight gain. It decreases with age in adults, even after correction for changes in fat-free mass. The sympathetic nervous system contributes to RMR by β-adrenergic receptor (β-AR) stimulation of energy metabolism, and RMR and β-AR support of RMR are greater in older adults who habitually exercise compared with sedentary older adults. Whether the source of this support is greater energy flux in habitually exercising older adults was determined.

Methods.—The study group was composed of 22 older adults (12 men and 10 women) aged 60 to 73 years. All the study subjects were determined to be healthy on the basis of history, physical examination, and electrocardiography and blood pressure at rest and during incremental exercise to exhaustion. All the subjects were nonsmokers and nonobese, with stable body mass over the previous 12-month period, and none was taking medication known to alter metabolism or cardiovascular function. Baseline energy flux, a reference to the absolute level of energy intake and expenditure under conditions of energy balance, was measured under conditions of regular daily exercise and usual energy intake determined over a consecutive 4-day period. Dietary intake was assessed from food diaries. The subjects were divided into an experimental group of 15 subjects who had maintained vigorous aerobic physical activity over the previous 2 years and a control group of 7 sedentary subjects. Participants in the experimental group had their energy expenditure and energy intake decreased by abstinence from exercise and feeding from a controlled diet. Data from 5 participants in the experimental group were subsequently excluded from the final analysis.

Results.—The 10 older adults regularly engaging in aerobic endurance exercise, compared with baseline, showed a reduction in energy flux (by abstention of exercise and proportional reduction in dietary intake) and decreased energy expenditure, energy intake, RMR, and skeletal muscle sympathetic nervous system activity. Significant β-AR support of RMR was observed at baseline but not during reduced energy flux. The change in RMR from baseline to reduced energy flux was related to the corresponding change in β-AR support of RMR. No changes were observed in the 7 control subjects who maintained energy flux.

Conclusions.—High energy flux is a vital component of elevated resting metabolic rate and β-AR support of RMR in habitually exercising older adults. The maintenance of high energy flux through regular exercise may be effective in maintaining energy expenditure and preventing age-associated obesity.

▶ These authors studied the augmented β-AR support of resting energy metabolism and determined this is a key contributing factor to the greater resting metabolic rate in older adults who habitually perform aerobic exercise compared with their sedentary peers.

R. C. Cantu, MD, MA

Impact of Self-reported Physical Activity Participation on Proportion of Excess Weight Loss and BMI Among Gastric Bypass Surgery Patients
Bond DS, Evans RK, Wolfe LG, et al (Virginia Commonwealth Univ, Richmond)
Am Surg 70:811-814, 2004   7–10

Background.—The International Obesity Task Force has estimated that 300 million people worldwide are obese. In the United States, the number of persons who are morbidly obese has quadrupled in the past 15 years. Obesity is identified as a significant risk factor, not only for all-cause mortality, but also for diseases such as diabetes mellitus, hypertension, and coronary artery disease. Dietary therapy, physical activity, behavior modification, and pharmacotherapy have been shown to produce modest initial decreases in body mass among obese persons and have been proved to be effective in combination with a comprehensive weight management program. The importance of habitual physical activity for nonsurgical weight loss and weight maintenance among overweight and obese persons has also been well established. Self-reported physical activity in relation to excess weight loss and body mass index (BMI) was investigated in patients who have undergone gastric bypass surgery.

Methods.—Physical activity (PA) participation was measured through self-reporting in 1585 patients who underwent gastric bypass surgery between 1988 and 2001. The patients were assigned to 2 groups, PA (1479 patients) and no PA (106 patients), and further stratified by presurgical BMI ($35\text{-}49$ kg/m^2, 897 patients; $50\text{-}70$ kg/m^2, 688 patients).

Results.—Patients who had undergone gastric bypass surgery and who reported PA participation were younger than those who reported no PA and had greater loss of excess body mass and a greater decrease in BMI (Table 3). Stratification by presurgical BMI showed that only physically active patients in the 50 to 70 kg/m^2 group had an increase in the percent loss of body mass, while both BMI groups had significant reductions in BMI at 2 years compared with patients who were not physically active.

Conclusions.—Physical activity had a beneficial effect on the percentage loss of body mass and BMI among patients who had undergone gastric bypass surgery at 2 years postsurgery. These findings are supportive of the inclusion of habitual physical activity in a comprehensive gastric bypass surgery postsurgical weight maintenance program.

TABLE 3.—Mean Values and Standard Deviations for Excess Weight Loss and Postsurgical Body Mass Index (BMI) Lost Among Self-Reported Physically Active (PA) and Sedentary (S) Gastric Bypass Surgery Patients with Presurgical BMIs of 35-49 kg/m² and 50-70 kg/m²

| | Presurgical BMI (35-49 kg/m²) | | | Presurgical BMI (50-70 kg/m²) | | |
	PA (n = 836)	S (n = 61)	P Value*	PA (n = 643)	S (n = 45)	P Value†
Age at surgery	40.7 ± 9.8	43.7 ± 10.4	0.0222	39.4 ± 3.3	44.8 ± 12.4	0.0005
Presurgical BMI kg/m²	44.5 ± 3.3	43.8 ± 3.3	0.1987	56.7 ± 5.1	57.5 ± 4.7	0.2611
Postsurgical BMI lost	16.0 ± 4.0	14.4 ± 4.0	0.0184	21.5 ± 6.0	19.7 ± 5.5	0.0221
% Excess weight loss	72.1 ± 17.1	68.3 ± 20.0	0.0849	63.2 ± 16.5	57.9 ± 17.3	0.0444

*By ANOVA.
†By ANOVA.
(Courtesy of Bond DS, Evans RK, Wolfe LG, et al: Impact of self-reported physical activity participation on proportion of excess weight loss and BMI among gastric bypass surgery patients. *Am Surg* 70:811-814, 2004.)

▶ The therapeutic value of exercise for obese patients has already received substantial documentation.[1,2] As can be seen from the presurgical BMIs, many of the patients involved in the present study were initially grossly obese. It is not clear how far patients were encouraged to exercise post-surgery. Nevertheless, there is an advantage to those who reported physical activity at any of their office visits when compared to those who did not. This is statistically significant in those with an initial BMI of 50 to 70 kg/m². The results merit repeating with a prospective randomized design.

R. J. Shephard, MD, PhD, DPE

References

1. Jakicic JM: Exercise in the treatment of obesity. *Endocrinol Metab Clin N Am* 32:967-980, 2003.
2. National Institutes of Health, National Heart, Lung, and Blood Institute: Clinical guidelines on the identification and treatment of overweight and obesity in adults—The evidence report. *Obes Res* 6:42S-86S, 1998.

Objective Evaluation of Small Bowel and Colonic Transit Time Using pH Telemetry in Athletes With Gastrointestinal Symptoms

Rao KA, Yazaki E, Evans DF, et al (Queen Mary and Westfield College, London; Barts and London School of Medicine)
Br J Sports Med 38:482-487, 2004   7–11

Introduction.—Long-distance runners, especially women, frequently experience gastrointestinal (GI) disturbances after prolonged high-intensity exercise. The effect of exercise on small bowel and colonic transit time were evaluated under fasted and normal ambulatory conditions to ascertain whether GI disturbances could be linked with alterations in GI motility.

Methods.—Small bowel and colonic transit times were determined with the use of pH telemetry in 11 female athletes 22 to 53 years of age. Six participants had lower GI symptoms during exercise. There were 2 experimen-

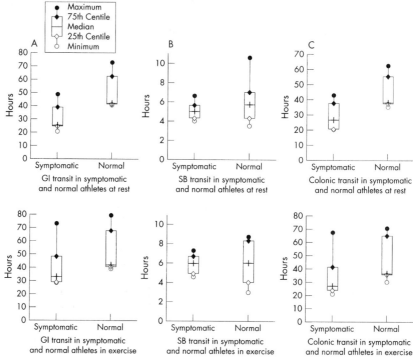

FIGURE 4.—Box and whisker plots of gut transit values during rest sessions (**top panels**) and exercise sessions (**bottom panels**) in symptomatic and control ("normal") athletes. (**A,**) Whole gut (GI) transit. (**B,**) Small bowel (SB) transit. (**C,**) Colonic transit. (Courtesy of Rao KA, Yazaki E, Evans DF, et al: Objective evaluation of small bowel and colonic transit time using pH telemetry in athletes with gastrointestinal symptoms. *Br J Sports Med* 38:482-487, 2004. Reprinted with permission from the BMJ Publishing Group.)

tal conditions: a control measurement in which the small bowel transit time was estimated during a rest period of 6 hours and an exercise session in which the small bowel transit time was determined during a 1-hour period of high intensity exercise (cross-country running) at greater than 70% $\dot{V}O_{2max}$. The colonic transit time was estimated indirectly from determinations of whole gut transit times with the use of a radio-opaque marker.

Results.—The small bowel transit time was 3.5 to 10.6 hours during rest and 3.0 to 8.7 hours during exercise in asymptomatic athletes compared with 4.0 to 6.6 hours during rest and 4.6 to 7.3 hours during exercise in symptomatic athletes (P = NS). The colonic transit time was 35.0 to 62.5 hours during rest and 30.5 to 70.9 hours during exercise in asymptomatic athletes compared with 20.4 to 42.9 hours during rest and 21.5 to 67.2 hours during exercise in symptomatic athletes (P = NS) (Fig 4).

Conclusion.—Small bowel and colonic transit times were similar in the 2 groups during the rest and exercise sessions. The diarrhea experienced by this cohort was not caused by accelerated colonic transit times.

▶ Abdominal cramps and diarrhea can be quite disabling, both for distance runners[1] and for men who have had irradiation of the lower abdomen for prostatic cancer. Moreover, an increase of physical activity is commonly advocated as a treatment for older individuals who have constipation, and hypothetical changes in colonic transit time have been invoked to explain the action of regular exercise in reducing the risk of developing a colonic cancer. However, empirical data concerning the impact of physical exercise on GI transit time are limited and conflicting. Some estimates of transit have been based on determinations of hydrogen in expired air after ingestion of lactulose; such data are a little suspect because this polysaccharide itself alters small bowel transit time.[2] The present study used 2 alternative and possibly more satisfactory approaches to the study of GI motility: radio-opaque markers and pH-sensitive radio-transmitters. No differences in overall transit times were found between those athletes with diarrhea and those who did not experience this problem. Colonic motility was not measured. Thus, a possible basis for the "trots" could be an increase in colonic segmental movement, propelling the intestinal contents into the rectum and causing an urgent need to defecate. Gravitational factors may also be involved, as diarrhea is not experienced by cyclists or swimmers.[3]

R. J. Shephard, MD, PhD, DPE

References

1. Riddoch C, Trinnick T: Gastro-intestinal disturbances in marathon runners. *Br J Sports Med* 22:71-74, 1988.
2. Bond JH, Levitt MD: Investigation of small bowel transit in man using pulmonary (H2) measurements. *J Lab Clin Med* 85:546-555, 1975.
3. Brouns F, Beckers E: Is the gut an athletic organ? Digestion, absorption and exercise. *Sports Med* 15:242-257, 1993.

Can Young Adult Patients With Proteinuric IgA Nephropathy Perform Physical Exercise?
Fuiano G, Mancuso D, Cianfrone P, et al (Univ Magna Graecia, Cantanzaro, Italy; Seconda Università di Napoli, Italy)
Am J Kidney Dis 44:257-263, 2004   7–12

Introduction.—Whether physical exercise increases daily proteinuria in patients with proteinuric nephropathies, therefore accelerating progression of the renal lesion, is not known. The effects of intense physical exercise on proteinuria were examined in young adults with immunoglobulin A (IgA) nephropathy.

Methods.—Changes caused by intense physical exercise on quantitative and qualitative proteinuria were assessed in basal conditions and after 10 days of ramipril therapy in 10 patients with IgA nephropathy, a normal glomerular filtration rate (GFR), proteinuria between 0.8 and 1.49 g every 24 hours, and "glomerular" microhematuria before and after completion of a maximal treadmill Bruce test (B-test). The basal evaluation was also performed in 10 age- and gender-matched healthy participants.

Results.—At rest, the GFR averaged 141 mL/min; it rose by 16.3% ($P <$ .005) and 7.1% at 60 and 120 minutes after the B-test, respectively. GFR-corrected proteinuria changed significantly during the test: urinary protein excretion averaged 0.76 mg/min per 100 mL GFR at rest; it rose to 1.55 mg/min per 100 mL GFR after 60 minutes ($P <$ .001) and diminished to 0.60 mg/min per 100 mL GFR at 120 minutes after completion of the B-test (Fig 1). The pattern of urinary proteins and microhematuria remained the same. Daily proteinuria did not vary from the basal value of the day of the B-test. After ramipril therapy, patients demonstrated a decrease in GFR but no

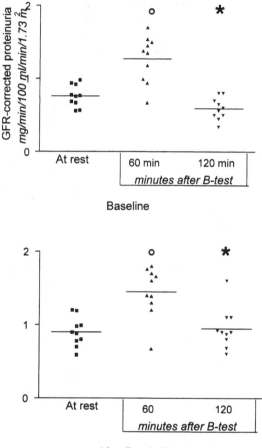

FIGURE 1.—GFR-corrected proteinuria at rest and 60 and 120 minutes after the end of physical exercise with and without ramipril. *Circles,* $P <$.05 versus basal proteinuria; *$P <$ .001 versus 60-minute proteinuria. *Abbreviations:* GFR, Glomerular filtration rate; B-test, Bruce treadmill test. (Courtesy of Fuiano G, Mancuso D, Cianfrone P, et al: Can young adult patients with proteinuric IgA nephropathy perform physical exercise? *Am J Kidney Dis* 44:257-263, 2004. Copyright National Kidney Foundation.)

change in daily GFR-corrected proteinuria, the pattern of urinary proteins, or hematuria.

Conclusion.—The increase in proteinuria after exercise was significant and lasted less than 120 minutes. It was not prevented by ramipril therapy. Decreasing intense physical activity in patients with nonnephrotic renal diseases does not seem to be necessary.

▶ Vigorous exercise causes marked proteinuria, even in healthy individuals.[1] Further, the rate of progression of some forms of renal disease is hastened by the reabsorption of glomerular filtered protein,[2]; thus, one might wonder about the wisdom of advocating exercise programs to those with renal disease. The study of Fuiano and colleagues suggests that the prognosis was not worsened in patients with nonnephrotic disease who adopted a physically active lifestyle, possibly because the exercise-induced proteinuria was of short duration. However, the follow-up period averaged only 14 months, and more longterm observations are needed before we can be entirely confident on this point.

R. J. Shephard, MD, PhD, DPE

References

1. Poortmans JR, Haggenmacher C, Vanderstraeten J: Postexercise proteinuria in humans and its adrenergic component. *J Sports Med Phys Fitness* 41:95-100, 2001.
2. Ruggenenti P, Remuzzi G: The role of protein traffic in the progression of renal disease. *Annu Rev Med* 51:315-327, 2000.

Sperm Characteristics of Endurance Trained Cyclists
Gebreegziabher Y, Marcos E, McKinon W, et al (Univ of Witwatersrand Med School, Parktown, South Africa)
Int J Sports Med 25:247-251, 2004   7–13

Background.—It has been well documented that exercise can be associated with menstrual cycle abnormalities in women. However, the effects of exercise on male reproductive functioning have not been as thoroughly investigated. Among the changes in the reproductive hormone profile associated with endurance exercise training is a reduction in total and free testosterone levels, changes in the pituitary pulsatile release of luteinizing hormone, and changes in pituitary hormone release in response to gonadotropin-releasing hormone. In addition, advances in andrology have suggested that prolonged exercise is one of the factors that negatively affect male fertility. The influence of cycling on sperm characteristics was evaluated in male endurance cyclists.

Methods.—The study group was composed of 10 long-distance competitive cyclists (median age, 25.5 years) and 10 sedentary control subjects (median age, 24.5 years). A questionnaire was used to obtain a history of training, health, nutrition, and life style. Semen analysis included a detailed

TABLE 3.—The Percentage of Spermatozoa With Different Morphological Features in the 2 Groups (Median, First, and Third Quartiles in Parentheses)

Sperm Morphology	Control ($n = 10$) (%)	Cyclists ($n = 10$) (%)	Group Difference
Normal	41.5 (34.8, 55.3)	19.5 (18.3, 30.8)	p<0.01
Tapered	4.5 (3.3, 6.0)	22.5 (13.3, 35.3)	p<0.01
Small acrosome	17.5 (8.0, 22.0)	15.0 (9.0, 19.8)	p>0.05
Double head	1.0 (0.0, 1.8)	0 (0, 0)	p>0.05
Immature forms	2.5 (0.3, 4.8)	1.0 (1.0, 5.5)	p>0.05
Other forms	0.0 (0.0, 0.8)	0 (0, 0)	p>0.05

(Courtesy of Gebreegziabher Y, Marcos E, McKinon W, et al: Sperm characteristics of endurance trained cyclists. *Int J Sports Med* 25:247-251, 2004. Copyright Georg Thieme Verlag.)

evaluation of sperm characteristics, including semen volume, sperm count, viability, motility, and morphological features.

Results.—In comparison with control subjects, the cyclists had a significantly lower proportion of spermatozoa with normal morphological features (median, 41.5% vs 19.5%) and a significantly higher proportion of morphologically abnormal tapered forms (median, 4.5% vs 22.5%) (Table 3). No significant differences were found between the 2 groups in semen volume or sperm motility, viability, and count.

Conclusions.—Endurance cycling seems to be associated with a significant alteration in sperm morphological features.

▶ Various factors could impair sperm functioning in long-distance cyclists, including the generally accepted decline in their testosterone levels,[1] the development of a negative energy balance,[2] substantial increases of body temperature during competition,[3] and mechanical trauma to the testes and their circulation. The changes in sperm morphological features observed in this article are at variance with earlier findings in 1 sample of professional cyclists.[4] It is unlikely that the amateurs engage in a greater volume of exercise, but, possibly, because of lower skill levels, they may subject their testes to greater mechanical trauma. Further studies seem warranted to determine whether the changes in morphological features are sufficient to have adverse consequences on the long-term fertility of cyclists.

R. J. Shephard, MD, PhD, DPE

References

1. Hacknet AC, Sinning WE, Bruot BC: Hypothalamic–pituitary–testicular axis function in endurance-trained males. *Int J Sports Med* 11:298-303, 1990.
2. Roberts AC, McClure RD, Weiner RI, et al: Overtraining affects male reproductive status. *Fertil Steril* 60:686-692, 1993.
3. Dewasness G, Botherell B, Hsuing K, et al: Human scrotal temperature during heat exposure associated with passive leg heating, in Zomgniottie AW (ed): *Temperature and Environmental Effects on the Testis*. New York, Plenum Press, 1991, pp 184-191.
4. Lucia A, Chicharro JL, Perez M, et al: Reproductive function in male endurance athletes: Sperm analysis and hormonal profile. *J Appl Physiol* 81:2627-2636, 1996.

A Clone of Methicillin-Resistant *Staphylococcus aureus* Among Professional Football Players

Kazakova SV, Hageman JC, Matava M, et al (Washington Univ, St Louis; BJC Med Group, St Louis; St Louis Rams Professional Football Team; et al)
N Engl J Med 352:468-475, 2005   7–14

Background.—Methicillin-resistant *Staphylococcus aureus* (MRSA) is an emerging cause of infections outside of health care settings. We investigated an outbreak of abscesses due to MRSA among members of a professional football team and examined the transmission and microbiologic characteristics of the outbreak strain.

Methods.—We conducted a retrospective cohort study and nasal-swab survey of 84 St. Louis Rams football players and staff members. *S. aureus* recovered from wound, nasal, and environmental cultures was analyzed by means of pulsed-field gel electrophoresis (PFGE) and typing for resistance and toxin genes. MRSA from the team was compared with other community isolates and hospital isolates.

Results.—During the 2003 football season, eight MRSA infections occurred among 5 of the 58 Rams players (9 percent); all of the infections developed at turf-abrasion sites. MRSA infection was significantly associated with the lineman or linebacker position and a higher body-mass index. No MRSA was found in nasal or environmental samples; however, methicillin-susceptible S. aureus was recovered from whirlpools and taping gel and from 35 of the 84 nasal swabs from players and staff members (42 percent). MRSA from a competing football team and from other community clusters and sporadic cases had PFGE patterns that were indistinguishable from those of the Rams' MRSA; all carried the gene for Panton-Valentine leukocidin and the gene complex for staphylococcal-cassette-chromosome mec type IVa resistance (clone USA300-0114).

Conclusions.—We describe a highly conserved, community-associated MRSA clone that caused abscesses among professional football players and that was indistinguishable from isolates from various other regions of the United States.

▶ MRSA has become a major problem in many North American hospitals, probably, in part, because of an unwise prescription of antibiotics. It is disturbing to read that antibiotic prescription for this group of football players was at 10 times the already excessive rate found in the general population. The patients most vulnerable to MRSA are those whose immune system has been compromised by old age or HIV infections. The transient immunosuppression associated with a bout of very strenuous exercise[1] may possibly have a similar effect upon the susceptibility of football players to MRSA. The strain of *Staphylococcus* detected in this report differed from that rampant in many hospitals. Disturbing features of the report are the high prevalence of carriers among apparently healthy people and the ability to transmit infection through such places as whirlpools. Factors contributing to the spread of infection seem to have included a lack of elementary hygiene (failure to shower before using whirlpools, and a lack of adequate hand hygiene by trainers treating the players). Precautions to reduce future infections include a tightening of hygiene recommendations, the treatment of known infections under isolated conditions, and the careful testing of microbial sensitivity in infected areas of skin before beginning the administration of antibiotics.

R. J. Shephard, MD, PhD, DPE

Reference

1. Shephard RJ: *Physical Activity, Training and the Immune Response*, Carmel, Ind, Cooper Publications, 1997.

Athletic Skin Injuries: Combating Pressure and Friction
Basler RSW, Hunzeker CM, Garcia MA (Univ of Nebraska, Omaha; Mercy Hosp, Pittsburgh, Pa)
Physician Sportsmed 32(5):33-40, 2004   7–15

Introduction.—Most of the skin problems that occur due to sports participation are caused by friction or pressure. Sports medicine physicians who regularly treat skin injuries can speed healing through a timely diagnosis, recommending effective treatment, and teaching prevention strategies. Common skin conditions treated by sports physicians were discussed.

Abrasions.—These lesion should initially be treated by flushing the wound and application of a hydrocolloid or semiocclusive hydrogel dressing. Prevention involves the use of protective equipment.

Chafing.—Treatment with lubricating ointment or 1% or 2.5% hydrocortisone ointment frequently relieves symptoms and helps prevent further chafing. Although annoying, chafing rarely necessitates modifying a training or competition schedule. The use of elasticized fabric or protective tape may be used to prevent chafing.

Calluses.—Asymptomatic calluses usually do not need treatment. A scalpel may be used for paring away the thickened skin. Use of a file, rasp, or pumice stone after soaking are also effective. Prevention involves properly fitting equipment or use of padding.

Blisters.—Small blisters do not require treatment. Large blisters should be drained and covered with a membrane to protect against additional friction. Prevention involves decreasing moisture and friction applied to the skin by gradually increasing the intensity of ones exercise regimen. Well-fitting shoes and acrylic socks can decrease friction and wick away perspiration.

Talon Noir.—This self-limited condition will resolve spontaneously over time. It does not impair athletic performance. For patients who seek medical attention, a scalpel can be used to gently pare the horny layer of affected skin to demonstrate to the patient that the black color is merely surface pigment.

Acne Mechanica.—Pressure, occlusion, and heat—common elements seen in friction—seem to be nearly universal under athletic apparel ranging from leotards to football helmets. The condition seems to be particularly prevalent among football players. Wearing a T-shirt under shoulder pads or leotards helps diminish all contributing factors. Especially helpful is removing sports apparel and showering.

Conclusion.—Well-informed sports medicine practitioners are as important in the care of cutaneous injuries as in other medical conditions. Most skin problems caused by the effects of friction and pressure can be prevented by thoughtful planning and preparation.

▶ These authors look at common skin conditions in athletes such as abrasions, chafing, calluses, blisters, talon noir, and acne mechanica. They find that timely diagnosis and effective treatment, as well as preventive measures, can speed healing of these common skin irritations caused by the pressure and friction of the specific sport.

R. C. Cantu, MD, MA

Dermatological Marks in Athletes of Artistic and Rhythmic Gymnastics
Biolcati G, Berlutti G, Bagarone A, et al (S Gallicano Dermatological Inst–IRCCS, Rome; Sport Sciences Inst, Rome)
Int J Sports Med 25:638-640, 2004   7–16

Introduction.—The authors present dermatological signs in: a) rhythmic gymnastics athletes, b) male artistic gymnastics athletes, compared to a control group of fitness athletes. Athletes from the artistic gymnastics group were observed twice. The signs they showed on their first examination (20 days previous to the competition) were two circular zones of thickening of the skin with relation to the radial epiphysis. In all of them, two zones of frictional alopecia were present, one on the dorsal face of the forearms, slantwise outlined, the other on the wrists. A noticeable thickening of the skin was present on the palms of the hands. On a second examination, at the beginning of the training, after about two months of inactivity, the alopecic area was replaced by hypertrichosis, although featuring different patterns in each athlete. Thickening of the skin was slightly smaller than that observed at the first examination. The authors describe onychopathology shown in its different forms in 94% of the athletes of the rhythmic group. Subsequently the authors discuss the pathogenesis of the above described signs.

▶ The skin and nail changes seen in gymnasts may be of interest to dermatologists; however, this study has little impact for most clinicians who work with gymnastic athletes. In rhythmic gymnastics, nail changes in the great toe and thickening of the skin on the upper aspect were common, which is in keeping with the nature of the foot movements when training on mats. In artistic gymnastics, alterations in forearm hair patterns and thickening of the skin over the radial epiphysis were the common features and once again reflect the likely sites of trauma when competing on parallel bars, pommel horse, rings, and high bar. The only surprising finding was that 94% of rhythmic gymnasts had fungal infections in skin of the big toe.

P. McCrory, MBBS, PhD

Diclofenac Patch for Topical Treatment of Acute Impact Injuries: A Randomised, Double Blind, Placebo Controlled, Multicentre Study

Predel HG, Koll R, Pabst H, et al (Deutsche Sporthochschule Cologne, Germany; Sports Medicine, Bergisch Gladbach, Germany; Sports Medicine, Grünwald, Germany; et al)
Br J Sports Med 38:318-323, 2004   7–17

Introduction.—Sports injuries need rapid treatment to relieve acute pain and decrease swelling in the injured area and to restore normal movement. A newly developed diclofenac patch formulation, containing 140 mg diclofenac sodium on an area of 140 cm^2, may fulfill these criteria. The clinical efficacy and safety of the recently developed diclofenac patch in the topical treatment of blunt impact injuries were examined in a placebo-controlled, double-blind, multicenter trial of 120 patients with traumatic blunt soft tissue injury.

Methods.—Within 3 hours of injury, participants of sports competitions and training camps were enrolled and treated daily with either the diclofenac or a placebo patch during a 7-day period. Participants were randomly assigned in 1:1 fashion to 2 parallel groups. Tenderness caused by pressure was defined as the amount of pressure (determined by a calibrated caliper at the center of the injury) that initially produced a pain reaction, as reported by the patient.

Results.—The primary efficacy variable was the area under the curve for tenderness during the first 3 days. The diclofenac patch was significantly more effective compared to placebo ($P < .0001$). The treatment effect was 64.7 kp h/cm^2 (95% confidence interval, 48.7-80.9) between diclofenac and placebo patches. These outcomes were supported by all secondary efficacy variables.

The diclofenac patch provided rapid pain relief, as reflected by the time to achieve resolution of pain at the injured site. This was significantly shorter with the diclofenac compared to placebo ($P < .0001$). Treatment with the diclofenac patch was well tolerated. The most commonly observed adverse events were local cutaneous adverse reactions (pruritis, rash) of minor severity that occurred with the same frequency as in control subjects.

Conclusion.—The newly developed diclofenac patch is effective and safe in the treatment of blunt impact injuries.

▶ This is a study of a new diclofenac patch for use in treatment of impact injuries. One hundred twenty patients were studied for efficacy as well as safety of this new product. The authors determined this is a safe and effective treatment for pain of blunt impact injuries.

R. C. Cantu, MD, MA

Case-Control Study of Lifetime Total Physical Activity and Prostate Cancer Risk

Friedenreich CM, McGregor SE, Courneya KS, et al (Alberta Cancer Board, Calgary, Alta, Canada; Univ of Alberta, Edmonton, Canada; Tom Baker Cancer Centre, Calgary, Alta, Canada; et al)
Am J Epidemiol 159:740-749, 2004   7–18

Background.—Physical activity may be inversely associated with prostate cancer risk. However, previous research on this possibility has yielded inconsistent results. A case-control study of lifetime total physical activity and prostate cancer risk was reported.

Methods.—Nine hundred eighty-eight patients with incident, histologically confirmed stage T2 or greater prostate cancer between 1997 and 2000 were frequency matched to 1063 population control subjects in Alberta, Canada. Occupational, household, and recreational activity levels from childhood until diagnosis were measured by means of the Lifetime Total Physical Activity Questionnaire.

Findings.—Total lifetime physical activity was not associated with prostate cancer risk. By activity type, risks were reduced for occupational and recreational activity, with odds ratios of 0.90 and 0.80, respectively, but increased for household activity (at 1.36) when the highest and lowest quartiles were compared. Activity in the first 18 years of life reduced the risk (odds ratio, 0.78). When activity intensity was compared, vigorous activity was found to reduce prostate cancer risk, with an odds ratio of 0.70 (Table 5).

Conclusion.—Overall, there was no correlation between total lifetime physical activity and prostate cancer risk. However, decreases in risk were observed for recreational activity, activity early and possibly also later in life, vigorous activity, and occupational activity when only duration and frequency were assessed.

▶ There is good evidence that regular physical activity offers protection against the development of certain forms of cancer, particularly tumors of the descending colon.[1,2] However, opinions about protection against prostatic cancer have been quite divergent. Some studies even find an increase of risk among physically active individuals.

The report of Friedenreich et al is based on a relatively large case-control study. Lifetime physical activity was assessed by a questionnaire of known reliability that had proven effective in a study of breast cancer. Multivariate analysis suggested benefit from both occupational and leisure activity but not from household activity, particularly if the activity was undertaken before 18 years of age. There are several plausible mechanisms that could account for the beneficial effects on the prostate, including depression of androgen levels, decrease in body fat, enhancement of immune function, and development of antioxidant defenses.[3]

R. J. Shephard, MD, PhD, DPE

TABLE 5.—Odds Ratios for Lifetime Physical Activity by Intensity of Activity

Hours/Week/Year Performed at Activity Intensity Level	Cases (no.) (n = 988)	Controls (no.) (n = 1,063)	Age Adjusted		Multivariable Adjusted*	
			OR	95% CI	OR	95% CI
Low intensity activity (<3 metabolic equivalent-hours/week/year)						
0-<5.85	262	266	1.0		1.0	
≥5.85-<17.5	277	266	0.96	0.75, 1.24	0.99	0.76, 1.29
≥17.5-<26.6	232	265	0.81	0.59, 1.10	0.81	0.58, 1.12
≥26.6	217	266	0.79	0.57, 1.11	0.83	0.58, 1.18
P_{trend}				0.40		0.44
Moderate intensity activity (3-6 metabolic equivalent-hours/week/year)						
0-<9.81	195	266	1.0		1.0	
≥9.81-<19.5	271	266	1.37	1.05, 1.77	1.32	1.00, 1.72
≥19.5-<32.4	285	265	1.30	0.97, 1.74	1.21	0.89, 1.65
≥32.4	237	266	0.97	0.69, 1.36	0.88	0.61, 1.26
P_{trend}				0.96		0.57
Vigorous intensity activity (>6 metabolic equivalent-hours/week/year)						
0-<0.48	275	266	1.0		1.0	
≥0.48-<1.63	228	266	0.86	0.67, 1.11	0.83	0.64, 1.07
≥1.63-<4.83	242	266	0.92	0.72, 1.17	0.88	0.68, 1.14
≥4.83	243	265	0.79	0.61, 1.03	0.70	0.54, 0.92
P_{trend}				0.62		0.64

Note: Participants included 988 cases and 1063 control subjects.

* Adjusted for age, region (4 urban vs rural areas in Alberta), education (highest level of education achieved), body mass index, waist/hip ratio, total caloric intake, average lifetime total alcohol intake, first degree family history of prostate cancer, number of times had prostate-specific antigen test done, and number of digital rectal examinations. Models for each level of intensity of activity were adjusted for the other levels of intensity of activity.

Abbreviations: OR, Odds ratio; CI, confidence interval.

(Courtesy of Friedenreich CM, McGregor SE, Courneya KS, et al: Case-control study of lifetime total physical activity and prostate cancer risk. *Am J Epidemiol* 159:740-749, 2004. Reprinted by permission of Oxford University Press.)

References

1. Shephard RJ, Futcher R: Physical activity and cancer: How may protection be maximized? *Crit Rev Oncog* 8:219-272, 1997.
2. Marrett LD, Theis B, Ashbury F, et al: Workshop report: Physical activity and cancer prevention. *Chronic Dis Can* 21:143-149, 2000.
3. Friedenreich CM, Thune I: A review of physical activity and prostate cancer risk. *Cancer Causes Control* 12:461-475, 2001.

Complex Regional Pain Syndrome: Redefining Reflex Sympathetic Dystrophy and Causalgia
Hayek SM, Mekhail NA (Cleveland Clinic Found, Ohio)
Physician Sportsmed 32(5):18-25, 2004   7–19

Background.—The sympathetic nervous system has a critical role in the protective and adaptive reflexes and adjustments in response to acute stress and impending pain. However, only within the last 50 years has the role of the sympathetic nervous system in the generation and maintenance of pain states been recognized. A considerable amount of research has been done in this area, and yet the exact mechanisms underlying pain syndromes with sympathetic nervous system involvement have not been elucidated. The term complex regional pain syndrome (CRPS) has been proposed to replace the old names (reflex sympathetic dystrophy, causalgia). This syndrome was defined and the findings of new studies reviewed that have provided insight into the contribution of the sympathetic nervous system to CRPS.

Overview.—CRPS is subdivided into types 1 and 2, with type 1 encompassing what was formerly referred to as reflex sympathetic dystrophy and type 2 encompassing causalgia as well as posttraumatic neuralgias. Unlike CRPS type 1, CRPS type 2 occurs after an injury to a specific nerve. In most cases of CRPS, an extremity is affected, but it may occur elsewhere in the body. CRPS has also been described in children, in whom the prognosis is more favorable. Most patients with CRPS have a history of soft tissue, bone, or nervous system trauma. The clinical signs of CRPS type 1 are variable, but the characteristic triad of signs and symptoms includes sensory abnormalities and autonomic and motor disturbances. These signs and symptoms may be present in varying combinations and intensities, depending on the severity and duration of the disorder. Pain after trauma that persists beyond the anticipated normal healing process is an early warning sign of type 1, and spontaneous burning pain and pain on light mechanical stimulation are prominent signs. Pain is usually not limited to the distribution of a specific peripheral nerve, and symptoms of CRPS often extend beyond the involved extremity. Dystonia affecting movement of the distal extremity is often noticed in patients with type 1, as is altered skin temperature in the hyperanalgesic region. Several modalities can be used to differentiate other disorders from CRPS, including thermography, triple-phase bone scan, quantitative sensory testing, and sympathetic blockade. Management is accomplished by providing physical therapy and rehabilitation; addressing psychological factors; and using adjuvant medications, sympathetic blockade, continuous infusion of drugs, and peripheral nerve stimulation.

Conclusions.—The International Association for the Study of Pain has proposed the term CRPS as a replacement for the terms reflex sympathetic dystrophy and causalgia. New studies of this syndrome have provided insight into the contribution of the sympathetic nervous system and have facilitated the reevaluation of the clinical features, diagnostic criteria, testing methods, and treatment of this syndrome.

▶ These authors discuss this new nomenclature for the previously defined reflex sympathetic dystrophy and causalgia. They describe symptoms and treatment for this pain syndrome.

R. C. Cantu, MD, MA

Kinesiophobia in Chronic Fatigue Syndrome: Assessment and Associations With Disability
Nijs J, De Meirleir K, Duquet W (Vrije Universiteit Brussel, Belgium)
Arch Phys Med Rehabil 85:1586-1592, 2004   7–20

Background.—Chronic fatigue syndrome (CFS) is a debilitating disease of unknown origin. Patients with CFS typically experience worsening of symptoms after previously well-tolerated levels of exercise. It has been speculated that avoidance of activity perpetuates the condition causing greater disability and providing a rationale for the incorporation of graded exercise and a cognitive behavioral approach to the management of CFS. The validity of the total scores of the Tampa Scale for Kinesiophobia (TSK), Dutch version, which was modified to allow its use in the assessment of the fear of movement (kinesiophobia) in patients with CFS (TSK-CFS) was investigated. This assessment tool was used to examine the associations between kinesiophobia, exercise capacity, and activity limitations and participation restrictions in patients with CFS.

Methods.—These prospective observational studies were conducted in an outpatient fatigue clinic. The first study was conducted in 40 patients who met the 1994 US Centers for Disease Control and Prevention (CDC) criteria for CFS. The study group for the second study was comprised of 51 CDC-defined patients with CFS. The main outcome measure in the first study was a series of questionnaires to assess physical activity and coping in patients with CFS, including the Dutch TSK-CFS. In the second study, all the patients answered 2 questionnaires and performed a maximal exercise stress test on a cycle ergometer. The heart rate was monitored continuously with an electrocardiograph. Spirometry was used to measure metabolic and ventilatory parameters.

Results.—In the first study, the Cronbach α coefficient for the individual item scores on the TSK-CFS was .80. The total scores on the Dutch TSK-CFS were indicative of a statistically significant correlation with both the avoidance/abide subscale of the Utrechtse Coping List and the total score of the

TABLE 2.—Correlation Analysis Between the Dutch TSK-CFS Scores and the Disability Parameters (n = 51)

	p Dutch TSK-CFS*	P Value†
CFS-APQ1‡	.39	.00*
CFS-APQ2§	.44	.00*
Illness duration	.02	.92
Exercise duration (min)	−.09	.55
HRpeak (bpm)	−.15	.29
Workload (W)	−.10	.51
Workload per body weight (w/kg)	−.09	.53
Vo₂peak (L/min)	−.07	.62
Vo₂peak/body weight (mL·kg⁻¹·min⁻¹)	−.10	.50
% functional aerobic impairment	.04	.76
RQpeak	−.03	.85
%THR	−.14	.33

*Total scores on the Dutch TSK-CFS range between 17 and 68; higher scores indicate a higher degree of kinesiophobia.
†Significant at .01.
‡A CFS-APQ1 score of 1 indicates no activity limitations or participation restrictions; 16 represents the maximum score.
§The CFS-APQ2 scores range between 1 and 4.
(Reprinted from Nijs J, De Meirleir K, Duquet W: Kinesiophobia in chronic fatigue syndrome: Assessment and associations with disability. *Arch Phys Med Rehabil* 85:1586-1592, 2004. Copyright 2004 with permission from The American Congress of Rehabilitation Medicine and the American Academy of Physical Medicine and Rehabilitation.)

Baecke Questionnaire. In the second study, the total scores on the Dutch TSK-CFS indicated a statistically significant correlation with the total scores on the CFE Activities and Participation Questionnaire (CFS-APQ). There were no statistically significant associations between the exercise capacity parameters and the total scores on the Dutch TSK-CFS (Table 2).

Conclusions.—These findings are supportive of the internal consistency and convergent and congruent validity of the scores obtained by use of the Dutch TSK-CFS. Kinesiophobia is apparently associated with activity limitations and participation restrictions but not with exercise capacity in patients with CFS.

▶ At least 1 previous report has suggested that exercise avoidance contributes to the progressive deterioration of function in CFS.[1] The criterion of avoidance behavior adopted in this study was a failure to reach 85% of the age-predicted maximal heart rate during a progressive cycle ergometer test. Another team of investigators noted that only 41% of their sample of CFS patients met the 85% predicted heart rate criterion.[2] Some avoidance scales use the word "pain" frequently, and in the current questionnaire the word "pain" was systematically replaced by "symptoms," in an attempt to give an avoidance score that was specific to CFS. A negative correlation was found between habitual physical activity and the avoidance score thus obtained; this seems logical, but the lack of correlation between the avoidance score and peak working capacity is surprising. Possibly, the range of peak oxygen consumptions was sufficiently wide and inconsistent (range, 6.6-31.8 mL/[kg·min]) that correlations were obscured by the variability in the data. The findings tend to support other recent reports, namely, that CFS patients should be treated by progressive exercise and therapy to reduce avoidance behavior. However, Nijs et al caution that such treatment may augment complement activation, an immune parameter sometimes associated with the severity of symptoms postexercise.[3] More work is thus needed on the long-term effectiveness of a progressive training regimen in CFS.

R. J. Shephard, MD, PhD, DPE

References

1. Fischler B, Dendale P, Michiels V, et al: Physical fatigability and exercise capacity in chronic fatigue syndrome: Association with disability, somatization and psychopathology. *J Psychosom Res* 42:369-378, 1997.
2. De Becker P, Roeykens J, Reynders M, et al: Exercise capacity in chronic fatigue syndrome. *Arch Intern Med* 160:3270-3277, 2000.
3. Sorensen B, Streib JE, Strand M, et al: Complement activation in a model of chronic fatigue syndrome. *J Allergy Clin Immunol* 112:397-403, 2003.

Physiological Responses During a Submaximal Cycle Test in Chronic Fatigue Syndrome
Wallman KE, Morton AR, Goodman C, et al (Univ of Western Australia, Crawely)
Med Sci Sports Exerc 36:1682-1688, 2004   7–21

Background.—Chronic fatigue syndrome (CFS) is a debilitating disorder, without known etiology or cure, whose primary symptom is debilitating fatigue. The physical functioning of patients with CFS was compared with that of healthy control subjects matched for gender, age, height, body mass and current physical activity levels.

Methods.—The study included 31 adult patients with CFS, as defined by Fukuda et al, matched to 31 healthy control subjects. Physical functioning was evaluated during a 1-week period, using a submaximal exercise test, the aerobic power index.

Results.—The averaged absolute values for heart rate (HR), oxygen intake and respiratory exchange ratio were not significantly different between the 2 groups. The only variable that was significantly different between the CFS patients and the healthy control subjects was the rating of perceived effort (RPE). RPE scores were significantly higher for patients with CFS for each level of work analyzed. The healthy control subjects were capable of greater power output than the CFS patients, as demonstrated by significantly higher end point scores for watts/kg, net lactate production, oxygen intake, respiratory exchange ratio, and HR values.

Conclusions.—Physiologic values recorded after submaximal exercise testing were similar for patients with CFS and healthy, matched control subjects; however, those with CFS rated perceived effort as higher. It is proposed that the reduced exercise tolerance associated with CFS can be attributed to an abnormal sense of effort and avoidance behaviors associated with a fear of relapse.

▶ This article is interesting in that care was taken to match CFS patients with control subjects who had an equally sedentary lifestyle, as assessed by the Exercise Status Inventory.[1] The patients were defined using the standard criteria of Fukuda and associates,[2] an important precaution in the poorly defined CFS. The only abnormality detected in the CFS patients at any given level of submaximal exercise was an increased rating of perceived exertion, suggesting that many manifestations of the syndrome arise from avoidance behavior and a fear of exacerbating symptoms.[3]

R. J. Shephard, MD, PhD, DPE

References

1. O'Brien-Cousins, S: An older adult exercise status inventory: Reliability and validity. *J Sport Behav* 19:288-302, 1996.
2. Fukuda K, Straus S, Hickie I, et al: The chronic fatigue syndrome: A comprehensive approach to its definition and study. *Ann Intern Med* 121:953-959, 1994.
3. Silver A, Haeney P, Vijayadurai D, et al: The role of fear of physical movement and activity in chronic fatigue syndrome. *J Psychosom Res* 52:485-493, 2001.

Randomised Controlled Trial of Graded Exercise in Chronic Fatigue Syndrome
Wallman KE, Morton AR, Goodman C, et al (Univ of Western Australia, Perth; Edith Cowan Univ, Perth, Western Australia)
Med J Aust 180:444-448, 2004   7–22

Introduction.—Maximal oxygen intake is the gold standard for determining cardiopulmonary functioning. Questions have been raised concerning the suitability of using an exercise test that necessitates maximal effort from individuals with debilitating fatigue, especially when this fatigue is exacerbated by physical activity. No trial has yet evaluated the effects of graded exercise on cognitive functioning in patients with chronic fatigue syndrome (CFS). Whether 12 weeks of graded exercise with pacing would improve specific physiologic, psychological, and cognitive functions in patients with CFS was determined in a randomized controlled trial.

Methods.—A total of 61 study participants (age range, 16-74 years) were randomly assigned to either graded exercise with pacing or relaxation–flexibility therapy performed twice daily for 12 weeks. The primary outcome measure was a change in any of the physiologic, psychological, or cognitive variables evaluated.

Results.—After 12 weeks of participation in a graded exercise intervention, scores were improved for resting systolic blood pressure ($P = .018$), work capacity ($P = .019$), net blood lactate production ($P = .036$), depression ($P = .027$), and performance on a modified Stroop Color Word test ($P = .029$). Ratings of perceived exertion scores, associated with an exercise test,

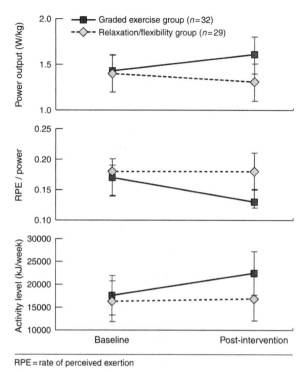

RPE = rate of perceived exertion

FIGURE 2.—Changes (95% CIs) in selected physiologic variables. *Abbreviation: RPE*, Rate of perceived exertion. (Courtesy of Wallman KE, Morton AR, Goodman C, et al: Randomized controlled trial of graded exercise in chronic fatigue syndrome. *Med J Aust* 180:444-448, 2004. Copyright 2004, the Medical Journal of Australia. Reproduced with permission.)

were lower after graded exercise ($P = .013$) (Fig 2). None of these changes were seen in the relaxation–flexibility group.

Conclusion.—Graded exercise was linked with improvements in physical work capacity and specific psychological and cognitive variables. Improvements may be linked with abandonment of avoidance behaviors.

► This article reports a substantial randomized controlled trial of graded exercise in the treatment of CFS. The symptoms of CFS are rather vague,[1] but all participants in the trial were required to meet the diagnostic criteria of Fukuda and associates.[2] The experimental design has the additional merit that the control group received an attentional placebo treatment (relaxation–flexibility training). The exercise group performed quite mild bouts of activity, beginning with 5 to 15 minutes every second day, progressing as fast as possible, but stopping at the sign of any relapse. Despite the moderate nature of this regimen, the individual's peak power output increased by some 10% over a 12-week period. On most physiologic and psychological tests, the exercise group fared better than did the controls, although the magnitude of the placebo effect is shown by the self-reported, improved clinical condition in most members of both treatment groups (29/32 vs 22/29). From an ethical perspective, it is unclear whether the placebo group was later given the option of participating in an equivalent exercise program, as most committees on human experimentation would now require.

R. J. Shephard, MD, PhD, DPE

References

1. Shephard RJ: Chronic fatigue syndrome: An update. *Sports Med* 31:167-194, 2001.
2. Fukuda K, Strauss S, Hickie I, et al: The chronic fatigue syndrome: A comprehensive approach to its definition and study. *Ann Intern Med* 121:953-959, 1994.

Exercise and Multiple Sclerosis
White LJ, Dressendorfer RH (Univ of Florida, Gainesville; Rocklin Physical Therapy and Wellness, Calif)
Sports Med 34:1077-1100, 2004   7–23

Introduction.—The pathophysiology of multiple sclerosis (MS) is characterised by fatigue, motor weakness, spasticity, poor balance, heat sensitivity and mental depression. Also, MS symptoms may lead to physical inactivity associated with the development of secondary diseases. Persons with MS are thus challenged by their disability when attempting to pursue an active lifestyle compatible with health-related fitness. Although exercise prescription is gaining favour as a therapeutic strategy to minimise the loss of functional capacity in chronic diseases, it remains under-utilised as an intervention strategy in the MS population. However, a growing number of studies indicate that exercise in patients with mild-to-moderate MS provides similar fitness and psychological benefits as it does in healthy controls.

We reviewed numerous studies describing the responses of selected MS patients to acute and chronic exercise compared with healthy controls. All training studies reported positive outcomes that outweighed potential adverse effects of the exercise intervention. Based on our review, this article highlights the role of exercise prescription in the multidisciplinary approach to MS disease management for improving and maintaining functional capacity. Despite the often unpredictable clinical course of MS, exercise programmes designed to increase cardiorespiratory fitness, muscle strength and mobility provide benefits that enhance lifestyle activity and quality of life while reducing risk of secondary disorders. Recommendations for the evaluation of cardiorespiratory fitness, muscle performance and flexibility are presented as well as basic guidelines for individualised exercise testing and training in MS. Special considerations for exercise, including medical management concerns, programme modifications and supervision, in the MS population are discussed.

▶ This review article tackles the issue of exercise prescription and training for a selected MS population from the perspective of physical therapy. It lacks a clinical neurologic input that would give a wider perspective of the range of problems and the range of clinical presentations that exist in this condition. As such, this article tends to take the "worst case" scenario of an ambulant MS patient with significant disability who is being prescribed exercise. The article's strengths, however, are that it provides a comprehensive summary of the major issues related to exercise in MS and the problems confronting a patient with MS who wants to exercise—namely, fatigue, motor weakness, spasticity, balance difficulty, lack of aerobic fitness, and heat sensitivity. The article provides generic advice in regard to exercise prescription in this population. While the article is a review article, it is not a critical one.

P. McCrory, MBBS, PhD

Six-Month and One-Year Followup of 23 Weeks of Aerobic Exercise for Individuals With Fibromyalgia

Gowans SE, DEHueck A, Voss S, et al (Univ of Toronto)
Arthritis Rheum 51:890-898, 2004   7–24

Objective.—To measure mood and physical function of individuals with fibromyalgia, 6 and 12 months following 23 weeks of supervised aerobic exercise.

Methods.—This is a followup report of individuals who were previously enrolled in 23 weeks of land-based and water-based aerobic exercise classes. Outcomes included the 6-minute walk test, Beck Depression Inventory (BDI), State-Trait Anxiety Inventory, Arthritis Self-Efficacy Scale (ASES), Fibromyalgia Impact Questionnaire (FIQ), tender point count, patient global assessment score, and exercise compliance. Outcomes were measured at the start and end of the exercise classes and 6 and 12 months later.

Results.—Analyses were conducted on 29 (intent-to-treat) or 18 (efficacy) subjects. Six-minute walk distances and BDI total scores were improved at followup (all analyses) (Fig 1). BDI cognitive/affective scores were improved at the end of 23 weeks of exercise (both analyses) and at the 12-month followup (efficacy analysis only). BDI somatic scores were improved at 6-month (both analyses) and 12-month followup (intent-to-treat only). FIQ and ASES function were improved at all followup points. ASES pain was improved in efficacy analyses only (all followup points). Tender points were unchanged after 23 weeks of exercise and at followup. Exercise duration at followup (total minutes of aerobic plus anaerobic exercise in the preceding week) was related to gains in physical function (6- and 12-month followup) and mood (6-month followup).

Conclusion.—Exercise can improve physical function, mood, symptom severity, and aspects of self efficacy for at least 12 months. Exercising at followup was related to improvements in physical function and perhaps mood.

▶ The authors of this report previously demonstrated some increases in 6-minute walk distance and an enhanced mood state resulting from exercise in a small 23-week controlled trial for patients with fibromyalgia.[1] The present ar-

Efficacy analysis

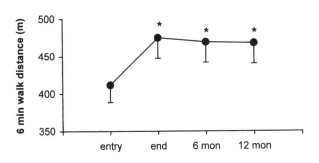

Intent-to-treat analysis

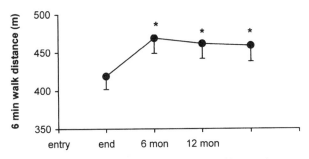

FIGURE 1.—Mean six-minute walk distances for subjects in the efficacy and intent-to-treat analysis. (Courtesy of Gowans SE, DEHueck A, Voss S, et al: Six-month and one-year followup of 23 weeks of aerobic exercise for individuals with fibromyalgia. *Arthritis Rheum* 51:890-898, 2004. Copyright American College of Rheumatology. Reprinted by permission of John Wiley & Sons, Inc.)

ticle indicates how well gains were maintained at a 12-month follow-up. Data for the former exercise group are supplemented by information from former controls, who subsequently elected to join the exercise program (this option is now required by many university Human Ethics Committees). Gains in both exercise performance and Beck depression scale scores were largely preserved to 12 months, but surprisingly exercise yielded little change in tender points or scores on the arthritis self-efficacy scale. Further, the changes in depression score were smaller than those seen when community exercise programs were organized for those with an uncomplicated depression.[2] Possibly, the subjects learned to exercise despite their disease. It is encouraging that more than half of the group were still exercising at 12 months.

R. J. Shephard, MD, PhD, DPE

References

1. Gowans SE, DEHueck A, Voss S, et al. A randomized, controlled trial of exercise and education for individuals with fibromyalgia. *Arthritis Care Res* 12:120-128, 1999.
2. Babyak M, Blumenthal JA, Herman S, et al: Exercise treatment for major depression: Maintenance of therapeutic benefit at 10 months. *Psychosom Med* 62:633-638, 2000.

Musculoskeletal Pain in Polio Survivors and Strength-matched Controls
Klein MG, Keenan MA, Esquenazi A, et al (Moss Rehabilitation Research Inst, Philadelphia; Albert Einstein Med Center; MossRehab Hosp; et al)
Arch Phys Med Rehabil 85:1679-1683, 2004   7–25

Objectives.—To determine whether a significant difference exists between musculoskeletal symptoms of polio survivors and those of older adults with no history of polio, and to determine if activity level and strength predict pain in either group.

Design.—Matched research design.

Setting.—A research laboratory in a rehabilitation setting.

Participants.—Fifty-four polio survivors and 54 adults with no history of polio were matched for gender, race, and bilateral knee extensor strength and selected from a cohort of 316 subjects who participated in a study on the relation between activity level and health status.

Interventions.—Not applicable.

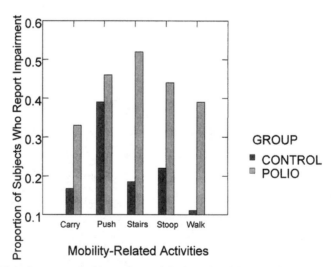

FIGURE 1.—Percentage of subjects reporting difficulty with mobility-related tasks. (Reprinted from Klein MG, Keenan MA, Esquenazi A, et al: Musculoskeletal pain in polio survivors and strength-matched controls. *Arch Phys Med Rehabil* 85:1679-1683, 2004. Copyright 2004 with permission from The American Congress of Rehabilitation Medicine and the American Academy of Physical Medicine and Rehabilitation.)

Main Outcome Measures.—Location and severity of musculoskeletal pain, activity frequency and intensity level, maximum voluntary isometric strength, and physical performance measures.

Results.—Polio survivors reported significantly more symptoms than the matched controls ($P < .05$) (Fig 1). Symptom status among the polio survivors was strongly associated with performance strain, perceived exertion, and activity intensity. Although the polio survivors had activity frequencies and habitual walking speeds that were similar to those from the matched controls, there was evidence that they performed activities at higher intensity levels.

Conclusions.—Activity level is a factor in the development of musculoskeletal symptoms in polio survivors. Polio survivors who perform at higher intensity levels are more likely to have moderate to severe pain and more mobility difficulties.

▶ There is evidence that polio survivors develop muscle and joint pain problems at a higher rate than age matched controls. This is due to the decreased strength levels of the polio survivors in the muscles affected by the virus, leaving them at higher risk for pain caused by overuse. No differences were noted in activity levels between the polio survivors and the controls, and the polio survivors performed activities at higher intensity levels than the controls. Since the polio survivors performed their activities at higher relative intensity levels, they experienced greater pain and mobility difficulties.

M. J. L. Alexander, PhD

A Diagnostic Cycle Test for McArdle's Disease
Vissing J, Haller RG (Rigshospitalet, Copenhagen; VA Med Ctr, Dallas)
Ann Neurol 54:539-542, 2003   7–26

Background.—Muscle glycogen is essential for working muscle early during exercise and at high work intensities. The absence of myophosphorylase activity in McArdle's disease typically results in the complete blocking of muscle glycogen breakdown. Thus, patients with McArdle's disease have severe exercise intolerance. Intense exercise in such patients provokes cramps, muscle injury, and myoglobinuria. Whether the second-wind phenomenon—a reduction in heart rate and perceived exertion during exercise—is pathognomonic for McArdle's disease was investigated.

Methods and Findings.—The study included 24 patients with McArdle's disease, 17 healthy persons, and 25 patients with other inborn errors of muscle metabolism. The participants were asked to cycle at a constant power output for 15 minutes. Heart rate in the patients with McArdle's disease was consistently reduced by a mean 35 beats per minute from minute 7 to 15 of exercise (Fig 2). In both control groups, heart rate increased progressively with exercise.

Conclusions.—A simple cycle ergometer test may be a useful diagnostic screening test for McArdle's disease, based on the presence or absence of the

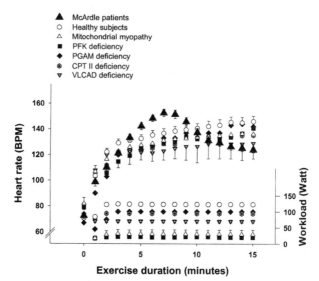

FIGURE 2.—Heart rate (7 upper curves) and workload (6 lower curves) during 15 minutes of constant workload exercise at 65% of VO$_{2max}$ in 17 healthy subjects, 14 patients with mitochondrial myopathy, 3 with phosphofructokinase (PFK) deficiency, 1 with phosphoglycerate mutase (PGAM) deficiency, 5 with carnitine palmitroyltransferase II (CPT II deficiency), and 2 patients with very long-chain acyl-CoA dehydrogenase (VLCAD) deficiency. The heart rate trace of the 24 patients with McArdle's disease is shown in the large, filled triangles for comparison. Values are mean ± SE. Where not shown, error bars are smaller than symbol size. (Courtesy of Vissing J, Haller RG: A diagnostic cycle test for MaArdle's disease. *Ann Neurol* 54: 539-542, 2003.)

second-wind phenomenon. In this series, the second-wind test was 100% sensitive and specific for detecting McArdle's disease.

▶ A final diagnosis of McArdle's disease depends on showing an absence of myophosphorylase activity in muscle biopsy specimens, but the test proposed by Vissing and Haller may allow a useful initial triage of patients. Nevertheless, I am a little nervous about calling the lack of heart-rate drift in patients with McArdle's disease evidence of a "second wind" associated with the enhanced delivery of extramuscular fuels. Lactate formation may also be less in the patient group, and a lower work rate may give rise to a smaller increase in core temperature; both of these factors could influence heart rate drift.

R. J. Shephard, MD, PhD, DPE

Multisegment Foot Motion During Gait: Proof of Concept in Rheumatoid Arthritis

Woodburn J, Nelson KM, Siegel KL, et al (Univ of Leeds, England; Dept of Health and Human Services, Bethesda, Md)

J Rheumatol 31:1918-1927, 2004   7–27

Objective.—To test a multisegment foot model for kinematic analysis during barefoot walking in patients with well established rheumatoid arthritis (RA) and foot impairments.

Methods.—Five healthy adult subjects and 11 RA patients with advanced disease were studied. Foot impairments were assessed using standardized outcomes and clinical examination techniques. A 6-camera 60 Hz video-based motion analysis system was used to measure motion of the shank, rearfoot, forefoot, and hallux segments and the vertical displacement of the navicular. Face validity and estimates of repeatability were determined. Motion patterns were calculated and comparisons were made between healthy subjects and patients with RA. Relationships between clinical impairment and abnormal motion were determined through inspection of individual RA cases.

Results.—Across the motion variables, the within-day and between-day coefficient of multiple correlation values ranged from 0.677 to 0.982 for the healthy subjects and 0.830 to 0.981 for RA patients. Based on previous studies, motion parameters for the healthy subjects showed excellent face validity. In RA patients, there was reduced range of motion across all segments and all planes of motion, which was consistent with joint stiffness. In the RA patients, rearfoot motion was shifted towards eversion and external rotation and peak values for these variables were increased, on average, by 7° and 11 degrees, respectively. Forefoot range of motion was reduced in all 3 planes (between 31% and 53%), but the maximum and minimum angles were comparable to normal. The navicular height, during full foot contact, was on average 3 mm lower in the RA patients in comparison to normal. The hallux was less extended in the RA subjects in comparison to normal (21° vs 33°) during the terminal stance phase. Individual cases showed abnormal patterns of motion consistent with their clinical impairments, especially those with predominant forefoot pain or pes planovalgus.

Conclusion.—In RA, multisegment foot models may provide a more complete description of foot motion abnormalities where pathology presents at multiple joints, leading to complex and varied patterns of impairment. This technique may be useful to evaluate functional changes in the foot and to help plan and assess logical, structurally based corrective interventions.

▶ Patients with RA suffer progressive degeneration of the small synovial joints of the foot, which leads to severe gait impairments. The site of the joint degeneration will often determine the exact type of gait impairment; for example, prolonged dorsiflexion is often indicative of forefoot impairments. A multisegment foot model was developed to compare RA foot movements during gait to those of healthy subjects. There was reduced range of motion in RA patients across all segments and all planes of motion; for example, forefoot motion was reduced between 30% and 50% in all 3 planes. This model was determined to be valuable in assessing foot deformities in RA patients and in assisting with corrective interventions.

M. J. L. Alexander, PhD

Comparison of Manual Therapy and Exercise Therapy in Osteoarthritis of the Hip: A Randomized Clinical Trial

Hoeksma HL, Dekker J, Ronday HK, et al (Leyenburg Hosp, The Hague, The Netherlands; Vrije Universiteit, Amsterdam; Cees Vel, PT, The Hague, The Netherlands; et al)
Arthritis Rheum 51:722-729, 2004   7–28

Background.—Osteoarthritis (OA) is a degenerative disease characterized by pain, loss of function, restriction of activities, and decreased quality of life (QOL). Conservative treatment includes both manual therapy (manipulation and stretching) and exercise therapy. The efficacy of manual therapy was compared with that of exercise therapy for the treatment of OA.

Study Design.—The study included 109 patients with OA who were randomly selected to undergo either outpatient manual therapy or exercise therapy. All patients received treatment twice weekly for 5 weeks for 9 treatments. Manual therapy consisted of stretching, followed by hip traction and traction manipulation. Exercise therapy focused on exercise to improve muscle function and joint motion. The primary outcome was improvement experienced by the patient, using a 6-point Likert scale. Health-related QOL was assessed by the Short form 36 (SF-36). Hip function was assessed by the

---

TABLE 2.—Differences Between the 2 Treatment Groups After 5 Weeks*

	Manual Therapy	Exercise Therapy	Main Comp Exercise Therapy	Main Comp Manual Therapy	Kellgren and Lawrence 0	1	2	3	Odds Ratio	95% CI
Worse	3	6	10 ± 15	23 ± 18	0	2	3	4		
Little worse	2	3	1 ± 8	22 ± 19	1	1	2	1		
Stable	5	16	4 ± 12	4 ± 12	2	0	6	13		
Improved	27	21	−12 ± 14	−20 ± 14	4	7	20	17		
Much improved	15	4	−34 ± 24	−35 ± 17	2	2	10	5		
Free of complaints	1	0	−18		0	0	1	0		
Improved (%)	43 (81)	25 (50)							1.92	1.30, 2.60
Not improved	10	25								

*Improvement of the main complaint (main comp; visual analog scale, analysis of covariance) on the basis of primary outcome; negative numbers indicate improvement. Primary outcome on the basis of Kellgren and Lawrence. Odds ratio for improvement of manual therapy versus exercise therapy.

Abbreviation: CI, Confidence interval.

(Courtesy of Hoeksma HL, Dekker J, Ronday HK, et al: Comparison of manual therapy and exercise therapy in osteoarthritis of the hip: A randomized clinical trial *Arthritis Rheum* 51: 722-729, 2004. Copyright 2004 American College of Rheumatology. Reprinted by permission of John Wiley & Sons, Inc.)

Harris Hip Score and a walking test. Results were evaluated by an observer blinded as to the treatment group.

Findings.—No significant differences were noted between the 2 groups at baseline. The primary outcome success rate after 5 weeks was 81% in the manual therapy group and 50% in the exercise group (Table 2). Patients in the manual therapy group had significantly better outcomes for pain, stiffness, hip function, and range of motion. These effects endured after 29 weeks.

Conclusions.—This randomized, single-blinded clinical trial found that manual therapy was superior to exercise therapy for the treatment of osteoarthritis. The effects of manual therapy persisted for 29 weeks.

▶ Most reports concerning the effects of exercise in chronic illness have shown a beneficial impact of an increase in physical activity, but in this article, patients with OA who were assigned to an exercise program appear to have fared significantly worse than a control group who received specific manual manipulations. The sample size was quite large, and the main criticism of this research (as the authors admit) is its relatively short time frame; in a person badly deconditioned by chronic joint pain, 9 exercise sessions spread over 5 weeks seems too short a program to anticipate much benefit. In view of previous more positive reports,[1] data on long-term outcomes are needed before exercise is abandoned in favor of passive manipulation.

R. J. Shephard, MD, PhD, DPE

Reference

1. Van Baar ME, Assendelft WJ, Dekker J, et al: The effectiveness of exercise therapy in patients with osteoarthritis of the hip or knee: A randomized clinical trial. *J Rheumatol* 25:2432-2439, 1998.

Muscle Dysfunction Versus Wear and Tear as a Cause of Exercise Related Osteoarthritis: An Epidemiological Update
Shrier I (SMBD-Jewish Gen Hosp, Montreal)
Br J Sports Med 38:526-535, 2004   7–29

Background.—Persons with osteoarthritis often are limited in their activities of daily living, such as climbing stairs and dressing, and these limitations can prevent younger persons from seeking employment. In the case of primary osteoarthritis—excluding causes such as genetic diseases, severe biomechanical abnormalities, postseptic arthritis—it is believed by many healthcare professionals that the major cause of osteoarthritis is wear and tear, the gradual thinning of the articular cartilage from repeated weight-bearing activity of the joints. Thus, osteoarthritis is caused and worsened by exercise. It has also been proposed that muscle dysfunction is the primary cause of osteoarthritis. The clinical literature to determine which hypothesis has the greatest support was reviewed.

Methods.—A systematic review was conducted of the MEDLINE and SportDiscus databases. The review was limited to exercise-related primary osteoarthritis and did not include studies that investigated osteoarthritis secondary to injury or previous surgery.

Results.—Twenty-three clinical articles (18 studies) related to exercise and osteoarthritis were retrieved. These articles investigated osteoarthritis and exposure to running, soccer, and elite team sports. Overall, the 3 cross-sectional running studies found that exercise is not associated with osteoarthritis, whereas the 3 case-control studies found mixed results but overall a suggestion that some higher intensity activities may be associated with the development of osteoarthritis. For the elite team sports, it was found that there was an increased risk of hip or knee disability, with an increase in osteoarthritis in all types of athletes. The greatest increase in osteoarthritis occurred in wrestling, weight lifting, soccer, and ice hockey. However, 3 of these sports do not involve impact, which would suggest that wear-and-tear is not a likely cause of osteoarthritis.

Conclusion.—This review of clinical studies of exercise-related osteoarthritis found greater support for the muscle dysfunction hypothesis over the wear-and-tear hypothesis.

▶ Ian Shrier presents a careful review of 18 published studies. The 1 weakness from a meta-analytic point of view suggested that running does not cause osteoarthritis[1]; problems have arisen only in sports where trauma has been applied to the joints. However, some studies of elite athletes have been less optimistic. Marti et al[2] found that there was a significant risk of joint injury in elite runners, and that this was better correlated with running pace than with mileage. The latter should reflect the number of impacts sustained by the joints. Shrier thus argues that a fast pace tires the muscle and limits its normal role in absorbing impact shock[3]. Muscle dysfunction may result not only from the fatigue of extreme competition, but also from exercising in the face of injury (strains) or loss of proprioception (anterior cruciate ligament tears). Adequate rehabilitation after injury is thus an important tactic in preventing osteoarthritis in athletes.

R. J. Shephard, MD, PhD, DPE

References

1. Lane NE, Bloch DA, Jones HH, et al: Long distance runners, bone density and osteoarthritis. *JAMA* 255:1147-1151, 1986.
2. Marti B, Knobloch M, Tschopp A, et al: Is excessive running predictive of degenerative hip disease? Controlled study of former elite athletes. *BMJ* 299:91-93, 1989.
3. Christina KA, White SC, Gilchrist LA: Effect of localized muscle fatigue on vertical ground reaction forces and ankle joint motion during running. *Hum Mov Sci* 20:257-276, 2001.

Bone Loss and Fracture Risk After Reduced Physical Activity

Nordström A, Karlsson C, Nyquist F, et al (Univ of Umeå, Sweden; Lund Univ, Malmö, Sweden)
J Bone Miner Res 20:202-207, 2005　　　　　　　　　　　　　　　　7–30

Introduction.—Former male young athletes partially lost benefits in BMD (g/cm²) with cessation of exercise, but, despite this, had a higher BMD 4 years after cessation of career than a control group. A higher BMD might contribute to the lower incidence of fragility fractures found in former older athletes ≥ 60 years of age compared with a control group. Physical activity increases peak bone mass and may prevent osteoporosis if a residual high BMD is retained into old age.

Materials and Methods.—BMD was measured by DXA in 97 male young athletes 21.0 ± 4.5 years of age (SD) and 48 controls 22.4 ± 6.3 years of age, with measurements repeated 5 years later, when 55 of the athletes had retired from sports. In a second, older cohort, fracture incidence was recorded in 400 former older athletes and 800 controls ≥ 60 years of age.

Results.—At baseline, the young athletes had higher BMD than controls in total body (mean difference, 0.08 g/cm²), spine (mean difference, 0.10 g/cm²), femoral neck (mean difference, 0.13 g/cm²), and arms (mean difference, 0.05 g/cm²; all $p < 0.001$). During the follow-up period, the young athletes who retired lost more BMD than the still active athletes at the femoral neck (mean difference, 0.07 g/cm²; $p = 0.001$) and gained less BMD at the total body (mean difference, 0.03 g/cm²; $p = 0.004$). Nevertheless, BMD was still higher in the retired young athletes (mean difference, 0.06-0.08 g/cm²) than in the controls in the total body, femoral neck, and arms (all $P < 0.05$). In the older cohort, there were fewer former athletes ≥ 60 years of age

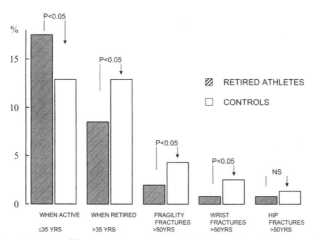

FIGURE 2.—Proportion of former athletes and controls ≥ 60 years of age with fractures. (Courtesy of Nordström A, Karlsson C, Nyquist F, et al: Bone loss and fracture risk after reduced physical activity. *J Bone Miner Res* 20:202-207, 2005. Reproduced with permission of the American Society for Bone and Mineral Research.)

than controls with fragility fractures (2.0% versus 4.2%; $p < 0.05$) and distal radius fractures (0.75% versus 2.5%; $p < 0.05$) (Fig 2).

Conclusions.—Although exercise-induced BMD benefits are reduced after retirement from sports, former male older athletes have fewer fractures than matched controls.

▶ Physical activity programs for children have been advocated in part on the grounds that they develop a "bank" of bone mass that protects those involved from osteoporosis during their declining years. However, earlier retrospective analyses by the same authors have not been encouraging in this regard,[1,2] and there have been few studies that have followed up subjects for long enough to test whether the basic hypothesis of a bone bank is valid. The present authors were only able to continue their prospective study for 4 to 5 years; during this time, the bone density remained higher in those who had ceased activity as ice-hockey or soccer players than in the controls. Perhaps more importantly, a parallel retrospective study showed that the incidence of fractures in those more than 60 years old was half as great among former athletes as in controls. One strength of the present analysis was a radiographic verification of the history of fracture in a subsample of the subjects. The extent of the protection against fractures is rather surprising, given the substantial loss of bone density within a few years of retiring from sport. One might wonder if the old age benefit reflected a continuing greater habitual physical activity on the part of the former athletes, but the authors of this report maintain that, during old age, former athletes and controls had similar lifestyles. Other possible explanations include inherited differences of bone strength or neuromuscular coordination. Such possibilities could only be excluded by a long-sustained, randomized, controlled prospective trial, and this would be very difficult to organize.

R. J. Shephard, MD, PhD, DPE

References

1. Karlsson MK, Johnell O, Obrant KJ: Is bone mineral density advantage maintained long-term in previous weight lifters? *Calcif Tiss Intern* 57:325-328, 1995.
2. Karlsson MK, Linden C, Karlsson C, et al: Exercise during growth and bone mineral density and fractures in old age. *Lancet* 355:469-470, 2000.

Protection of Bone Mass by Estrogens and Raloxifene During Exercise-induced Weight Loss
Gozansky WS, Van Pelt RE, Jankowski CM, et al (Univ of Colorado, Denver)
J Clin Endocrinol Metab 90:52-59, 2005   7–31

Introduction.—The aim of this study was to determine whether estrogen and/or raloxifene help to conserve bone mineral density (BMD) during moderate weight loss. Postmenopausal women (n = 68) participated in a 6-month weight loss program that consisted primarily of supervised exercise training. Another 26 women were studied over 6 months of weight stability. All participants were randomized to three treatment arms: placebo, raloxi-

TABLE 3.—Changes in Body Composition in Response to 6 Months of Exercise Training (Weight Loss Group) or Observation (Weight-Stable Group) in Women Randomized to Placebo, Raloxifene, or HT

	Placebo	Treatment Group Raloxifene	HT
Weight loss group			
Weight (kg)[a]	−4.0 ± 3.2	−4.4 ± 3.8	−4.0 ± 3.2
Fat mass (kg)[a]	−4.0 ± 2.7	−4.2 ± 4.3	−4.0 ± 3.2
Fat-free mass (kg)[b]	0.0 ± 1.4	−0.2 ± 1.5	0.0 ± 1.1
Total BMC (g)[c]	−30 ± 58	−21 ± 108	54 ± 75
Weight-stable group			
Weight (kg)[a]	1.6 ± 1.9	0.0 ± 2.4	0.9 ± 2.8
Fat mass (kg)[a]	1.2 ± 1.4	−0.1 ± 1.5	−0.1 ± 2.8
Fat-free mass (kg)[b]	0.4 ± 0.8	0.1 ± 1.3	1.0 ± 1.4
Total BMC (g)[c]	79 ± 134	37 ± 170	50 ± 123

*Note:*There were no significant main effects of drug treatment for any of the variables.
[a]Weight loss vs weight stable: main effect, *P* < 0.001.
[b]Weight loss vs weight stable: main effect, *P* = 0.055.
[c]Weight loss vs weight stable: main effect, *P* = 0.025.
Abbreviation: HT, Hormone therapy.
(Courtesy of Gozansky WS, Van Pelt RE, Jankowski CM, et al: Protection of bone mass by estrogens and raloxifene during exercise-induced weight loss. *J Clin Endocrinol Metab* 90:52-59, 2005. Copyright The Endocrine Society.)

fene (60 mg/d), or hormone therapy (HT; conjugated estrogens, 0.625 mg/d; trimonthly medroxyprogesterone acetate, 5 mg/d for 13 d, for women with a uterus). Changes in body weight (mean ± SE) averaged 0.8 ± 0.5 kg in the weight-stable group and −4.1 ± 0.4 kg in the weight loss group (Table 3). Across all measured skeletal sites, average changes in BMD in weight stable women were −0.6 ± 1.1% (n = 7), 0.9 ± 0.6% (n = 9), and 3.0 ± 0.7% (n = 10) in the placebo, raloxifene, and HT groups, respectively; comparable BMD changes in the weight loss groups were −1.5 ± 0.5% (n = 22), −0.5 ± 0.5% (n = 23), and 1.1 ± 0.4% (n = 23). There were no significant interactions between weight loss and drug treatment on changes in BMD, but there were significant main effects of weight loss on lumbar spine (*P* = 0.022), total hip (*P* = 0.010), and trochanter BMD (*P* < 0.001). These findings suggest that weight loss, even when modest in magnitude and induced by exercise training, causes a reduction in BMD, particularly in women not taking raloxifene or HT. It is not known whether reductions in BMD of this magnitude increase the risk for osteoporotic fracture.

▶ Progressive moderate exercise is probably the most effective method of reducing body mass in older women, particularly if advisors ensure the patient does not compensate by an increased food intake. The present study began with the idea that exercise might also help in conserving BMD relative to dieting alone. However, it is important to keep in mind that a low energy intake such as that adopted periodically in the study of Gozansky et al is unlikely to provide the patient with the necessary minimum quantities of either calcium or Vitamin D.[1] Thus, a shortage of these nutrients may explain the bone loss seen in those patients who did not also receive HT. Before advocating HT (which has other, undesired, side effects), it would seem necessary to test the extent of bone loss if a similar exercise and diet program was undertaken with provision of adequate calcium and vitamin supplements.

R. J. Shephard, MD, PhD, DPE

Reference

1. Tiidus P, Shephard RJ, Montepare W: Overall intake of energy and key nutrients: Data for middle-aged and older middle-class adults. *Can J Sport Sci* 14:173-177, 1989.

Effects of Exercise Training and Detraining On Oxidized Low-density Lipoprotein–Potentiated Platelet Function in Men

Wang J-S, Chow S-E (Chang Gung Univ, Taoyuan, Taiwan)
Arch Phys Med Rehabil 85:1531-1537, 2004   7–32

Objective.—To investigate how exercise training and detraining affect oxidized low-density lipoprotein (Ox-LDL)-potentiated platelet function in men.

Design.—Cohort study.

Setting.—Department of physical medicine and rehabilitation.

Participants.—Ten sedentary men (mean age ± standard error of the mean, 21.6±0.2 y) who did not engage in any regular physical activity for at least 1 year before the study.

Interventions.—Subjects cycled on an ergometer at about 50% of maximal oxygen consumption for 30 minutes daily, 5 days a week, for 8 weeks, then detrained for 12 weeks.

Main Outcome Measures.—During the experimental period, blood samples from the subjects were collected before and immediately after a progressive exercise test (ie, strenuous, acute exercise) every 4 weeks. The following measurements were taken when the subjects were at rest and immediately after exercise: plasma lipid profile, plasma Ox-LDL level, and platelet aggregation and intracellular calcium concentration ($[Ca^{2+}]_i$) elevation induced by adenosine disphosphate (ADP) alone or simultaneous ADP and Ox-LDL addition.

Results.—Analytical results indicated that: (1) plasma total cholesterol and LDL levels were reduced after exercise training from 151±7 mg/dL and 58±2 mg/dL to 133±6 mg/dL and 46±2 mg/dL ($P < .05$), respectively, whereas the plasma Ox-LDL level remained unchanged; (2) platelet aggregation and $[Ca^{2+}]_i$ elevation promoted by 100 µg/mL of Ox-LDL were significantly increased from 70%±5% and 91%±7% of resting level to 108%±4% and 125%±3% after strenuous, acute exercise ($P < .05$); (3) exercise training decreased resting and postexercise 100 µg/mL Ox-LDL-potentiated platelet aggregation (ie, 31%±4% and 82%±4%, respectively; $P < .05$) and $[Ca^{2+}]_i$ elevation (ie, 35%±6% and 71%±4%, respectively; $P < .05$); (4) detraining reversed the training effects on lipid profile and platelet function; and (5) treating the platelet with L-arginine-inhibited Ox-LDL-potentiated platelet activation during the experimental period.

Conclusions.—Our results suggest that 8 weeks of exercise training decreased the plasma LDL level, but failed to influence production of plasma Ox-LDL. Importantly, resting and exercise-induced Ox-LDL-potentiated platelet activation was decreased by exercise training. However, this was reversed by detraining to the pretraining level.

▶ Risk of cardiovascular disease (CVD) is reduced in physically active adults. One mechanism by which exercise may reduce CVD risk is through alteration of platelet function. Chronic exercise may also decrease levels of oxidized LDL. This training-detraining study showed that 8 weeks of cycling ergometer exercise (30 minutes per session, 5 sessions per week, 50% $\dot{V}O_{2max}$) lowered LDL-cholesterol, but failed to reduce oxidized LDL levels. Exercise-induced platelet activation (potentiated by oxidized LDL) was decreased by exercise training, with this benefit erased after 12 weeks of detraining. The authors concluded that exercise training protects people against platelet activation from oxidative stress, thereby decreasing the risk of vascular thrombosis during exercise.

D. C. Nieman, DrPH

Reduced Exercise Endurance in Interleukin-6-Deficient Mice
Fäldt J, Wernstedt I, Fitzgerald SM, et al (Sahlgrenska Univ, Gothenberg, Sweden; Gothenberg Univ, Sweden)
Endocrinology 145:2680-2686, 2004   7–33

Introduction.—Interleukin (IL)-6 is produced and released in large amounts from skeletal muscle during prolonged exercise in mice and humans. There are few data that demonstrate the biological significance of this finding. IL-6 produces metabolic effects, including stimulating energy expenditure and decreasing body fat mass. The effects of IL-6 deficiency on exercise endurance and energy were evaluated in preobese and obese IL-6–deficient (IL-6-/-) mice.

Methods.—Four-month-old preobese and 7-month-old obese IL-6-/- male mice backcrossed to C57BL/6 and their littermate control animals were evaluated. All animals were exercised on a treadmill and energy expenditure was measured as oxygen consumption via indirect calorimetry.

Results.—The preobese IL-6-/- mice were significantly leaner compared to control animals. As expected, obesity developed in the older IL-6-/- mice. At rest, young, not older, IL-6-/- animals had an elevated respiratory exchange ratio (RER), indicating that they oxidize carbohydrates versus fat for energy utilization. During exercise, both young and older IL-6-/- mice had diminished endurance (Fig 3) and a progressive reduction in oxygen consumption compared to control animals. There was no difference in RER in young IL-6-/- mice, whereas RER was enhanced in older IL-6-/- animals during exercise.

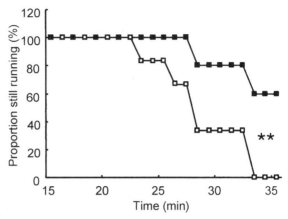

FIGURE 3.—Endurance capacity in 4-month-old preobese IL-6-/- (*white squares*) and wild type (*black squares*) mice. The mice started on the treadmill at an inclination of 20° and a speed of 10 m/min, with an incremental increase in speed until exhaustion. The results are shown as a Kaplan-Meier survival curve, and the comparison of the groups was performed using the log-rank test, n = 5-6. *Double asterisk* indicates P < .01. (Courtesy of Fäldt J, Wernstedt I, Fitzgerald SM, et al: Reduced endurance in interleukin-6-deficient mice. *Endocrinology* 145(6):2680-2686, 2004. Copyright 2004, The Endocrine Society.)

Conclusion.—IL-6–deficient mice have diminished endurance and energy expenditure during exercise, indicating that IL-6 is needed for normal exercise capacity.

▶ Cytokines such as IL-6 are proteins of low molecular weight that mediate a variety of different functions relevant to the immune system and to all other organs and tissue systems. It is becoming increasingly clear that IL-6 has multiple functions and is secreted by many cell types. During intense and prolonged exercise, the muscle tissue releases large quantities of IL-6, and the plasma concentration of IL-6 increases to high levels.[1] Other cells from the liver, brain, adipose, and immune system release IL-6 during exercise, but the relative contribution from the various tissues is not known.

IL-6 may be released from immune cells during exercise because of muscle cell damage and inflammation, but evidence suggests IL-6 also has a metabolic role in influencing lipolysis and glucose metabolism. The data from this study of IL-6–deficient mice indicate that they have reduced exercise endurance (Fig 3) and that energy expenditure is decreased compared to control mice. This suggests that the increase in IL-6 production during exercise is critical to support underlying metabolic pathways.

D. C. Nieman, DrPH

Reference

1. Pedersen BK, Steensberg A, Fischer C, et al: The metabolic role of IL-6 produced during exercise: Is IL-6 an exercise factor? *Proc Nutr Soc* 63:263-267, 2004.

Exercise-induced Apoptosis of Lymphocytes Depends On Training Status
Mooren FC, Lechtermann A, Völker K (Univ Hosp Münster, Germany)
Med Sci Sports Exerc 36:1476-1483, 2004   7–34

Purpose.—To investigate the effect of training status on lymphocyte apoptosis as well as the expression of cell death receptors and ligands after a marathon run, and to compare these data with the alterations after treadmill exercise tests.

Methods.—Sixteen volunteers successfully finished the 2002 Munster marathon. Venous blood samples were drawn before and 0, 3, and 24 h after the race. After cell isolation, cell-based apoptosis markers annexin V, Fas receptor, and Fas ligand were measured by flow cytometry. The same parameters were investigated in a group of 10 subjects before, and 0 and 1 h after both an exhaustive (ExT) and a low-intensity (LoT) treadmill test.

Results.—The percentage of apoptotic cells after the marathon changed in a biphasic manner. An early increase 3 h after the run was followed by a significant decrease 1 d later. Interestingly, the increase in apoptotic cells was not observed in highly trained athletes, whereas it was significantly more pronounced in badly trained athletes. ExT induced a lymphocyte apoptosis similar to the marathon, whereas no change in apoptosis was observed after the LoT. Both Fas receptor and ligand were increased after the marathon with different kinetics. Whereas the Fas receptor peaked at 1 h, Fas ligand was increased 3 h after the run. After the treadmill tests Fas receptor expression was enhanced in both groups, whereas Fas ligand increased only after the ExT.

Conclusions.—Endurance exercise like a marathon is able to induce apoptosis in lymphocytes. Thereby, apoptosis sensitivity seems to be related to training status in an inverse relationship. The increased expression levels of death receptors and ligands might indicate the high apoptosis inducing potential of this type of exercise.

▶ There is increasing evidence that high-intensity, long-duration exercise induces lymphocyte apoptosis and may partly explain postexercise lymphopenia.[1,2] Data from this study support this finding and also show that moderate-intensity exercise does not induce lymphocyte apoptosis. Surface expression of the proapoptotic Fas ligand did not fully explain why apoptosis occurred after exercise. The authors reason that following intensive exercise workrates "the involvement of apoptosis makes sense since it terminates and confines the inflammation-like activation of the immune system."

D. C. Nieman, DrPH

References

1. Mars M, Govender S, Weston A, et al: High intensity exercise: A cause of lymphocyte apoptosis? *Biochem Biophys Res Commun* 19:366-370, 1998.
2. Quadrilatero J, Hoffman-Goetz L: N-acetyl-L-cysteine inhibits exercise-induced lymphocyte apoptotic protein alterations. *Med Sci Sports Exerc* 37:53-56, 2005.

Sonographic Evaluation of Spleen Size in Tall Healthy Athletes

Spielmann AL, DeLong DM, Kliewer MA (Vancouver Gen Hosp, BC, Canada)
AJR 184:45-49, 2005   7–35

Objective.—The purpose of this study was to establish the range of spleen sizes in tall healthy athletes.

Subjects and Methods.—Sonographic measurements of spleen size and left renal length were performed on 129 college athletes (82 men, 47 women). Length, width, and thickness of the spleen and left renal length were obtained. In addition, the height, weight, and age of each athlete were recorded. Pearson's product moment correlation coefficients were calculated, and linear regression analysis was used to create a model for calculating normative values.

Results.—The mean body height for men was 74.3 (189 cm) ± (SD) 3.7 inches (9 cm) and for women was 69.3 (176 cm) ± 3.7 inches (9 cm). Spleen length was greater than 12 cm in 31.7% of the men (mean spleen length, 11.4 ± 1.7 cm) and in 12.8% of the women (mean spleen length, 10.3 ± 1.3 cm). In women, height correlated with spleen length ($r = 0.3$, $p = 0.05$), width ($r = 0.4, p = 0.01$), and volume ($r = 0.3, p = 0.02$) but not with thickness ($r = 0.08, p = 0.6$). Spleen length did correlate with left renal length ($r = 0.5, p = 0.0005$). In men, height correlated with spleen length ($r = 0.4, p = 0.0003$), width ($r = 0.5, p = 0.0001$), and volume ($r = 0.4, p = 0.0002$) and less with thickness ($r = 0.3, p = 0.01$). Spleen length and left renal length were poorly correlated ($r = 0.2, p = 0.04$). Regression analysis showed that in women taller than 5 ft 6 inches (168 cm), the mean splenic length of 10 cm increased by 0.1 cm for each 1-inch incremental increase in height. In men taller than 6 ft (180 cm), the mean splenic length of 11 cm increased by 0.2 cm for each 1-inch incremental increase in height.

Conclusion.—Spleen size correlates with height in tall healthy athletes. Nomograms from this data can be used to gauge the risk of returning to play after episodes of acute splenomegaly, as with infectious mononucleosis.

▶ The accurate estimation of spleen size in athletes, particularly those who are taller than average, is a matter of considerable importance in the diagnosis and management of a number of medical disorders. Most clinicians will be familiar with the real dilemma of determining recovery from infectious mononucleosis and the normalization of splenic size before contact sports can be resumed. This study is an important addition to the literature that characterizes normative data in an athletic population. Interestingly, spleen size correlates with height in healthy athletes.

P. McCrory, MBBS, PhD

N-Acetyl-L-Cysteine Inhibits Exercise-Induced Lymphocyte Apoptotic Protein Alterations

Quadrilatero J, Hoffman-Goetz L (Univ of Waterloo, Ont, Canada)

Med Sci Sports Exerc 37:53-56, 2005

7–36

Purpose.—To investigate the effect of strenuous exercise and antioxidant administration on pro- and antiapoptotic protein expression in intestinal lymphocytes.

Methods.—Female C57BL/6 mice ($N = 52$) were randomly assigned to receive N-acetyl-L-cysteine (NAC; 1 g·kg^{-1}) or saline (SAL) 30 min before treadmill exercise (EX) for 90 min and 2 degrees slope (30 min at 22 m·min^{-1}, 30 min at 25 m·min^{-1}, and 30 min at 28 m·min^{-1}) and sacrificed immediately (Imm) or 24 h (24h) after exercise. Control mice were exposed to treadmill noise and vibration without running (nonexercised). Intestinal lymphocytes (IL) were isolated and pro- and antiapoptotic protein expression was evaluated by Western blot analysis.

Results.—IL protein levels of proapoptotic (caspase 3 and cytosolic cytochrome c) and antiapoptotic (Bcl-2) were significantly different among groups. Relative to nonexercised mice, protein levels of caspase 3 ($P < 0.001$) and cytosolic cytochrome c ($P < 0.005$) were significantly elevated, whereas Bcl-2 ($P < 0.05$) was significantly lower immediately after exercise in mice receiving saline (EX + SAL + Imm) but not in animals receiving NAC (EX + NAC + Imm) or both 24h postgroups (EX + SAL + 24h and EX + NAC + 24h).

Conclusion.—These results suggest that oxidative stress acting through a mitochondrial pathway may play a role in intestinal lymphocyte apoptosis after strenuous exercise.

▶ Virtually no data were available before this publication on exercise-induced changes in IL and apoptosis, and underlying mechanisms. This study showed that 90 minutes of intense exercise by mice reduced the total number of IL 24 hours after exercise, that this loss was in part caused by apoptosis, and that an exercise-induced increase in oxidative stress was a primary mechanism.

D. C. Nieman, DrPH

Epinephrine Infusion Increases Adipose Interleukin-6 Gene Expression and Systemic Levels in Humans

Keller P, Keller C, Robinson LE, et al (Univ Hosp of Copenhagen, Denmark)

J Appl Physiol 97:1309-1312, 2004

7–37

Background.—Plasma epinephrine levels are significantly increased in response to physical activity, and exercise is known to affect several metabolic genes at both the mRNA and plasma levels. However, it is not possible to determine whether the exercise-induced metabolic effects are mediated via epinephrine or muscle contraction-induced factors. It has been suggested in recent studies that the cytokine IL-6, which is substantially enhanced during exercise, may play an important metabolic role. The exercise-induced increase in systemic levels of IL-6 is thought to originate in contracting skeletal muscles; however, adipose tissue may also be a contributing factor because IL-6 mRNA expression is increased by exercise. The possible role of epinephrine in the induction of IL-6 in adipose tissue was investigated.

Methods.—Subcutaneous adipose tissue biopsies and blood samples were obtained from 8 healthy men in response to epinephrine infusion or saline infusion. The study participants had a mean age of 27 years, a mean height of 1.84 m, and a mean body mass of 83 kg. The rate of epinephrine infusion was such that circulating epinephrine concentrations mimicked that typically seen during exercise.

Results.—The level of IL-6 mRNA in subcutaneous adipose tissue increased 26-fold at 3 hours of epinephrine infusion compared with that of control subjects. An increase in plasma levels of IL-6 in response to epinephrine infusion was also noted. However, epinephrine did not affect the IL-6 receptor mRNA.

Conclusion.—IL-6 mRNA levels in subcutaneous adipose tissue and circulating IL-6 levels were increased acutely in healthy men with infusion of epinephrine.

▶ Prolonged and intensive physical exercise increases plasma IL-6 levels significantly above resting levels. Muscle tissue is a major source of IL-6 during exercise, but other cells may produce IL-6, including adipose tissue.[1] This study showed that infusion of epinephrine to levels seen during exercise increased IL-6 gene expression in adipose tissue, leading to a modest elevation of plasma IL-6. Muscle-derived IL-6, however, is not induced by epinephrine, and countermeasures designed to lower epinephrine during exercise (eg, carbohydrate ingestion) do not have an appreciable effect on tissue IL-6 gene expression or plasma IL-6 levels through this pathway.

D. C. Nieman, DrPH

Reference

1. Keller C, Keller P, Marshal S, et al: IL-6 gene expression in human adipose tissue in response to exercise-effect of carbohydrate ingestion. *J Physiol* 550:927-931, 2003.

Effects of Oat β-Glucan on Innate Immunity and Infection After Exercise Stress

Davis JM, Murphy EA, Brown AS, et al (Univ of South Carolina, Columbia)
Med Sci Sports Exerc 36:1321-1327, 2004   7–38

Background.—It has been shown that physical exercise can alter many aspects of immune system function and can increase the susceptibility to infection. Studies have generally supported the hypothesis that exhaustive exercise stress may lead to immunosuppression and increased risk of infection, including upper-respiratory tract infection (URTI); however, the strength of the evidence in this area is not convincng. Oat β-glucan is a mild immune system enhancer that may offset immune suppression-associated exercise stress. The effects of oat β-glucan (OβG) on respiratory infection, macrophage antiviral resistance, and natural killer (NK) cytotoxicity were assessed.

Methods.—Mice were randomly assigned to 1 of 4 groups: Ex-water, Ex-OβG, Con-water, or con-OβG. OβG was fed in the drinking water for 10 days before intranasal inoculation of herpes simplex virus type 1 (HSV-1) or sacrifice. Exercise consisted of running on a treadmill to volitional fatigue (approximately 140 minutes) for 3 consecutive days. A group of 24 mice were intranasally inoculated with a standardized dose of HSV-1 15 minutes after the last bout of exercise or rest. Mice were monitored twice daily for morbidity and mortality. Additional mice were sacrificed after exercise; peritoneal macrophages were obtained via intraperitoneal lavage and assayed for antiviral resistance to HSV-1 (18 mice), and spleens were harvested and assayed for natural killer (NK) cell cytotoxicity (12 mice).

Results.—Exercise stress resistance was associated with a 28% increase in morbidity and an 18% increase in mortality. Ingestion of OβG before infection prevented the increases in morbidity and mortality. Exercise stress was associated with a decrease in macrophage antiviral resistance, which was blocked by the ingestion of OβG. No effects of exercise or OβG were noted on NK cytotoxicity.

Conclusion.—The daily ingestion of OβG may offset the increased risk of URTI associated with exercise stress, which may be mediated in part by an increase in macrophage antiviral resistance.

► Intense and prolonged exertion is a significant stressor, leading to an elevation in stress hormones and profound alterations in immune function in multiple compartments of the body. Is it possible to ingest nutritional supplements that help counter exercise-induced immune changes? This study provides important animal data that OβG abrogates the increase in morbidity and mortality after intranasal inoculation of HSV-1 in mice running for about 140 minutes, 3 days in a row, and may operate via increase macrophage viral resistance. Additional studies in humans are warranted to determine if this nutritional strategy is effective in athletes and war-fighters.

D. C. Nieman, DrPH

Vitamin E and Immunity After the Kona Triathlon World Championship
Nieman DC, Henson DA, McAnulty SR, et al (Appalachian State Univ, Boone, NC; Vanderbilt Univ, Nashville, Tenn; Kronos The Optimal Health Company, Phoenix, Ariz)
Med Sci Sports Exerc 36:1328-1335, 2004   7–39

Background.—The production of free radicals and reactive oxygen species is increased in bouts of intense exercise through several pathways, including oxidative phosphorylation, increase in catecholamines, prostanoid metabolism, xanthine oxidase, and reduced nicotinamide adenine dinucleotide phosphate (NADPH) oxidase. Most reactive oxygen species are neutralized by a sophisticated antioxidant defense system that consists of a variety of enzymes and nonenzymatic antioxidants, including vitamins A, E, and C, glutathione, ubiquinone, and flavonoids. However, intensive and sustained physical activity can create an imbalance between reactive oxygen species and antioxidants, leading to oxidative stress. The primary function of vitamin E is of a nonspecific, chain-breaking antioxidant that prevents the propagation of lipid peroxidation. The effects of vitamin E ingestion oxidative stress and immune changes in response to the Triathlon World Championship in Kona, Hawaii were determined.

Methods.—The study included 38 triathletes who were selected randomly to receive either vitamin E (800-IU/d α-tocopherol) or placebo capsules in a double-blind fashion for 2 months before the triathlon. Blood, urine, and saliva samples were collected the day before the race, 5 to 10 minutes after the race, and 1.5 hours after the race.

Results.—No difference was noted in race times between the vitamin E and placebo groups, and both groups maintained an intensity of approximately 80% of maximal heart rate during the cycling and running legs of the triathlon. The mean plasma α-tocopherol levels were approximately 75% higher in the vitamin E versus the placebo group prerace (24.1 vs 13.8 μmol/L) and postrace. The mean plasma F2-isoprostane levels increased 181% versus 97% postrace in the vitamin E versus placebo groups. The mean IL-6 level was 89% higher (166 vs 88 pg/mL), and the mean IL-1ra level was 107% higher in the vitamin E versus placebo groups (4848 vs 2341 pg/mL). The mean IL-8 level was also 41% higher postrace in the vitamin E versus the placebo group (26.0 vs 18.4 pg/mL), respectively).

Conclusion.—Vitamin E (800 IU/d for 2 months) compared with placebo ingestion before a competitive triathlon race event appeared to promote lipid peroxidation and inflammation during exercise.

▶ Before this study, my research team had conducted 2 double-blinded placebo-controlled studies with vitamin C and found that 1000 to 1500 mg/d for a week before heavy exertion did not counter exercise-induced oxidative stress or alterations in immune parameters. [1,2] We reasoned that vitamin E had a higher potential to serve as an effective countermeasure to oxidative stress and immune changes after prolonged and intense exercise because it prevents the propagation of lipid peroxidation, in contrast to vitamin C, which provides antioxidant protection primarily as an aqueous-phase peroxyl. To our surprise, a 2-month supplementation regimen of vitamin E in high doses (800 IU/d) exacerbated oxidative stress and increased plasma levels of inflammatory cytokines in triathletes competing in the Triathlon World Championship race in Kona, Hawaii. There is increasing evidence that vitamin E ingestion in high doses (≥400 IU/d) and under certain conditions acts in a pro-oxidative manner and increases all-cause mortality rates. [3] In general, athletes should avoid high-dose vitamin E supplements until more is known.

D. C. Nieman, DrPH

References

1. Nieman DC, Henson DA, McAnulty SR, et al: Influence of vitamin C supplementation on oxidative and immune changes following an ultramarathon. *J Appl Physiol* 92:1970-1977, 2002.
2. Nieman DC, Henson DA, Butterworth DE, et al: Vitamin C supplementation does not alter the immune response to 2.5 hours of running. *Int J Sports Nutr* 7:173-184, 1997.
3. Miller ER III, Pastor-Barriuso R, Dalal D, et al: Meta-analysis: High-dosage vitamin E supplementation may increase all-cause mortality. *Ann Intern Med* 142:37-46, 2005.

8 Women, Children, and Aging

Gender Differences in Viral Infection After Repeated Exercise Stress
Brown AS, Davis JM, Murphy EA, et al (Univ of South Carolina, Columbia)
Med Sci Sports Exerc 36:1290-1295, 2004   8–1

Introduction.—Fatiguing exercise can increase susceptibility to respiratory infection after intranasal inoculation with herpes simplex virus-1 (HSV-1) in male mice. Although gender differences in susceptibility to certain pathogens do exist, it is unknown whether female mice will respond differently than males in response to strenuous exercise and HSV-1 infection.

Purpose.—To test the effects of gender on susceptibility to HSV-1 respiratory infection after repeated exhaustive exercise.

Methods.—Male (N = 86) and female (N = 89) CD-1 mice (approximately 60 d old) were randomly assigned to exercise (Ex) or control (C) groups. Exercise consisted of 3 d of treadmill running at 36 m/min at 8% grade until volitional fatigue (135 ± 5 min). Fifteen minutes after the last bout of exercise, Ex and C mice were inoculated intranasally with a standard dose (LD30) of HSV-1. Mice were monitored for 21 d for morbidity (time to sickness and symptom severity) and mortality.

Results.—Run time to fatigue was significantly longer in females than males ($P = 0.027$). Significant gender differences in susceptibility to infection were found after exercise stress. In males, exercise stress resulted in increased morbidity (66%, $P < 0.05$) and mortality (30%, $P < 0.05$) whereas in females, exercise stress only resulted in increased morbidity (66%, $P < 0.05$).

Conclusion.—Results suggest that although males and females have similar morbidity rates after infection and exercise stress, females recover to a greater extent and are ultimately better protected from death.

▶ Human studies suggest that females compared to males develop a stronger immune response after infection. Males are more susceptible to certain types of respiratory infections, whereas females are more prone to autoimmune diseases. Do genders differ in immune and infection responses to intense exercise training? In previous studies, my research team has reported no differences in respiratory infection rates and immune perturbations following marathon and ultramarathon race events.[1,2] In this interesting study, male and female mice exercised intensely for over 2 hours 3 days in a row, and were then inoculated with HSV-1. Morbidity rates were similar between the male and female groups, but the male mice had a higher mortality rate. The authors speculated that the sex difference may be related to differences in macrophage antiviral activity and/or inflammatory responses.

D. C. Nieman, DrPH

References

1. Nieman DC, Dumke CL, Henson DA, et al: Immune and oxidative changes during and following the Western States Endurance Run. *Int J Sports Med* 24:541-547, 2003.
2. Nieman DC, Henson DA, Fagoaga OR, et al: Change in salivary IgA following a competitive marathon race. *Int J Sports Med* 23:69-75, 2002.

Relationship of Physical Fitness vs Body Mass Index With Coronary Artery Disease and Cardiovascular Events in Women
Wessel TR, Arant CB, Olson MB, et al (Univ of Florida, Gainesville; Univ of Pittsburgh, Pa; Atlanta Cardiovascular Research Inst, Ga; et al)
JAMA 292:1179-1187, 2004   8–2

Context.—Individual contributions of obesity and physical fitness (physical activity and functional capacity) to risk of coronary heart disease in women remain unclear.

Objective.—To investigate the relationships of measures of obesity (body mass index [BMI], waist circumference, waist-hip ratio, and waist-height ratio) and physical fitness (self-reported Duke Activity Status Index [DASI] and Postmenopausal Estrogen-Progestin Intervention questionnaire [PEPI-Q] scores) with coronary artery disease (CAD) risk factors, angiographic CAD, and adverse cardiovascular (CV) events in women evaluated for suspected myocardial ischemia.

Design, Setting, and Participants.—The National Heart, Lung, and Blood Institute-sponsored Women's Ischemia Syndrome Evaluation (WISE) is a multicenter prospective cohort study. From 1996-2000, 936 women were enrolled at 4 US academic medical centers at the time of clinically indicated coronary angiography and then assessed (mean follow-up, 3.9 [SD, 1.8] years) for adverse outcomes.

Main Outcome Measures.—Prevalence of obstructive CAD (any angiographic stenosis ≥50%) and incidence of adverse CV events (all-cause death or hospitalization for nonfatal myocardial infarction, stroke, congestive heart failure, unstable angina, or other vascular events) during follow-up.

Results.—Of 906 women (mean age, 58 [SD, 12] years) with complete data, 19% were of nonwhite race, 76% were overweight (BMI ≥25), 70% had low functional capacity (DASI scores <25, equivalent to ≤7 metabolic equivalents [METs]), and 39% had obstructive CAD. During follow-up, 337 (38%) women had a first adverse event, 118 (13%) had a major adverse event, and 68 (8%) died. Overweight women were more likely than normal weight women to have CAD risk factors, but neither BMI nor abdominal obesity measures were significantly associated with obstructive CAD or adverse CV events after adjusting for other risk factors ($P=.05$ to.88). Conversely, women with lower DASI scores were significantly more likely to have CAD risk factors and obstructive CAD (44% vs 26%, $P<.001$) at baseline, and each 1-MET increase in DASI score was independently associated with an 8% (hazard ratio, 0.92; 95% confidence interval, 0.85-0.99; $P=.02$) decrease in risk of major adverse CV events during follow-up.

Conclusions.—Among women undergoing coronary angiography for suspected ischemia, higher self-reported physical fitness scores were independently associated with fewer CAD risk factors, less angiographic CAD, and lower risk for adverse CV events. Measures of obesity were not independently associated with these outcomes.

▶ Findings from this study help to elucidate the independent contributions of obesity and physical fitness to cardiovascular health or disease in women. Participants (N = 906) were part of a multicenter trial, WISE, to improve diagnostic testing for CAD. A woman had to have chest discomfort, suspected myocardial ischemia, or both, to qualify for enrollment. Two questionnaires were used to assess fitness: DASI to evaluate physical fitness, and PEPI-Q to assess physical activity. Both tests have been shown to be significantly correlated to treadmill functional capacity measure in METS, although the correlations are moderate (DASI, $r = 0.31$; PEPI-Q, $r = 0.27$). Obstructive CAD was determined as any luminal diameter stenosis of greater than 50%, and severe as greater than 70%. Four-year follow-up data were available on 880 (97%) of the women. No significant hazard ratios were found between any of the anthropometric data (BMI, waist circumference, waist-to-hip ratio, waist-to-height ratio) and all adverse events or major adverse events. However, the 2 fitness assessments were found to be significant independent predictors for all adverse events. For women, these findings suggest fitness levels may be more important than obesity for risk of cardiovascular disease. The actual cardiovascular risk of obesity for women may be partially explained by the association to low fitness. Further research is needed to determine the independent roles of obesity and physical fitness.

C. F. Sanborn, PhD

Body Fat Distribution of Overweight Females With a History of Weight Cycling
Wallner SJ, Luschnigg N, Schnedl WJ, et al (Med Univ of Graz, Austria; Karl-Franzens-Univ of Graz, Austria)
Int J Obes 28:1143-1148, 2004   8–3

Introduction.—Weight cycling may cause a redistribution of body fat to the upper body fat compartments. We investigated the distribution of subcutaneous adipose tissue (SAT) in 30 overweight women with a history of weight-cycling and age-matched controls (167 normal weight and 97 overweight subjects). Measurements of SAT were performed using an optical device, the Lipometer. The SAT topography describes the thicknesses of SAT layers at 15 anatomically well-defined body sites from neck to calf. The overweight women with a history of weight cycling had significantly thicker SAT layers on the upper body compared to the overweight controls, but even thinner SAT layers on their legs than the normal weight women. An android fat pattern was attributed to overweight females and, even more pronounced, to the weight cyclers. The majority of normal weight women showed a gynoid fat pattern. Using stepwise discriminant analysis, 89.0% of all weight cyclers and overweight controls could be classified correctly into the two groups. These findings show the importance of normal weight maintenance as a health-promoting factor.

▶ An issue that also needs to be examined when determining the adverse health consequences of being overweight is the history of weight cycling and the distribution of the body fat (android vs gynoid). Often overweight individuals will have a pattern of dieting, losing weight, and then regaining the weight lost. Although not conclusive, there is evidence to suggest that weight cycling is related to cardiovascular morbidity and mortality. The possible explanation for this relationship is that weight cycling may result in a redistribution of body fat to the upper body compartments. The authors examine the body fat distribution of 3 groups of women: overweight weight cyclers, overweight individuals, and controls. Overweight was not defined in the study, but the average body mass index (kg/m^2) was 32, 30, and 21 for the overweight weight cyclers, overweight individuals, and controls, respectively. Weight cycling was defined as a weight loss of more than 4 kg at least 3 times. SAT was determined using an optical device, the Lipometer, on 15 sites from the neck to the calf. There was a wide range of coefficient of variation (range, 2.2%-12.2%) using the Lipometer, which may be problematic in using this device in long-term obesity studies but is appropriate for the current cross-sectional design. The overweight cyclers were found to have an android patterning of upper body obesity in contrast to the gynoid fat patterning of the overweight group. The 2 overweight groups were correctly classified (85%) using a set of 5 body sites (triceps, lateral chest, hip, front thigh, and calf). The authors also present a factor plot examining the relative health risk of upper body fat versus lower body fat. While preliminary, an android versus gynoid factor plot may become an indicator of health risk and obesity.

C. F. Sanborn, PhD

Central Adiposity, Aerobic Fitness, and Blood Pressure in Premenopausal Hispanic Women

Afghani A, Abbott AV, Wiswell RA, et al (Univ of Southern California, Los Angeles; California State Univ, Northridge; Cerritos College, Calif)
Int J Sports Med 25:599-606, 2004   8–4

Introduction.—Hispanics comprise one of the fastest-growing segments of the U.S. population. Mexican-American adults are more likely to be overweight, physically inactive, diabetic, and to have higher levels of hypertension than are white adults. However, studies addressing the relationship between physical fitness and coronary artery disease (CAD) risk factors among Mexican-Americans are much less conclusive. Therefore, understanding the etiology of factors influencing resting systolic (SBP) and diastolic blood pressure (DBP) in Hispanic women was the aim of this investigation. SBP, DBP, peak oxygen uptake (peak VO_2), weekly physical activity, waist (WC) and hip circumference, blood glucose, and levels of plasma lipids (triglyceride, total cholesterol, low-density lipoprotein-cholesterol, high-density lipoprotein-cholesterol) of 39 Hispanic women age 22-51 years were measured. Factors with significant correlation to SBP were age, WC, sagittal diameter, and weight. Similarly, significant correlations were observed between anthropometric indices, age, and DBP. Peak VO_2 ($r = -0.53$, $p < 0.01$) and heart rate at maximal effort ($r = -0.34$, $p \leq 0.05$) were inversely associated to DBP. There was also a strong inverse correlation ($r = -0.53$, $p < 0.01$) between peak VO_2 and CAD risk profile (created from one or the combination of: hypertension, obesity, hyperglycemia, dyslipidemia, smoking). Stepwise multiple linear regression revealed that 33% of the variance in SBP is attributed to age (25%), and WC (8%), while DBP is explained by WC alone (26%). The addition of peak VO_2 did not make significant contributions to the variances in SBP or DBP. The findings of this study suggest that central adiposity is an important predictor of resting blood pressure in Hispanic women. The inverse association between aerobic fitness and diastolic blood pressure as well as CAD risk factors suggests that recommendations regarding prevention of hypertension in this population should be based on the interrelationships between physical fitness and obesity.

▶ The researchers provide a descriptive study of 39 Latino women recruited from a low-income Hispanic community in Los Angeles. Peak aerobic power (VO_2 peak) was determined using a continuous incremental treadmill protocol. The criteria were a respiratory exchange ratio greater than 1.05 and a heart rate within ±10 beats/min of the age-predicted maximal heart rate (HR_{max}; no participants met the criteria of a plateau in VO_2 with increasing workrates. On average, the Hispanic women were obese (body mass index >30), had a low aerobic power (26.4 mL/[kg·min]), and had elevated levels of total cholesterol (239 mg/dL) and triglycerides (157 mg/dL). WC and sagittal diameter of the abdomen were significantly correlated to both SBP and DBP ($r = 0.37$-0.56). These preliminary findings stress the importance of developing appropriate strategies for physical fitness and weight management for the Hispanic population.

C. F. Sanborn, PhD

Lifestyle Factors and the Development of Bone Mass and Bone Strength in Young Women
Lloyd T, Petit MA, Lin H-M, et al (Penn State Univ, Hershey, Pa; Johns Hopkins Univ, Baltimore, Md)
J Pediatr 144:776-782, 2004   8–5

Introduction.—Bone mineral density (BMD) (expressed as grams per centimeter^2) is used extensively as a surrogate for risk fracture, but it is not a direct measurement of bone strength. Specific measurements of bone strength and geometric properties (ie, section modulus, cross-sectional area, subperiosteal width, and cortical thickness) provide clinically relevant measurement of bone strength. Longitudinal data from healthy white females, aged 12 to 22 years, was used to obtain a comprehensive view of how modifiable determinants of bone health (ie, calcium intake, oral contraceptive use, and exercise) are linked to the development of peak bone mass and the development of young adult hip bone bending strength.

Methods.—Eighty white females participating in 10 years of the Penn State Young Women's Health Study underwent measurements of BMD and body composition by dual energy x-ray absorptiometry and estimated proximal femur section modulus (bone bending strength). Calcium intake was ascertained from 45 days of prospectively documented food records completed at regular intervals between ages 12 and 22 years. Exercise history and oral contraceptive use were evaluated by questionnaire.

Results.—Calcium use ranged between 500 to 1900 mg/d and was not significantly correlated with bone gain or bone strength. Oral contraceptive use during adolescence was not associated with bone or body composition measurements. Femoral neck BMD did not change between ages 17 to 22 years; section modulus increased 3% ($P < .05$). Only exercise during adolescence was significantly linked with increased BMD and bone bending strength.

Conclusion.—Adolescent lifestyle patterns can affect young bone strength in white females. Exercise was the predominant lifestyle determinant of bone strength in this population.

▶ In this 10-year study, girls between the ages of 12 and 16 years gained 850 g of bone mineral or 40% of their adult skeleton. The most important correlate of bone mass and strength in these study participants was sport-exercise, with no significant relationship found with average daily calcium intake across the range of 500 to 1900 mg/d. Thus, during the critical adolescent years, load-bearing physical activities have the greatest impact on the mass and strength of the rapidly growing skeleton.

D. C. Nieman, DrPH

Interaction Between Calcium Intake and Menarcheal Age on Bone Mass Gain: An Eight-Year Follow-up Study From Prepuberty to Postmenarche

Chevalley T, Rizzoli R, Hans D, et al (Univ Hosps, Geneva)

J Clin Endocrinol Metab 90:44-51, 2005   8–6

Introduction.—Both late menarcheal age and low calcium intake (Ca intake) during growth are risk factors for osteoporosis, probably by impairing peak bone mass. We investigated whether lasting gain in areal bone mineral density (aBMD) in response to increased Ca intake varies according to menarcheal age and, conversely, whether Ca intake could influence menarcheal age. In an initial study, 144 prepubertal girls were randomized in a double-blind controlled trial to receive either a Ca supplement (Ca-suppl.) of 850 mg/d or placebo from age 7.9-8.9 yr. Mean aBMD gain determined by dual energy x-ray absorptiometry at six sites (radius metaphysis, radius diaphysis, femoral neck, trochanter, femoral diaphysis, and L2-L4) was significantly ($P = 0.004$) greater in the Ca-suppl. than in the placebo group (27 *vs.* 21 mg/cm^2). In 122 girls followed up, menarcheal age was recorded, and aBMD was determined at 16.4 yr of age. Menarcheal age was lower in the Ca-suppl. than in the placebo group ($P = 0.048$). Menarcheal age and Ca intake were negatively correlated ($r = -0.35$; $P < 0.001$), as were aBMD gains from age 7.9-16.4 yr and menarcheal age at all skeletal sites (range: $r = -0.41$ to $r = -0.22$; $P < 0.001$ to $P = 0.016$). The positive effect of Ca-suppl. on the mean aBMD gain from baseline remained significantly greater in girls below, but not in those above, the median of menarcheal age (13.0 yr). Early menarcheal age (12.1 ± 0.5 yr): placebo, 286 ± 36 mg/cm^2; Ca-suppl., 317 ± 46 ($P = 0.009$); late menarcheal age (13.9 ± 0.5 yr): placebo, 284 ± 58; Ca-suppl., 276 ± 50 ($P > 0.05$). The level of Ca intake during prepuberty may influence the timing of menarche, which, in turn, could influence long-term bone mass gain in response to Ca supplementation. Thus, both determinants of early menarcheal age and high Ca intake may positively interact on bone mineral mass accrual.

▶ Is there a window of opportunity during childhood for enhancing peak bone mass with exercise or nutrition intervention? This question has been raised in regards to physical activity or specifically, bone-loading activities. Regarding bone-loading activity, Khan and associates[1], in their overview, suggest that although exercise is important for any age, during childhood it appears that bone may be more responsive to bone loading. The possible role of Ca supplementation during prepubescence on bone accrual is examined by the authors in their follow-up study. In the original study, the participants were 8 years of age, and the experimental group, who received 48 weeks of Ca supplementation (850 mg/d), had a significantly greater mean aBMD than the control group. Eight years later, the postmenarcheal girls (16 years of age) were reexamined. There was no difference between the 2 postmenarcheal groups in mean aBMD. Thus, the premenarcheal bone gains in the Ca-suppl. group were not maintained. A weak but significant correlation ($r = -0.32$; $P < .001$) was observed between menarcheal age and mean aBMD. Whether Ca supplementation during the prepubertal years might influence menarche and thus bone accrual needs further investigation.

C. F. Sanborn, PhD

Reference

1. Khan K, McKay HA, Kannus P, et al: *Physical Activity and Bone Health*. Champaign, Human Kinetics, 2001.

Exercise Effects on Menopausal Risk Factors of Early Postmenopausal Women: 3-yr Erlangen Fitness Osteoporosis Prevention Study Results

Kemmler W, von Stengel S, Weineck J, et al (Univ of Erlangen, Germany)
Med Sci Sports Exerc 37:194-203, 2005   8–7

Purpose.—To determine the impact of multipurpose exercise training on bone, body composition, blood lipids, physical fitness, and menopausal symptoms in early postmenopausal women with osteopenia.

Methods.—Forty-eight fully compliant (more than two sessions per week for 38 months) women (55.1 ± 3.3 yr) without any medication or illness affecting bone metabolism took part in the exercise training (EG); 30 women (55.5 ± 3.0 yr) served as the nontraining control group (CG). Both groups were individually supplemented with calcium and vitamin D. Bone mineral density (BMD) at various sites (lumbar spine, hip, forearm, calcaneus) was measured by dual x-ray absorptiometry (DXA) and quantitative ultrasound (QUS). Maximal isometric and dynamic strength, maximal oxygen consumption ($\dot{V}O_{2max}$), CHD risk factors (blood lipids, body composition), and menopausal symptoms were determined.

Results.—After 38 months, significant differences between EG and CG were observed for the BMD at the lumbar spine (0.7% vs −3.0%) and the femoral neck (−0.7% vs −2.6%), body composition (waist circumference, waist-to-hip ratio), blood lipids (total cholesterol, triglycerides), and menopausal symptoms (insomnia, migraines, mood changes). Maximal isometric strength increased significantly by 10-36% in the EG, whereas, with one exception, changes in the CG were all negative. One-repetition maximum increased significantly at all sites measured (15-43%, $P < 0.001$). $\dot{V}O_{2max}$ of the EG increased throughout the study with a significant 13.9 ± 15.6% net increase after 3 yr. No significant changes after 3 yr could be observed in the CG.

Conclusions.—Our mixed high-intensity exercise program effectively compensates for most negative changes related to the menopausal transition.

▶ The hypoestrogenic effects of menopause are quickly observed in the early postmenopausal years. Declines are observed in bone loss and strength along with negative changes in blood lipids and body composition. The researchers present the third-year results from their 5-year exercise trial in early postmenopausal women. At baseline, 86 women were in the EG and 51 in the CG. All women were supplemented with vitamin D and calcium based on individual nutritional needs. A potential limitation to the study is that the participants were not randomized to the 2 groups; however, this aspect should not deter from the overall findings of the longitudinal study. The 3-year results are presented for the exercisers who were compliant (n = 48) and the CG (n = 30). The exercise program occurred 4 days per week, with 2 supervised and 2 unsupervised home sessions. The emphasis of the exercise program was geared towards maintenance of BMD and reduction of risk factors and early menopausal symptoms. Warm-up consisted of 10 minutes of aerobic activity followed by bone-loading exercises (jump roping and resistance training). The home exercises were changed every 12 weeks to reduce boredom, and their intensity was increased. As reported by the authors, the central results of the exercise program are that exercise appears to stop early postmenopausal bone loss along with increasing physical fitness, decreasing CHD risk factors, and positively changing body composition. Most importantly, these benefits have been maintained over the 3-year exercise program. Whether the positive outcomes will continue for the next 2 years, over the course of the 5-year exercise intervention, will be extremely interesting.

C. F. Sanborn, PhD

Fasting Ghrelin Levels in Physically Active Women: Relationship With Menstrual Disturbances and Metabolic Hormones
De Souza MJ, Leidy HJ, O'Donnell E, et al (Univ of Toronto; Penn State Univ, University Park, Pa; Univ of California, Davis)
J Clin Endocrinol Metab 89:3536-3542, 2004   8–8

Introduction.—Recent findings support a role for ghrelin in the regulation of energy homeostasis and possibly reproductive function. The primary purpose of this study was to test whether differences in fasting ghrelin levels exist in exercising women with differing menstrual and metabolic status. Menstrual cycle status was defined as sedentary ovulatory (SedOvul; n = 10, cycles = 26), exercising ovulatory (ExOvul; n = 11, cycles = 22), exercising luteal phase defect/anovulatory (ExLPD/Anov; n = 11, cycle = 27), and exercising amenorrheic (ExAmen; n = 8, cycle = 16). Subjects were 27.7 ± 1.2 yr of age, weighed 60.2 ± 3.3 kg, and had menstrual cycle lengths of 28.4 ± 0.9 d. Blood was collected during the follicular phase (d 2-9) of each menstrual cycle and analyzed for total ghrelin, insulin, total T_3, and leptin. Ghrelin was significantly elevated by approximately 85% in the ExAmen category (725.5 ± 40.8 pmol/liter) when compared with all other categories ($P < 0.001$; SedOvul = 393.6 ± 32.0 pmol/liter, ExOvul = 418.9 ± 34.8 pmol/liter, and ExLPD/Anov = 381.1 ± 314 pmol/liter). Leptin levels were lower in all groups vs. SedOvul ($P < 0.001$). Insulin was lower in both the ExLPD/Anov and ExAmen categories vs. SedOvul and ExOvul ($P < 0.018$), and total T_3 was lower in ExAmen compared with all other groups ($P < 0.001$), with concentrations in ExLPD/Anov and ExOvul exceeding those in SedOvul ($P < 0.05$). These data clearly indicate a metabolic hormonal profile consistent with chronic energy deficiency in exercising women across a range in menstrual status and introduces ghrelin as a potential supplementary indicator that uniquely discriminates amenorrheic athletes from athletes with other menstrual disturbances.

▶ The cause of amenorrhea among athletes has been identified as low energy availability. The amenorrheic athlete is in a state of inadequate energy availability, expending more calories through exercise than she is consuming or restricting her food intake, or a combination of the two. The direct causal relationship between disruptions in energy homeostasis and menstrual dysfunction is not known. Recently, ghrelin has been suggested as having a possible role in the suppression of reproductive function in amenorrheic athletes. An overview of ghrelin is provided by the authors to support a potential link between ghrelin, energy deficiency, and reproductive dysfunctions. Ghrelin is primarily produced in the stomach and gastrointestinal tract and is a peripheral metabolic signal of energy homeostasis. Fasting ghrelin levels have been found to be elevated in patients with anorexia nervosa. The authors also provide background research to suggest that ghrelin may have a direct role in reproductive function and luteinizing hormone pulsatility. The researchers conducted a prospective study to determine whether there were differences in fasting ghrelin in exercising women with menstrual disturbance. Elevated ghrelin levels were only observed in the athletic amenorrheic group. No differences were observed in athletes who had subtle menstrual disturbances (luteal phase deficiency and anovulation). These preliminary findings suggest a possible role of ghrelin in athletic amenorrhea and warrant further research.

C. F. Sanborn, PhD

Collegiate Athletic Trainers' Confidence in Helping Female Athletes With Eating Disorders
Vaughan JL, King KA, Cottrell RR (Northern Kentucky Independent District Health Dept, Edgewood; Univ of Cincinnati, Ohio)
J Athl Train 39:71-76, 2004   8–9

Objective.—To examine college athletic trainers' confidence in helping female athletes who have eating disorders.

Design and Setting.—We mailed a 4-page, 53-item survey to head certified athletic trainers at all National Collegiate Athletic Association Division IA and IAA institutions (N = 236). A 2-wave mailing design was used to increase response rate.

Subjects.—A total of 171 athletic trainers returned completed surveys for a response rate of 77%. Eleven institutions either did not identify their head athletic trainer or did not have an identifiable mailing address. Two surveys were undeliverable because of incorrect mailing addresses.

Measurements.—The survey consisted of 4 subscales: (1) efficacy expectation, (2) outcome expectation, (3) outcome value, and (4) experience in dealing with eating disorders. Content validity was established by review from a national panel of experts. Reliability ranged from .66 to .73 for the subscales.

Results.—Although virtually all athletic trainers (91%) had dealt with a female athlete with an eating disorder, only 1 in 4 (27%) felt confident identifying a female athlete with an eating disorder, and only 1 in 3 (38%) felt confident asking an athlete if she had an eating disorder. One in 4 athletic trainers (25%) worked at an institution that did not have a policy on handling eating disorders. Almost all athletic trainers (93%) felt that increased attention needs to be paid to preventing eating disorders among collegiate female athletes.

Conclusions.—Collegiate athletic programs are encouraged to develop and implement eating-disorder policies. Continuing education on the prevention of eating disorders among athletes is also strongly recommended.

▶ Some female athletes and physically active women are at risk for the female athlete triad: eating disorders, amenorrhea, and osteoporosis. The mechanism behind these 3 interrelated clinical disorders is low energy availability (expending more energy through exercise than consuming).[1,2] The cascading events typically begin with an energy imbalance. The athlete can slide along an energy balance continuum to disordered eating to a frank eating disorder, resulting in amenorrhea and a loss in bone mass. The American College of Sports Medicine is currently revising the original female athlete position stand.[3] The revised position stand clarifies that each disorder has a continuum from health to disease: energy balance to reduced energy availability to eating disorders/low energy imbalance; eumenorrhea to subclinical menstrual disorders to amenorrhea; and bone health to osteopenia to osteoporosis.[4] The key to prevention and treatment is early detection of athletes who may be vulnerable to developing an eating disorder. For collegiate athletes, the athletic trainer has a primary responsibility in maintaining the athlete's health. The athletic trainer has a vital role in helping to identify athletes with eating disorders. For treatment to be successful, the university needs to have an eating disorder policy and a "team" of professionals identified to work with the athlete. Findings from this study clearly indicated that athletic trainers need more formal education regarding eating disorders. Another problem is that not all institutions have policies and procedures in place for eating disorders.

C. F. Sanborn, PhD

References

1. Loucks AB, Thuma JR: Luteinizing hormone pulsatility is disrupted at a threshold of energy availability in regularly menstruating women. *J Clin Endocrinol Metab* 88:297-311, 2003.
2. Loucks AB, Verdun M, Heath EM: Low energy availability, not the stress of exercise, alters LH pulsatility in exercising women. *J Appl Physiol* 84:37-46, 1998.
3. Yeager KK, Agostini R, Nattiv A, et al: The female athlete triad: Disordered eating, amenorrhea, osteoporosis (commentary). *Med Sci Sports Exerc* 25:775-777, 1993.
4. Nattiv A, Sundgot-Borgen J, Loucks A, et al: The female athlete triad position stand: 2004 update. ACSM Annual Meeting, San Francisco, 2004.

The Cardiovascular Effects of Chronic Hypoestrogenism in Amenorrhoeic Athletes: A Critical Review

O'Donnell E, De Souza MJ (Univ of Toronto)
Sports Med 34:601-627, 2004   8–10

Introduction.—In premenopausal women, the most severe menstrual dysfunction is amenorrhoea, which is associated with chronic hypoestrogenism. In postmenopausal women, hypoestrogenism is associated with a number of clinical sequelae related to cardiovascular health. A cardioprotective effect of endogenous oestrogen is widely supported, yet recent studies demonstrate a deleterious effect of hormone replacement therapy for cardiovascular health. What remain less clear are the implications of persistently low oestrogen levels in much younger amenorrhoeic athletes. The incidence of amenorrhoea among athletes is much greater than that observed among sedentary women. Recent data in amenorrhoeic athletes demonstrate impaired endothelial function, elevated low- and high-density lipoprotein levels, reduced circulating nitrates and nitrites, and increased susceptibility to lipid peroxidation. Predictive serum markers of cardiovascular health, such as homocysteine and C-reactive protein, have not yet been assessed in amenorrhoeic athletes, but are reportedly elevated in postmenopausal women. The independent and combined effects of chronic hypoestrogenism and exercise, together with subclinical dietary behaviours typically observed in amenorrhoeic athletes, warrants closer examination. Although no longitudinal studies exist, the altered vascular health outcomes reported in amenorrhoeic athletes are suggestive of increased risk for premature cardiovascular disease. Future research should focus on the presentation and progression of these adverse cardiovascular parameters in physically active women and athletes with hypoestrogenism to determine their effects on long-term health.

▶ The article is an excellent critical review of the current research examining the potential cardiovascular risk of an amenorrheic athlete. The authors compile research that was published between 1966 and 2003. The findings are detailed into the following headings: total cholesterol, low-density lipoproteins, high-density lipoproteins, triglycerides, lipid peroxidation, nitric oxide, endothelin, homocysteine, and C-reactive protein. Each section provides a brief overview regarding the cardiovascular mechanism along with the research summary for postmenopausal women and amenorrheic athletes. Since there is a lack of research findings for amenorrheic athletes, the authors extrapolate from conclusions drawn from postmenopausal women and patients with anorexia nervosa to conjecture the potential impact of hypoestrogenism in athletes. Intuitively, the overwhelming evidence of the cardiovascular risks associated with the hypoestrogenic state in postmenopausal and anorectic women should also occur in the amenorrheic athlete. The problem is a lack of research and thus, evidence to support an increased risk of cardiovascular disease among amenorrheic athletes. Obviously, research is needed. Whether cardiovascular risk should be added to the female athlete triad is not clear. A consensus panel should be convened to provide recommendations.

C. F. Sanborn, PhD

Relationship Between Sex Hormones and Anterior Knee Laxity Across the Menstrual Cycle
Shultz SJ, Kirk SE, Johnson ML, et al (Univ of North Carolina, Greensboro; Univ of Virigina, Charlottesville; United States Naval Hosp, Okinawa, Japan)
Med Sci Sports Exerc 36:1165-1174, 2004   8–11

Purpose.—To comprehensively quantify through daily, serial measures changes in knee laxity as a function of changing sex-hormone levels across one complete menstrual cycle.

Methods.—Twenty-five females, 18–30 yr, body mass index ≤30, who reported normal menstrual cycles (28–32 d) over the past 6 months participated. Participants were tested daily across one complete menstrual cycle; 5–7 cc of venous blood were withdrawn to assay serum levels of estradiol, progesterone, and testosterone. Knee laxity was measured as the amount of anterior tibial displacement at 133 N, using a standard knee arthrometer. To evaluate the relationship of knee laxity to changes in sex hormone concentrations, a multiple linear regression model with the possibility of a time delay was performed on each individual subject and the group as a whole.

Results.—Individual regression equations revealed an average of 63% of the variance in knee laxity was explained by the three hormones and their interactions. All three hormones significantly contributed to the prediction equation, and the amount of variance explained was substantially greater when a time delay was considered. On average, knee laxity changed approximately 3, 4, and 4.5 d after changes in estradiol, progesterone, and testosterone, respectively. When females were analyzed as a group, only 8% of the variance in knee laxity was explained by sex-hormones levels.

Conclusion.—Changes in sex hormones mediate changes in knee laxity across the menstrual cycle. However, the strength of this relationship, the relative contribution of each hormone, and the associated time delay are highly variable between women. This individual variability is consistent with the variability in menstrual cycle characteristics among women.

▶ Anterior cruciate ligament injuries are 2 to 10 times higher in female athletes than in male athletes. Females have a greater knee joint laxity (anterior knee joint displacement with an anterior directed force) as a result of menstrual hormones, especially estrogen, compared with men. The researchers examined the relationship of estrogen, progesterone, and testosterone to knee laxity across a menstrual cycle in regularly menstruating nonathletes. As noted by the authors, the finding that testosterone added to the prediction of knee laxity is puzzling. The major finding of this study was the extremely large variability among the women, which makes the overall mean outcomes difficult to interpret. More research needs to be conducted before the role of sex hormones in anterior crucial ligament injury risk can be identified.

C. F. Sanborn, PhD

Knee Laxity Does Not Vary With the Menstrual Cycle, Before or After Exercise

Belanger MJ, Moore DC, Crisco JJ III, et al (Harvard Med School, Pawtucket, RI; Brown Med School, Providence, RI)
Am J Sports Med 32:1150-1157, 2004   8–12

Background.—An intriguing explanation for the disproportionately high rate of anterior cruciate ligament injury in female athletes is that the structural properties of the anterior cruciate ligament are affected by the menstrual hormones. Whether this actually occurs, however, is the subject of ongoing debate.

Hypotheses.—(1) Anterior cruciate ligament laxity is different in the follicular, ovulatory, and luteal phases of the menstrual cycle, and (2) exercise exacerbates the difference in anterior cruciate ligament laxity in the 3 phases.

Methods.—Over the course of 10 weeks, repeated knee laxity measurements were taken on 27 high-level female athletes, before and after exercise. Point in the menstrual cycle was determined with charts of waking temperature and menstruation. The independent effects of menstrual phase and exercise were evaluated using generalized estimating equations.

Results.—Data from 18 participants were included in the final analysis. There were no significant differences in anterior cruciate ligament laxity in any of the 3 menstrual phases, before or after exercise.

Conclusions.—Anterior cruciate ligament laxity is not significantly different during the follicular, ovulatory, and luteal phases of the menstrual cycle, and bicycling exercise does not exacerbate or create any differences in anterior cruciate ligament laxity.

▶ The possible mechanisms for the increased rate of anterior cruciate ligament (ACL) injuries in female athletes compared with male athletes has been hypothesized to result from gender-related differences in anatomy, physiology, training, and conditioning. It has been shown that the tissue material properties of the ACL are affected by hormonal fluctuations during the menstrual cycle. Further, ACL injuries have been reported to occur more frequently during the ovulatory phase of the menstrual cycle.[1] The authors have provided a well-written study that examines whether ACL laxity is different during the menstrual cycle phases (follicular, ovulatory, and luteal) or impacted by exercise. They found that ACL laxity was not different throughout the menstrual phase and with exercise. The authors speculate that menstrual hormonal changes may have an indirect role in increasing ACL injuries by altering neuromuscular performance, but not a direct role by causing laxity in the ligament.

C. F. Sanborn, PhD

Reference

1. Wojtys EM, Huston LJ, Boynton MD, et al: The effect of the menstrual cycle on anterior cruciate ligament injuries in women as determined by hormone levels. *Am J Sports Med* 30:182-188, 2002.

Urinary Incontinence, Pelvic Floor Dysfunction, Exercise and Sport

Bø K (Norwegian Univ, Oslo, Norway)
Sports Med 34:451-464, 2004   8–13

Introduction.—Urinary incontinence is defined as "the complaint of any involuntary leakage of urine" and is a common problem in the female population with prevalence rates varying between 10% and 55% in 15- to 64-year-old women. The most frequent form of urinary incontinence in women is stress urinary incontinence, defined as "involuntary leakage on effort or exertion, or on sneezing or coughing". The aim of this article is to systematically review the literature on urinary incontinence and participation in sport and fitness activities with a special emphasis on prevalence and treatment in female elite athletes. Stress urinary incontinence is a barrier to women's participation in sport and fitness activities and, therefore, it may be a threat to women's health, self-esteem and well-being. The prevalence during sports among young, nulliparous elite athletes varies between 0% (golf) and 80% (trampolinists). The highest prevalence is found in sports involving high impact activities such as gymnastics, track and field, and some ball games. A 'stiff' and strong pelvic floor positioned at an optimal level inside the pelvis may be a crucial factor in counteracting the increases in abdominal pressure occurring during high-impact activities. There are no randomised controlled trials or reports on the effect of any treatment for stress urinary incontinence in female elite athletes. However, strength training of the pelvic floor muscles has been shown to be effective in treating stress urinary incontinence in parous females in the general population. In randomised controlled trials, reported cure rates, defined as <2g of leakage on pad tests, varied between 44% and 69%. Pelvic floor muscle training has no serious adverse effects and has been recommended as first-line treatment in the general population. Use of preventive devices such as vaginal tampons or pessaries can prevent leakage during high impact physical activity. The pelvic floor muscles need to be much stronger in elite athletes than in other women. There is a need for more basic research on pelvic floor muscle function during physical activity and the effect of pelvic floor muscle training in female elite athletes.

▶ Stress urinary incontinence is a common problem among women and also female athletes. Stress urinary incontinence is embarrassing and can lead to withdrawal from sports and physical activity. The author provides a detailed background of urinary incontinence pathophysiology and pelvic floor muscle function. The review of the current literature highlights the lack of information on stress urinary incontinence, especially among female athletes. As discussed, the first line of treatment should be conservative such as pelvic floor muscle training versus surgery. Alarmingly, only 11 of 843 reports on the effect of surgery on incontinence were randomized trials. Further, the quality of the nonrandomized, prospective studies were poor. No reports have examined the effect of surgery in young, nulliparous elite athletes; however, surgery would not be recommended. The efficacy and adverse events from surgery are also poorly examined and reported. Education is the key for prevention and coping with urinary incontinence.

C. F. Sanborn, PhD

Physical Activity Levels Among Breast Cancer Survivors
Irwin ML, McTiernan A, Bernstein L, et al (Yale School of Medicine, New Haven, Conn; Fred Hutchinson Cancer Research Ctr, Seattle; Univ of Southern California, Los Angeles; et al)
Med Sci Sports Exerc 36:1484-1491, 2004   8–14

Introduction.—Obesity and weight gain are negative prognostic factors for breast cancer survival. Physical activity (PA) prevents weight gain and may decrease obesity. Little information exists on PA levels among cancer survivors. We assessed PA, including the proportion of breast cancer survivors engaging in recommended levels, by categories of adiposity, age, disease stage, and ethnicity in 806 women with stage 0-IIIA breast cancer participating in the Health, Eating, Activity, and Lifestyle Study.

Methods.—Black, non-Hispanic white, and Hispanic breast cancer survivors were recruited into the study through Surveillance Epidemiology End Results registries in New Mexico, Western Washington, and Los Angeles County, CA. Types of sports and household activities and their frequency and duration within the third yr after diagnosis were assessed during an in-person interview.

Results.—Thirty-two percent of breast cancer survivors participated in recommended levels of PA defined as 150 min·wk^{-1} of moderate- to vigorous-intensity sports/recreational PA. When moderate-intensity household and gardening activities were included in the definition, 73% met the recommended level of PA. Fewer obese breast cancer survivors met the recommendation than overweight and lean breast cancer survivors ($P < 0.05$). Fewer black breast cancer survivors met the recommendation compared with non-Hispanic white and Hispanic breast cancer survivors ($P < 0.05$).

Conclusions.—Most of the breast cancer survivors were not meeting the PA recommendations proposed for the general adult population. Efforts to encourage and facilitate PA among these women would be an important tool to decrease obesity, prevent postdiagnosis weight gain, and improve breast cancer prognosis.

▶ As a cancer survivor of 10 years, I can confirm that PA is not encouraged during cancer treatment or rehabilitation. The authors first reported that women with diagnosed breast cancer were significantly less physically active within their first year after diagnosis than 1 year before diagnosis. In this study, new information is presented regarding PA and body composition assessments 3 years after diagnosis of 806 women breast cancer survivors. Overall, PA increased and returned to the prediagnosed levels. The problem was that the majority of obese women with breast cancer (BMI >30) did not increase their PA levels after 3 years. Further, fewer black breast cancer survivors met the recommendations for PA than non-Hispanic white and Hispanic breast cancer survivors. PA is important in all stages of our lives and stages of illness or diseases. Health care providers should include PA as a part of their prescription and treatment for breast cancer patients and breast cancer survivors.

C. F. Sanborn, PhD

Therapeutic Exercise for Individuals With Heart Failure: Special Attention to Older Women With Heart Failure
Haykowsky MJ, Ezekowitz JA, Armstrong PW (Univ of Alberta, Edmonton, Canada)
J Card Fail 10:165-173, 2004   8–15

Background.—A cardinal feature of heart failure (HF) is the reduced peak aerobic power (VO_{2peak}) secondary to alterations in cardiovascular and musculoskeletal function.

Methods and Results.—During the last decade, a number of randomized trials have examined the role that exercise training plays in attenuating the HF-mediated decline in VO_{2peak} and muscle strength. The major finding of these investigations was that aerobic or strength training was an effective intervention to increase VO_{2peak}, muscular strength, distance walked in 6 minutes, and quality of life without negatively altering left ventricular systolic function. Despite these benefits, a limitation of these investigations was the primary focus on males <60 years with impaired left ventricular systolic function. Thus the role that exercise training may play in attenuating the HF-mediated decline in VO_{2peak} in women ≥ 65 years of age remains unknown.

Conclusion.—Older women with HF have a VO_{2peak} that is below the minimal threshold level required for independent living. Moreover, older women with HF have greater disability then men and are less likely to be referred to an exercise rehabilitation program. Accordingly, future exercise intervention trials are required to examine the role that exercise training may play in attenuating the HF-mediated decline in cardiorespiratory and musculoskeletal fitness and disability in older women with HF.

▶ The authors review studies that have been conducted over the past decade examining exercise training in individuals with congestive HF (CHF). A table is compiled of 37 investigations detailing the age, gender, exercise intervention overview, and major findings. Exercise training can improve aerobic power without negatively altering left ventricular systolic function in individuals with HF. A concern raised by the authors was a lack of representation of women older than 65 as study participants. The authors then explore the limited evidence and examine the possible role that exercise training may have in reducing the functional capacity (VO_{2peak}) associated with CHF. Older women with CHF may have the most to gain from an exercise program because their functional disability is greater than men, and has been shown to be below minimal levels required for independent living. Aerobic training has been shown to increase VO_{2peak} in both sexes, but the mechanism may be dissimilar between older men and women with CHF. The most effective exercise intervention for women with CHF may be a program that incorporates aerobic and strength training. Future research is needed to examine the role of exercise prescription in attenuating the decline in VO_{2peak} and functional disability in older women with CHF.

C. F. Sanborn, PhD

Exercise for Health for Early Postmenopausal Women: A Systematic Review of Randomised Controlled Trials
Asikainen T-M, Kukkonen-Harjula K, Miilunpalo S (UKK Inst for Health Promotion Research, Tampere, Finland; Satakunta Central Hosp, Pori, Finland)
Sports Med 34:753-778, 2004   8–16

Introduction.—Women who pass menopause face many changes that may lead to loss of health-related fitness (HRF), especially if sedentary. Many exercise recommendations are also relevant for early postmenopausal women; however, these may not meet their specific needs because the recommendations are based mainly on studies on men. We conducted a systematic review for randomised, controlled exercise trials on postmenopausal women (aged 50 to 65 years) on components of HRF. HRF consists of morphological fitness (body composition and bone strength), musculoskeletal fitness (muscle strength and endurance, flexibility), motor fitness (postural control), cardiorespiratory fitness (maximal aerobic power, blood pressure) and metabolic fitness (lipid and carbohydrate metabolism). The outcome variables chosen were: bodyweight; proportion of body fat of total bodyweight (F%); bone mineral density (BMD); bone mineral content (BMC); various tests on muscle performance, flexibility, balance and coordination; maximal oxygen consumption (VO_{2max}); resting blood pressure (BP); total cholesterol (TC); high-density lipoprotein-cholesterol; low-density lipoprotein-cholesterol; triglycerides; blood glucose and insulin.

The feasibility of the exercise programme was assessed from drop-out, attendance and injury rates. Twenty-eight randomised controlled trials with 2646 participants were assessed. In total, 18 studies reported on the effects of exercise on bodyweight and F%, 16 on BMD or BMC, 11 on muscular strength or endurance, five on flexibility, six on balance or coordination, 18 on VO_{2max}, seven on BP, nine on lipids and two studies on glucose an one on insulin. Based on these studies, early postmenopausal women could benefit from 30 minutes of daily moderate walking in one to three bouts combined with a resistance training programme twice a week. For a sedentary person, walking is feasible and can be incorporated into everyday life. A feasible way to start resistance training is to perform eight to ten repetitions of eight to ten exercises for major muscle groups starting with 40% of one repetition maximum. Resistance training initially requires professional instruction, but can thereafter be performed at home with little or no equipment as an alternative for a gym with weight machines. Warm-up and cool-down with stretching should be a part of every exercise session. The training described above is likely to preserve normal bodyweight, or combined with a weight-reducing diet, preserve BMD and increase muscle strength. Based on limited evidence, such exercise might also improve flexibility, balance and coordination, decrease hypertension and improve dyslipidaemia.

▶ This well-written article is an excellent review of exercise for early postmenopausal women. I would recommend this review for 5 major reasons:

1. The detailed table of randomized controlled trials of early postmenopausal women with health-related outcome measures
2. The recommended exercise prescription for early postmenopausal women
3. The methodololgy used to conduct a critical review of the literature
4. Characteristics of a quality exercise intervention study
5. Future research in the area of exercise and health for early postmenopausal women.

Approximately 1500 studies were identified that matched the key words (women and exercise); however, only 21 randomized controlled trials met the criteria and were detailed in the table. The majority of the selected studies were found using the Cochrane Central Register of Controlled Trials. The authors noted that some randomized controlled trials failed to provide the following data, which are critical components of a study: randomization protocols, power calculations, and procedures for "blinding." Some suggested future research topics for early postmenopausal interventions include the effects of training on flexibility, motor fitness, balance and coordination, BP, and lipid and glucose levels.

C. F. Sanborn, PhD

A Pilot Study Comparing Pedometer Counts With Reported Physical Activity in Elementary Schoolchildren
Cardon G, De Bourdeaudhuij I (Ghent Univ, Belgium)
Pediatr Exerc Sci 16:355-367, 2004   8–17

Background.—In an increasingly sedentary society, children continue to be more active than adults; however, there is evidence to suggest that some children are insufficiently active and that physical activity in children declines from 8 to 18 years of age. Regular physical activity during childhood and adolescence is associated with improvements in many physiological and psychological variables and is being promoted as an objective for disease prevention, so all children and adolescents should be encouraged to engage in moderate-to-vigorous physical activity (MVPA) for at least 60 minutes and up to several hours daily. Numerous studies have shown the pedometer to be a cost effective, valid, reliable measure of physical activity in children, adolescents, and adults. The use of pedometers has become increasingly popular among adults, largely through the promotion of the 10,000 daily steps recommendation for adults. However, it is unclear how many steps equate to the "Healthy 2010" recommendation of 1 hour of MVPA per day for children and adolescents. The daily step counts in Belgian school children were evaluated and pedometer counts were compared with reported minutes of MVPA engagement.

Methods.—Pedometer counts were recorded for 6 consecutive days for 92 children in Flanders, Belgium, with a mean age of 9.5 years (range, 6.5-12.7 years). Findings in these children were compared with the number of minutes per day in which the study participants engaged in MVPA. The minutes of MVPA for each child were determined by use of diaries completed with the help of children's parents.

Results.—The average daily step count was significantly higher in boys than in girls, although there was no significant sex difference in the average daily MVPA engagement in minutes. On the basis of the regression equations used in this study, 60 minutes of MVPA was equivalent to 15,340 step counts in boys, 11,317 step counts in girls, and 13,130 step counts when results for boys and girls were combined. There was moderate correlation between pedometer step counts and reported minutes of MVPA.

Conclusions.—There is a weak relationship between recommendations based on step counts and recommendations based on minutes of engagement in moderate-to-vigorous physical activity. Additional study is needed to validate pedometer step-count standards before using them for promotion and quantification of daily MVPA engagement in children.

▶ Pedometers may prove useful not only for measuring physical activity but also as motivating devices in exercise intervention programs. This study of young children provides useful "normative" data on step counts in this age group. The finding of only a moderate correlation between step counts and minutes of moderate activity by diary/questionnaire led the authors to caution the use of pedometer step counts for prediction and promotion of activity in this age group. It is possible, however, that the limitations in accuracy of activity measurement might lie in the parent-assisted activity diary rather than pedometer measures of step counts.

T. Rowland, MD

Fundamental Movement Skills and Habitual Physical Activity in Young Children

Fisher A, Reilly JJ, Kelly LA, et al (Yorkhill Hosps, Glasgow, Scotland; Glasgow City Council, Scotland; Univ of Glasgow, Scotland)
Med Sci Sports Exerc 37:684-688, 2005   8–18

Purpose.—To test for relationships between objectively measured habitual physical activity and fundamental movement skills in a relatively large and representative sample of preschool children.

Methods.—Physical activity was measured over 6 d using the Computer Science and Applications (CSA) accelerometer in 394 boys and girls (mean age 4.2, SD 0.5 yr). Children were scored on 15 fundamental movement skills, based on the Movement Assessment Battery, by a single observer.

Results.—Total physical activity (r = 0.10, $P < 0.05$) and percent time spent in moderate to vigorous physical activity (MVPA) (r = 0.18, $P < 0.001$) were significantly correlated with total movement skills score. Time spent in light-intensity physical activity was not significantly correlated with motor skills score (r = 0.02, $P > 0.05$).

Conclusions.—In this sample and setting, fundamental movement skills were significantly associated with habitual physical activity, but the association between the two variables was weak. The present study questions whether the widely assumed relationships between motor skills and habitual physical activity actually exist in young children.

▶ It has often been assumed that fundamental motor skills such as throwing, jumping, and skipping are related to habitual activity in very young children. By this concept, those who are more capable of performing activities will be more likely to engage in regular exercise. Consequently, promoting acquisition of motor skills has been considered to be important in not only developing athletic abilities but also promoting an active lifestyle in children. This study challenges this concept. Fundamental motor skills and habitual physical activity were found to be related in a group of preschool children, but the association was weak. The results support the suggestion of other authors that an excessive emphasis on motor skill acquisition in children may be inappropriate.

T. Rowland, MD

Physical Activity Among Children Attending Preschools

Pate RR, Pfeiffer KA, Trost SG, et al (Univ of South Carolina, Columbia; Kansas State Univ, Manhattan; Gerber Products Co, Parsippany, NJ)
Pediatrics 114:1258-1263, 2004   8–19

Objectives.—Obesity rates are increasing among children of all ages, and reduced physical activity is a likely contributor to this trend. Little is known about the physical activity behavior of preschool-aged children or about the influence of preschool attendance on physical activity. The purpose of this study was to describe the physical activity levels of children while they attend preschools, to identify the demographic factors that might be associated with physical activity among those children, and to determine the extent to which children's physical activity varies among preschools.

Methods.—A total of 281 children from 9 preschools wore an Actigraph (Fort Walton Beach, FL) accelerometer for an average of 4.4 hours per day for an average of 6.6 days. Each child's height and weight were measured, and parents of participating children provided demographic and education data.

Results.—The preschool that a child attended was a significant predictor of vigorous physical activity (VPA) and moderate-to-vigorous physical activity (MVPA). Boys participated in significantly more MVPA and VPA than did girls, and black children participated in more VPA than did white children. Age was not a significant predictor of MVPA or VPA.

Conclusions.—Children's physical activity levels were highly variable among preschools, which suggests that preschool policies and practices have an important influence on the overall activity levels of the children the preschools serve.

▶ It is increasingly evident that for some children obesity can begin well before school age. Consequently, influences on physical activity and food intake in the life of the preschool child are taking on increasingly important meaning. In this study, considerable variation in daily physical activity was observed in various preschool settings. It would seem, then, that assuring that the structured preschool experience include adequate time to optimize physical activity is important in this young age group. Other influences in the preschool population, particularly introduction to regular consumption of fast foods deserve attention as well.

T. Rowland, MD

Scaling or Normalising Maximum Oxygen Uptake to Predict 1-Mile Run Time in Boys
Nevill A, Rowland T, Goff D, et al (Univ of Wolverhampton, Walsall, England)
Eur J Appl Physiol 92:285-288, 2004   8–20

Introduction.—There is still considerable debate and some confusion as to the most appropriate method of scaling or normalizing maximum oxygen uptake ($\dot{V}O_{2max}$) for differences in body mass (m) in both adults and children. Previous studies on adult populations have demonstrated that although the traditional ratio standard $\dot{V}O_{2max}$ (ml kg^{-1} min^{-1}) fails to render $\dot{V}O_{2max}$ independent of body mass, the ratio standard is still the best predictor of running performance. However, no such evidence exists in children. Hence, the purpose of the present study was to investigate whether the ratio standard is still the most appropriate method of normalising $\dot{V}O_{2max}$ to predict 1-mile run speed in a group of 12-year-old children ($n = 36$). Using a power function model and log-linear regression, the best predictor of 1-mile run speed was given by: speed (m s^{-1}) = 55.1 $\dot{V}O_{2max}$$^{0.986}m^{-0.96}$. With both the $\dot{V}O_{2max}$ and body mass exponents being close to unity but with opposite signs, the model suggest the best predictor of 1-mile run speed is almost exactly the traditional ratio standard recorded in the units $(ml\,kg^{-1}\,min^{-1})$. Clearly, reporting the traditional ratio standard $\dot{V}O_{2max}$, recorded in the units $(ml\,kg^{-1}\,min^{-1})$, still has an important place in publishing the results of studies investigating cardiovascular fitness of both children and adults.

▶ An appropriate means of expressing physiologic and performance measures to body size is particularly critical in growing children. The use of the traditional ratio standard, or mass[1.00], as a normalizing denominator has been criticized for producing spurious results, and for physiologic functions allometrically derived exponents of body mass in most cases appear instead to be more accurate. However, this study demonstrates that at least for 1 performance measure, the 1.6-km (1-mile) run, the ratio standard (or "per kg body mass") is the most appropriate size-normalizing factor. This points out that different measures may require specific forms of adjustments for differences in body size.

T. Rowland, MD

Energy Costs of Physical Activities in Children and Adolescents
Harrell JS, McMurray RG, Baggett CD, et al (Univ of North Carolina, Chapel Hill; Univ of Utah, Salt Lake City)
Med Sci Sports Exerc 37:329-336, 2005   8–21

Purpose.—The primary aim was to determine the energy expenditure (EE: $kcal\cdot kg^{-1}\cdot h^{-1}$) in terms of caloric cost and metabolic equivalents of activities commonly performed by children and adolescents. Secondary aims were to determine at what age and pubertal developmental stage values approach those of adults.

Methods.—In this descriptive study, 295 volunteer youth 8-18 yr of age completed 18 common physical activities (including rest) while EE was measured continuously with a portable metabolic system. Three sets of activities were assigned in random order for each subject. Activities ranged from television viewing and video game play to running and rope skipping. Pubertal development was estimated from a self-report questionnaire.

Results.—At rest, $\dot{V}O_2$ and EE were highest in the youngest children and decreased with advancing age and higher pubertal stage in both genders. The age-adjusted and puberty-adjusted energy expenditure values were generally lower than the compendium MET values for sedentary and moderate activities but were more varied for high-intensity activities. However, the ratio of activity EE to REE was comparable in children and adults.

Conclusions.—Energy expenditure per kilogram of body mass at rest or during exercise is greater in children than adults and varies with pubertal status, thus using the definition of a MET in the compendium of physical activities without adjustment is inadequate for energy estimation in children, until a child reaches Tanner Stage 5. However, the ratio of activity EE to resting EE in children appears to be similar or slightly less than in the compendium, suggesting that the compendium MET increments used with our adjusted EE values more closely approximate the true EE of activities in children than present adult norms.

▶ This is a long-awaited compendium that catalogues typical EE of youth of various ages performing common forms of physical activity. It thus supplements similar previous studies in adults and provides us with a more population-wide estimate of the energy cost of these activities. As expected, the authors found that EE related to body mass is greater in children. For this reason, use of the metabolic equivalent (MET) as described for adults is inappropriate until the end of puberty is reached.

T. Rowland, MD

The Effect of Office-Based Physician's Advice on Adolescent Exercise Behavior
Ortega-Sanchez R, Jimenz-Mena C, Cordoba-Garcia R, et al (Centro de Salud Santa Bárbara, Toledo, Spain; Centro de Salud Telde, Gran Canaria, Spain; Centro de Salud Delicias Sur, Zaragoza, Spain; et al)
Prev Med 38:219-226, 2004   8–22

Background.—This study examines whether the adolescents' current levels of physical activity are increased by their physicians' advice provided in the office, in accordance with the American Medical Association recommendation.

Methods.—The first adolescent (12-21 years old) of whichever age and gender, passing through six family physicians' offices during a 6-month period was assigned to the intervention group, and the second adolescent of the same age and gender was assigned to the control group. Each patient was classified as active, partially active, and inactive, according to how they answered the questions about their physical activity levels, and patients in the intervention group were then provided with reinforcement, increase, or initiation counseling, respectively. Identical procedures were repeated at the 6- and 12-month office visits. Changes in prevalence of activity, as well as, duration, frequency, and intensity of exercise and/or sports were verified at each visit.

Results.—Of the 87.5% of the original sample that completed the survey, 6- and 12-month data were available for 70.1%. Among the 392 adolescents that finished the study, those provided with counseling had 41.5% more active adolescents, as well as 26.8%, 38.0% and 26.2% higher duration, frequency and intensity, respectively, than the control group.

Conclusions.—The proportion of active adolescents, as well as, the duration, frequency and intensity of leisure time exercise and/or sports are increased by physician advice.

▶ Primary care health providers for youth are in an ideal setting for encouraging improved physical activity habits in sedentary children. Whether this is truly feasible, given the heavy time demands in the busy pediatric office, has not yet been clearly determined. This study is at least encouraging. The authors found that providing office-based exercise advice improved reported activity levels in a significant proportion of patients compared with a nonencouraged group. Still, it needs to be recognized that activity was assessed by questionnaire, improvements were only modest, and retention of increased activity over the long-term was not assessed. Moreover, 3 of the original 10 physicians dropped out of the study because they thought that they had insufficient time to provide exercise counseling.

T. Rowland, MD

Influence of Changes in Sedentary Behavior on Energy and Macronutrient Intake in Youth
Epstein LH, Roemmich JN, Paluch RA, et al (State Univ of New York, Buffalo; Brown Univ, Providence, RI)
Am J Clin Nutr 81:361-366, 2005   8–23

Background.—Changes in sedentary behavior may be related to changes in energy intake.

Objective.—The purpose of this study was to investigate how experimental changes in the amount of sedentary behaviors influence energy intake.

Design.—Sixteen nonoverweight 12–16-y-old youth were studied in a within-subject crossover design with three 3-wk phases: baseline, increasing targeted sedentary behaviors by 25-50% (increase phase), and decreasing targeted sedentary behaviors by 25-50% (decrease phase). Repeated 24-h recalls were used to assess energy and macronutrient intakes during targeted sedentary behaviors. Accelerometers were used to assess activity levels.

Results.—Targeted sedentary behaviors increased by 81.5 min/d (45.8%) and decreased by 109.8 min/d (-61.2%) from baseline (both: $P < 0.01$). Girls increased sedentary behaviors significantly more than did boys (107.3 and 55.8 min/d, respectively; $P < 0.01$) in the increase phase. Energy intake decreased (-463.0 kcal/d; $P < 0.01$) when sedentary behaviors decreased: the decrease in fat intake was -295.2 kcal/d ($P < 0.01$). No significant changes in energy intake were observed when sedentary behaviors were increased. Youth also increased their activity by 102.4 activity counts $\cdot$ min^{-1} $\cdot$ d^{-1} (estimated at 113.1 kcal) when sedentary behaviors were decreased ($P < 0.05$).

Conclusions.—Decreasing sedentary behaviors can decrease energy intake in nonoverweight adolescent youth and should be considered an important component of interventions to prevent obesity and to regulate body weight.

▶ Decreasing a child's time spent in sedentary activities such as television watching and playing video games may play an important role in obesity management and prevention. This study provides further documentation of the potential efficacy of this approach. A reduction in time spent in sedentary behavior was associated with both a reduction in food intake as well as a shift in time spent being more physically active. It was interesting that making children more sedentary did not alter either caloric intake or level of daily physical activity.

T. Rowland, MD

Cardiovascular Fitness and Exercise as Determinants of Insulin Resistance in Postpubertal Adolescent Females

Kasa-Vubu JZ, Lee CC, Rosenthal CC, et al (Univ of Michigan, Ann Arbor)
J Clin Endocrinol Metab 90:849-854, 2005   8–24

Background.—The epidemic of obesity in the United States and recent reports of the increased prevalence of type 2 diabetes in children in this country have highlighted the need for prevention. The most frequently identified risk factors for the onset of type 2 diabetes in youth are puberty, obesity, and evidence of insulin resistance. It is thought that a sedentary lifestyle and heavy consumption of high-energy foods and beverages are driving the obesity epidemic among children of all ages. The relative contributions of diet and exercise as risk factors for obesity and type 2 diabetes are open to debate. There is a significant decline in physical activity in girls as they mature through puberty, and this decrease in physical activity has been associated with a steady increase in body mass index (BMI). In adults, obesity is a strong determinant of insulin resistance; however, recent studies have found that an elevated BMI by itself may not be predictive of the degree of insulin resistance. The hypothesis that BMI, relative fat mass, and cardiovascular fitness would be predictors of insulin resistance was investigated in adolescent women across the weight and fitness spectra.

Methods.—The study group was composed of 53 healthy adolescent and young women ages 16 to 21 years with a BMI between the 10th and 95th percentiles for age. The subjects were studied at a minimum of 2 years after menarche. Body composition was measured by total-body dual x-ray absorptiometry. Self-reported weekly frequency of aerobic exercise for 1 hour (RDE) was recorded, and maximal oxygen intake (VO_2max) was measured. Insulin sensitivity was estimated by the homeostasis model assessment index for insulin resistance ($HOMA_{IR}$), which has been used as a surrogate measure for insulin resistance and validated in adolescents.

Results.—BMI was not related to $HOMA_{IR}$. RDE showed a marginal relationship to $HOMA_{IR}$, while percent body fat and VO_2max were significantly related to $HOMA_{IR}$. Multiple regression modeling showed that VO_2max was a more critical determinant of insulin resistance than percent body fat or RDE.

Conclusions.—BMI had a poor predictive value for insulin resistance in postpubertal adolescent females, while cardiovascular fitness was a predictor of $HOMA_{IR}$, even after adjusting for percent body fat. Thus, physical inactivity may be a greater metabolic risk than obesity alone for insulin resistance in girls and young women.

▶ This is an interesting study in older adolescent females, in whom the authors have attempted to parcel out the relative contributions of aerobic fitness (VO_2max/kg) and percent body fat to levels of insulin resistance. In a multiple regression model, they found that VO_2max accounted for more of the variance in insulin resistance than body fat content. It was, therefore, considered that adiposity was not as important in these subjects as aerobic fitness in predicting insulin resistance. This study supports the idea that both reductions in body fat and improvements in activity/fitness may be independent and important strategies for managing and preventing type 2 diabetes mellitus.

T. Rowland, MD

Adolescent Growth Spurts in Female Gymnasts

Thomis M, Claessens AL, Lefevre J, et al (Katholieke Universiteit Leuven, Belgium; Ghent Univ, Belgium; Tarleton State Univ, Stephenville, Tex)
J Pediatr 146:239-244, 2005   8–25

Objectives.—Three questions were addressed: (1) Do female gymnasts have adolescent growth spurts in height, sitting height, and leg length? (2) Are the sequence and magnitude of spurts comparable with female adolescent non-athletes? (3) How do the data compare with other female gymnasts and with short girls?

Study Design.—Height and sitting height were measured annually on 15 Belgian gymnasts from 8.7 ± 1.5 to 15.5 ± 1.5 years. The gymnasts trained, on average, approximately 15 h/wk. Leg length was estimated as height minus sitting height. The Preece-Baines Model I was fitted to individual growth records to estimate ages at peak velocity and peak velocities for the three dimensions. Age at menarche and skeletal age were also assessed.

Results.—Gymnasts have clearly defined adolescent spurts in height, estimated leg length, and sitting height that occur approximately 1 year later and are slightly less intense than in nonathletic adolescent girls. Age at menarche and skeletal age are consistent with later somatic maturation. The pattern of adolescent growth and maturation is similar to that of other gymnasts, short normal late-maturing girls, and late-maturing girls with short parents.

Conclusions.—The results emphasize a primary role for constitutional factors in the selection process of female gymnasts at relatively young ages.

▶ Some believe that intensive gymnastics training can delay growth and sexual maturation, particularly in girls. This study provides ammunition for the viewpoint that growth patterns and biological development in female gymnasts mimic those of other short, late-maturing girls. This means that the trends of sexual development and somatic growth in gymnasts represent constitutional factors which are preselected in those with gymnastics talent. The findings suggest that regular training in itself does not affect timing of growth spurt nor speed of sexual maturation. The potential influence of undernutrition during training in elite-level gymnasts on these factors, however, remains problematic.

T. Rowland, MD

Recovery During High-Intensity Intermittent Anaerobic Exercise in Boys, Teens, and Men

Zafeiridis A, Dalamitros A, Dipla K, et al (Univ of Thessaloniki, Greece)
Med Sci Sports Exerc 37:505-512, 2005   8–26

Purpose.—This study examined the effects of age on recovery of peak torque of knee extensors (PTEX) and flexors (PTFL), and total work (TW) during high-intensity intermittent 30-s (HI30) and 60-s (HI60) exercise in boys ($N = 19$; age, 11.4 ± 0.5 yr), teens ($N = 17$; age, 14.7 ± 0.4 yr), and men ($N = 18$; age, 24.1 ± 2.0 yr).

Methods.—Each age group's subjects were subdivided to participate in an HI30 or an HI60 protocol. The HI30 involved 4×18 maximal knee extensions and flexions (1-min rest between sets), and the HI60 comprised of 2×34 reps (2-min rest). PTEX ($N \cdot m \cdot kg^{-1}$), PTFL ($N \cdot m \cdot kg^{-1}$), and TW ($J \cdot kg^{-1}$) were recorded at each set. The percent recovery of PTEX, PTFL, and TW was calculated as percent of the value achieved in the first set.

Results.—In HI60, the percent recovery for PTEX, PTFL, and TW after the first set was higher in boys compared with teens and men ($P < 0.01$). In HI30, the percent recovery for PTEX, PTFL, and TW was higher in boys compared with men in all sets ($P < 0.01$), and in teens compared with men in the last two sets ($P < 0.05$). The percent recovery of PTFL and TW was higher in boys compared with teens in the last two sets ($P < 0.05$). Lactate increase was most pronounced in men, less pronounced in teens, and least pronounced in boys ($P < 0.01$). Heart rate recovered faster in boys compared with teens and men in both protocols ($P < 0.05$).

Conclusions.—The recovery was faster in boys than in teens and men during HI30 and HI60, as evident by the greater percent recovery in boys for a given time. Furthermore, it appears that the rate of recovery during HI30 and HI60 anaerobic exercise is maturity dependent.

▶ This study measured various biochemical and performance markers in boys, adolescents, and adult men during recovery from intense brief anaerobic exercise. Although there was some variability in the findings, most supported earlier investigations indicating that boys recover more rapidly in these measures than do teenagers or adults. The explanation for this influence of biologic maturation on recovery from anaerobic work is not clear. One possible idea is that anaerobic metabolic processes are different before puberty (ie, lower glycolytic capacity). These findings may have implications for designing training regimens for children in sports that involve short-burst activities.

T. Rowland, MD

Comparison of Thermoregulatory Responses to Exercise in Dry Heat Among Prepubertal Boys, Young Adults and Older Males

Inbar O, Morris N, Epstein Y, et al (Wingate Inst, Israel; Griffith Univ, Gold Coast, Australia; Tel Aviv Univ, Israel)
Exp Physiol 89:691-700, 2004

8–27

Introduction.—The purpose of this investigation was to compare the thermoregulatory responses during exercise in a hot climate among three age categories. Eight prepubertal (PP), eight young adult (Y) and eight elderly (O) male subjects cycled at an intensity of $50 \pm 1\%$ of their maximum oxygen uptake ($\dot{V}O_{2peak}$) for 85 min (three 20 min bouts with three 7 min rest periods) in hot and dry conditions ($41 \pm 0.67°C$, $21 \pm 1\%$ relative humidity). During the exercise-in-heat protocol, rectal temperature (T_{re}) skin temperatures (T_{sk}), heart rate (HR), $\dot{V}_{O2}$, $\dot{V}_{CO2}$, $\dot{V}_E$, RER, sweat rate, and the number of heat activated sweat glands (HASG) were determined. Despite highest and lowest end-exposure T_{re} in the Y and O groups, respectively, the rise in rectal temperature (accounting for differences in baseline T_{re}) was similar in all age groups. Changes in body heat storage (ΔS), both absolute and relative to body mass, were highest in the Y and O groups and lowest in the PP group. While end-session as well as changes in mean skin temperature were similar in all three age groups, HR (absolute and percentage of maximum) was significantly lower for the O compared with the PP and Y groups. Total body as well as per body surface sweating rate was significantly lower for the PP group, while body mass-related net metabolic heat production ($(M - W)$ kg^{-1}) and heat gained from the environment were highest in the PP and lowest in the O group. Since mass-related evaporative cooling (E_{sk} kg^{-1}) and sweating efficiency (E_{sk}/M_{sw} kg^{-1}) were highest in the PP and lowest in the O group, the mass-dependent heat stored in the body (ΔS kg^{-1}) was lowest in the PP (1.87 ± 0.03 W kg^{-1}) and highest in Y and O groups (2.19 ± 0.08 and 1.97 ± 0.11 W kg^{-1}, respectively). Furthermore, it was calculated that while the O group required only 4.1 ± 0.5 W of heat energy to raise their body core temperature by 1°C, and the Y group needed 6.9 ± 0.9 W $(1°C)^{-1}$, the PP group required as much as 12.3 ± 0.7 W to heat up their body core temperature by 1°C. These results suggest that in conditions similar to those imposed during this study, age and age-related characteristics affect the overall rate of heat gain as well as the mechanisms through which this heat is being dissipated. While prepubertal boys seem to be the most efficient thermoregulators, the elderly subjects appear to be the least efficient thermoregulators.

▶ Abundant research has confirmed that prepubertal boys sweat less than postpubertal boys during exercise. Conceptually, this should place children at higher risk for hyperthermia and injury when exercising in very hot environments, when body cooling relies principally on sweat evaporation. Yet, surprisingly, most studies do not indicate a greater rise in core temperature in children in such conditions, nor has a higher risk of heat injury been documented in child athletes. This study provides some interesting data that might explain this paradox. The findings suggest that children may be more efficient thermoregulators, with lower amounts of heat storage relative to body mass compared to older individuals. The authors proposed that although sweat production was relatively less in the children, cooling by sweating efficiency might be greater because smaller sweat drops could result in more evaporative cooling than larger drops, which tend to coalesce and drip.

T. Rowland, MD

Temperature Regulation During Rest and Exercise in the Cold in Premenarcheal and Menarcheal Girls
Klentrou P, Cunliffe M, Slack J, et al (Brock Univ, St Catharines, Ont, Canada; McMaster Univ, Hamilton, Ont, Canada; Univ of Toronto)
J Appl Physiol 96:1393-1398, 2004   8–28

Background.—Temperature regulation in cold weather has been linked to age, adiposity, and sex. Although the thermoregulatory response of adult women to heat or cold exposure is indicative of menstrual phase-related differences, the effect of the ovarian hormones on temperature regulation during cold exposure during growth and development is unclear. Both estrogen and progesterone influence temperature regulation in women, so the fluctuations of these hormones during the different phases of the menstrual cycle can affect temperature regulation. The use of synthetic hormones in birth control pills has provided investigators with the ability to manipulate the menstrual cycle and explore the influence of the menstrual hormones on thermoregulation in women. This relationship was investigated and whether any thermoregulatory differences are solely a function of geometric differences or whether they reflect maturation-related differences in the thermogenic and vasoconstrictive responses was determined.

Methods.—Temperature regulation during exercise in the cold was examined in 13 adolescent girls and young women aged 13 to 18 years. The subjects were divided into a eumenorrheic menarcheal (EM) group (6 girls) and a premenarcheal group (PM) group (7 girls). At the first visit, maximal oxygen intake ($VO_{2\,max}$), height, body mass, and percent body fat were measured. The second visit included a determination of metabolic rate in thermoneutrality (21°C), consisting of a 10-minute rest period and 20 minutes of cycling (30% of $VO_{2\,max}$), and a cold test (5°C, 40% humidity, <0.3 m/s air velocity) involving a 20-minute rest period and 40 minutes of cycling.

Results.—Heat production per kilogram in thermoneutrality and in the cold was significantly higher in the PM group than in the EM group. However, subjects in the PM group had a significantly lower core temperature in the cold than the EM group. Girls in the PM group also had a significantly higher body surface area-to-mass ratio compared with girls in the EM group. The difference in percent body fat between the groups was not significant, but within the PM group, percent body fat explained 79% of the variance in the decrease in core temperature.

Conclusions.—Young premenarcheal girls showed an altered thermoregulatory response during cold exposure compared with eumenorrheic menarcheal young women, most likely as a result of differences in their hormonal milieu. The absence of reproductive hormones may have an effect on the thermoregulatory responses of women in the cold, and the effects of exogenous hormones on temperature control in both younger and older women are indicative of the differences that an altered menstrual status may have on thermoregulatory responses.

▶ Most studies of maturational differences in thermoregulation during exercise have been performed in the heat. This study demonstrated that children's responses to exercise in the cold may differ from that of postpubertal subjects. Specifically, during cycling in a 5°C environment, premenarcheal girls had a higher heat production relative to body mass. However, their core temperature fell to a greater extent than that of postpubertal females. The most obvious explanation is geometric—the young girls had a higher body surface area-to-mass ratio, allowing greater loss of heat from the skin. So this is one reason, at least, why prepubertal girls should not compete in the Iditarod.

T. Rowland, MD

Behavioral and Psychological Factors Related to the Use of Nutritional Ergogenic Aids Among Preadolescents
Pesce C, Donati A, Magrì L, et al (Univ Inst of Motor Sciences, Piazza, Rome; Italian Natl Olympic Committee, Rome; Univ Tor Vergata, Rome)
Pediatr Exerc Sci 16:231-249, 2004   8–29

Background.—The use of ergogenic aids, in the form of creatine and amino acids, has become common practice in sports, even among preadolescent athletes. However, most reviews of the literature have reported equivocal results concerning the potential benefits and long-term side effects of creatine supplementation. The relationship between preadolescent use of ergogenic aids and gender, age, athletic participation, and sport-relevant psychological factors (sport success motivation, task and ego orientation, and self-efficacy) were investigated.

Methods.—The study was conducted among 2450 boys and girls aged 11 to 13 years at middle schools in Rome. All of the study subjects completed a closed-response questionnaire anonymously. The questionnaire included questions about the children's knowledge of and use of creatine and amino acids and their daily practices concerning sports. Also included were abbreviated versions of several psychological tests. Of the 2450 subjects included in the study, data from 326 subjects were excluded from the final analysis due to incomplete or inconsistently completed questionnaires.

Results.—Survey responses indicated that there is an increase in substance abuse with age, particularly among male preadolescents, that gender differences are more pronounced among older preadolescents, and that a high commitment to sport training is a risk factor for ergogenic supplementation only when it is associated with specific psychological dispositions, such as a high ego orientation and a low task orientation. It was also clear from the findings that preadolescents' use of creatine or amino acids is associated, particularly in males, with the use of vitamin and mineral supplements in a kind of dietary "polysupplementation habit."

Conclusions.—These results were consistent with recent evidence regarding the use of creatine among children who engage in sport activity. However, these findings also indicate that the use of creatine and amino acids is relatively common among preadolescents engaged in low-intensity, educational school sport.

▶ The use of inappropriate ergogenic aids in child and adolescent athletes is certainly a disturbing trend. Efforts to understand factors that lead to such use would be helpful in preventive strategies. This study identifies some psychological characteristics of athletes who might be more prone to take supplements such as creatine and amino acids. In particular, a high commitment to sport training and success was linked to use of ergogenic aids only when associated with certain psychological features, such as a high ego orientation and low task orientation. One surprising finding was that high confidence levels increased rather than reduced the probability of supplement use. Clearly, much more needs to be learned.

T. Rowland, MD

Moderate Physical Exercise Increases Cardiac Autonomic Nervous System Activity in Children With Low Heart Rate Variability

Nagai N, Hamada T, Kimura T, et al (Kyoto Univ, Japan; Okayama Prefectural Univ, Japan)
Childs Nerv Syst 20:209-214, 2004   8–30

Object.—Our objective was to investigate the effect of a long-term moderate exercise program on cardiac autonomic nervous system (ANS) activity in healthy children.

Methods.—Three hundred and five children aged 6-11 years participated in a 12-month school-based exercise training program (130-140 bpm, 20 min/day, 5 days/week). Cardiac ANS activities were measured using heart rate variability (HRV) power spectral analysis in resting conditions. Following the first measurement, 100 children from the lowest total power (TP) HRV were chosen as experimental samples and the same number of age-, height-, and weight-matched controls (CG) was randomly selected from the remaining children.

Results.—In the low group (LG), all the frequency components of the HRV were significantly increased after the training period, whereas only low-frequency power was augmented in the control group (CG).

Conclusion.—Our data suggest that the 12-month moderate exercise training has a positive effect on cardiac ANS activity in the children who initially had low HRV.

▶ Increasing research evidence indicates a role of autonomic activity on the health of children as well as adults. This study revealed favorable changes in HRV after a period of exercise training in children in those who initially had low variability. Although the relationship of markers of HRV and sympathetic and parasympathetic activity have not been validated in the pediatric age group, the findings can be considered supportive of salutary effects of exercise training in children.

T. Rowland, MD

Left Ventricular Function in Endurance-Trained Children by Tissue Doppler Imaging
Nottin S, Nguyen L-D, Terbah M, et al (Lab of Cardiovascular Adaptations to Exercise, Avignon, France; Regional Hosp Ctr, Orléans, France)
Med Sci Sports Exerc 36:1507-1513, 2004   8–31

Introduction.—In children and adults, endurance training increases resting stroke volume, mainly as a result of an increase in left ventricular (LV) filling.

Purpose.—To evaluate whether the LV morphologic and functional alterations responsible for this increase in cardiac filling are similar in children and young adults.

Methods.—Standard echocardiography (LV morphology and function) and tissue Doppler imaging (LV relaxation properties) were assessed in 10 adult cyclists, 13 age-matched sedentary controls, 12 boy cyclists, and 11 untrained boys.

Results.—In our endurance-trained adults, LV morphological adaptations included increase in LV internal diameters, wall thickness, and mass. However, effects associated with training on LV morphology were different in children because no true cardiac hypertrophy was observed in our child cyclists compared with age-matched nonactive boys. Effects related training on LV systolic and diastolic function assessed by TDI were similar in boys and men. The LV diastolic function was improved in trained subjects (i.e., increased transmitral early to late filling velocities) as a result of an increase in LV relaxation properties. However, LV filling pressures, estimated from TDI, were similar in trained individuals compared with age-matched controls.

Conclusion.—In both children and adults, an increase in LV relaxation properties and normal LV filling pressures in endurance-trained subjects might be taken as additional indicators for a physiologic or "normal" hypertrophy. However, further investigations are needed to evaluate whether the specific LV morphological adaptation observed in trained-children reflects a blunted trained-induced cardiac hypertrophy before puberty.

▶ As children and young adolescents become increasingly involved in high-intensity athletic training, it will be important to recognize any maturation differences in cardiovascular features in the growing years. Most studies have indicated, as does this one, that anatomic and functional cardiac characteristics of highly trained prepubertal endurance athletes differ from their nontrained peers in ways that are similar to those observed in adults. In this report, however, adult athletes had greater hypertrophy than the prepubertal cyclists. It remains to be seen to what extent these cardiac features of athletes reflect genetic endowment versus the effects of endurance training.

T. Rowland, MD

Strength Adaptations and Hormonal Responses to Resistance Training and Detraining in Preadolescent Males
Tsolakis CK, Vagenas GK, Dessypris AG (Univ of Athens, Greece)
J Strength and Cond Res 18:625-629, 2004   8–32

Background.—The physiological muscle-growth changes in boys in early puberty are attributable mainly to the increase in androgen levels. These changes are usually observed after the age of 11. At about this same age, many children begin participation in systematic resistance-training programs that can lead to an increase in muscular strength, provided all basic principles of design and safety are followed. These programs can also improve health and prevent possible exercise-related injuries attributed to muscle weakness and muscle-strength imbalance during development. The influence of a brief, supervised progressive resistance-training program with isotonic equipment and a 2-month detraining program on strength adaptations, serum hormones testosterone (T), sex hormone-binding globulin (SHBG), and free androgen index (FAI) was investigated in a cohort of Greek preadolescents who had no previous training experience.

Methods.—Nineteen untrained high school boys (11-13 years old) were randomly assigned to an experimental group (9 boys) and a control group (10 boys). All of the subjects were given a medical evaluation before testing to exclude those with chronic diseases or other inhibiting factors.

Results.—There were significant posttraining increases in isometric force (17.5%) and mean T and FAI values in the strength-training group compared with the control group. At the end of the detraining period, the mean hormonal concentrations in the strength-training group were not significantly different from the posttraining concentrations, while there was a significant decrease in strength. There was significant correlation between the relative postdetraining hormonal responses and the respective isometric strength changes.

Conclusions.—Resistance training in preadolescent boys induced changes in muscle force independent of the changes in the anabolic and androgenic activity in these boys. There is a need for additional research into the physiological mechanisms that underlie the strength training and detraining processes.

► In the past, prepubertal children were considered incapable of improving muscle strength with resistance training because of lack of circulating testosterone. An abundance of contemporary studies have found this to be untrue—boys and girls before puberty (that is, lacking circulating anabolic hormones) are as capable of improving strength with weight training as postpubertal subjects. This study confirms the obvious conclusion: strength training improvements in peak muscle force are not related to changes in anabolic and androgen hormonal influences in prepubertal boys. Neurologic adaptive influences remain the most likely explanation for strength gains with training before puberty.

T. Rowland, MD

Mechanical Efficiency of Normal-Weight Prepubertal Boys Predisposed to Obesity
Weinstein Y, Kamerman T, Berry E, et al (Wingate Inst, Israel; Ohalo Colege, Katzerin, Israel; Hadassah Med School, Jerusalem)
Med Sci Sports Exerc 36:567-573, 2004   8–33

Purpose.—To compare 1) energy expenditure during rest and during submaximal exercise, and 2) the mechanical efficiency of normal-weight boys liable to obesity with normal-weight boys who are not liable to obesity.

Methods.—Two groups of prepubertal boys, aged 9-12 yr were compared, one with both parents of normal weight (NP, $20 \leq BMI \leq 27$, $N = 20$) and the other ($N = 20$) with one obese parent (OP, $BMI \geq 30$).

Results.—No significant differences were found between the two groups in the anthropometric measurements (means ± SD): body mass (32.9 ± 5.4 and 31.5 ± 3.1 kg, NP and OP, respectively), stature (141.0 ± 6.2 and 140.0 ± 5.5 cm, NP and OP, respectively), and body fat (16.6 ± 3.5 and $15.1 \pm 3.5\%$, NP and OP, respectively). Likewise, there were no differences in the reported physical activity habits. No differences were observed in the resting metabolic rate values between the two groups (5.071 ± 0.351 and 4.956 ± 0.386 MJ·d^{-1}, NP and OP, respectively). Submaximal $\dot{V}O_2$ at 30, 45, and 60 W was similar in the two groups (0.63 ± 0.05, 0.78 ± 0.06, and 0.92 ± 0.08; and 0.63 ± 0.06, 0.78 ± 0.08, and 0.95 ± 0.08 L·min^{-1}, NP and OP, respectively). Likewise, the mechanical efficiency, calculated at 30, 45, and 60 W was similar in both groups (19.5 ± 2.3, 21.8 ± 2.2, $23.4 \pm 2.5\%$; and 19.5 ± 3.0, 21.9 ± 2.9, $22.6 \pm 2.5\%$, NP and OP, respectively. No differences were found between groups in their $\dot{V}O_{2peak}$ (38.4 ± 3.8 and 40.4 ± 4.9 mL·kg^{-1}·min^{-1}, NP and OP, respectively).

Conclusion.—These data suggest that energy expenditure during rest and exercise may not be used to predict future obesity in normal-weight prepubertal boys predisposed to obesity.

▶ The search continues for the critical factors responsible for the energy imbalance that is leading to increasing frequency of obesity in youth. Although the usual suspects, excessive caloric intake and diminished activity habits, are intuitively attractive, it is not clear how much these are etiologic (ie, primary determinants) or secondary manifestations of increased body bulk. This study examined an alternative possibility that obesity might be an outcome of individual differences in cellular energy use during exercise (ie, mechanical efficiency). This was examined before development of obesity in groups that were considered based on family history to be at different risk for gaining excessive body fat. The results suggest that individual differences in energy use are not responsible for excessive adiposity in youth.

T. Rowland, MD

Are Changes in Distance-Run Performance of Australian Children Between 1985 and 1997 Explained by Changes in Fatness?
Olds T, Dollman J (Univ of South Australia, Underdale)
Pediatr Exerc Sci 16:201-209, 2004   8–34

Background.—It has been well established that children in many developed countries, including Australia, are getting fatter. There is also evidence to indicate that the performance of children on aerobic fitness tests has declined in Australia and in other developed countries. It could be assumed from these data that the increase in fatness has caused the decline in fitness performance among children. However, it has also been argued that fitness has declined among children because they are less active today than children in the past. The decrease in moderate to vigorous physical activity has resulted in a reduced training effect, and thus fitness has been reduced. If the decline in fitness is to be reversed, it is vital to determine whether the decline is solely attributable to increases in fatness or whether declines in physical activity are also involved. Fitness performance in samples of children tested in 1985 and 1997 was compared to determine whether declines in fitness levels are attributable to increases in fatness or decreases in vigorous physical activity.

Methods.—The study groups consisted of 279 10- to 12-year-old children tested in 1985 as part of a national survey in Australia. These subjects were matched for age, sex, body mass index, and triceps skin-fold thickness with 279 children from a 1997 survey. Average speeds on the 1.6 km walk/run test were compared. If there were no performance differences between the matched samples, then declines in fitness could be attributed to increases in fatness. However, if there were residual differences in fitness despite the matching procedure, then it would be likely that factors other than changes in fatness were contributing to reduced fitness in children.

Results.—Children from the 1997 performed significantly worse than their matched peers from the 1985 survey. The decline in performance was evident among both girls and boys and persisted in an overall comparison of all children. There were also significant relationships between the sum of skin folds and running speed for boys, girls, and all children. Running speed declined by .047 m/s in boys and by .032 m/s in girls for every 1-mm increase in triceps skin-fold thickness. Matching the 2 cohorts for fatness reduced performance differences by approximately 61% in boys and 37% in girls.

Conclusions.—The declines in fitness performance in the 1997 cohort of Australian children have not been due entirely to increases in fatness. The residual decline in performance may be attributable to decreases in vigorous physical activity among children.

▶ Performance in weight-bearing exercise is inversely related to body fat content. One would expect, then, that the current epidemic of childhood obesity would be paralleled by a decline over time in performance in activities such as distance run times. In this study of Australian youth, the authors found this was true, but increases in body fat accounted for only about half of the decline in fitness performance. As they concluded, decreases in regular physical activity per se might also be playing a role.

T. Rowland, MD

Lipid-Lipoproteins in Children: An Exercise Dose-Response Study
Tolfrey K, Jones AM, Campbell IG (Manchester Metropolitan Univ, England)
Med Sci Sports Exerc 36:418-427, 2004   8–35

Purpose.—To study the effect of exercise volume on pre- and early-pubertal children's lipid-lipoprotein profile.

Methods.—Thirty-four children (15 girls) completed 12 wk of exercise training, preceded by a 12-wk control period. Sixteen (7 girls and 9 boys) expended an additional 422 ± 5 kJ·kg BM (LOW, 100 kcal·kg), whereas 18 (8 girls and 10 boys) expended an additional 586 ± 7 kJ·g (MOD, 140 kcal·kg) as a result of the training program. They all exercised on three nonconsecutive days per week at $80 \pm 1\%$ HR_{peak}. Exercise duration was individualized to match energy expenditure targets. Plasma TG, TC, and HDL-C were measured precontrol, pretraining, and posttraining. LDL-C, TC/HDL-C, and LDL-C/HDL-C were also calculated.

Results.—Group mean lipid-lipoprotein concentrations did not change as a result of training energy expenditure in either of the groups ($P > 0.05$). Dietary composition, habitual physical activity, and body composition were also relatively stable over the intervention period ($P > 0.05$). In the LOW, but not the MOD group, peak $\dot{V}O_2$ (mL·kg·min) tended to increase over the intervention period ($P = 0.07$). Pearson's product moment correlation analyses indicated that pretraining concentrations of TG, TC, LDL-C, TC/HDL-C, and LDL-C/HDL-C were all related to the small changes seen in the lipid-lipoprotein profile ($P < 0.01$).

Conclusion.—Additional energy expenditure of 422 or 586 kJ·kg, as a direct result of aerobic exercise training over a 12-wk period, did not cause significant alterations in the lipid-lipoprotein profile in pre- and early-pubertal children. This may indicate that the exercise volume was insufficient, the lipoprotein profiles of the majority of children in this study were classified as "desirable," or more likely a combination of these factors.

▶ This study confirms what has been consistently reported before: a short-term (< 12 weeks) program of intense aerobic training does not alter serum lipoprotein profile in healthy normolipemic children. This is a bit of a mystery, because (1) an improved lipid profile, particularly increases in HDL-cholesterol, is observed in adults with aerobic training, and (2) prepubertal athletes tend to show more "favorable" serum lipid concentrations than nonathletes. The authors of this study suggest 2 possible explanations: Training studies in children are too short in duration to effect lipid changes, and/or lipid changes with training in this age group are not to be expected if pretraining levels are normal to start with. This whole issue does raise interesting questions regarding the mechanism of lipid changes with exercise training and how this might be affected by level of sexual maturation.

T. Rowland, MD

Effects of Anaerobic Training in Children With Cystic Fibrosis: A Randomized Controlled Study

Klijn PHC, Oudshoorn A, van der Ent CK, et al (Univ Med Ctr, Utrecht, The Netherlands)
Chest 125:1299-1305, 2004   8–36

Background.—Children's physical activity patterns are characterized by short-term anaerobic activities. Anaerobic exercise performance in children with cystic fibrosis (CF) has received little attention compared to aerobic performance. This study investigated the effects of anaerobic training in children with CF.

Design and Methods.—Twenty patients were randomly assigned to the training group (TG) [11 patients; mean (± SD) age, 13.6 ± 1.3 years; mean FEV_1, 75.2 ± 20.7% predicted] or the control group (CG) [9 patients; mean age, 14.2 ± 2.1 years; FEV_1, 82.1 ± 19.1% predicted]. The TG trained 2 days per week for 12 weeks, with each session lasting 30 to 45 min. The training program consisted of anaerobic activities lasting 20 to 30 s. The control subjects were asked not to change their normal daily activities. Body composition, pulmonary function, peripheral muscle force, habitual physical activity, aerobic and anaerobic exercise performance, and quality of life were reevaluated at the end of the training program, and again after a 12-week follow-up period.

Results.—Patients in the TG significantly improved their anaerobic performance, aerobic performance, and quality of life. No significant changes were seen in other parameters, and no improvements were found in CG. After the follow-up period, only anaerobic performance and quality of life in TG were significantly higher compared to pretraining values.

Conclusions.—Anaerobic training has measurable effects on aerobic performance (although not sustained), anaerobic performance, and health-related quality of life in children with CF. Therefore, anaerobic training could be an important component of therapeutic programs for CF patients.

▶ The role of exercise interventions in youth with chronic disease is just beginning to be explored. In many types of illnesses there is, in fact, growing evidence that regular physical activity can reap both physical and psychosocial benefits. In this study, exercise training of early adolescent patients with CF was demonstrated to favorably influence exercise function and, importantly, quality of life. Considering the physical incapacity and emotional impact that this disease can impose, this is a noteworthy report. The findings support the concept that regular exercise (in this case, anaerobic) should be a component of therapeutic regimens for youth with CF.

T. Rowland, MD

Reproducibility of the Jumping Mechanography as a Test of Mechanical Power Output in Physically Competent Adult and Elderly Subjects
Rittweger J, Schiessl H, Felsenberg D, et al (Institut für Physiologie, FU Berlin; Novotec Med, Pforzheim, Germany; Universitätsklinikum Benjamin Franklin, FU Berlin; et al)
J Am Geriatr Soc 52:128-131, 2004   8–37

Objectives.—To compare the reproducibility of the newly developed jumping mechanography with other physical tests.

Design.—Study 1: Repeated testing with an interval of 2 weeks to assess the short-term repetition error. Study 2: Testing on 5 successive days to assess learning effects.

Setting.—Geriatric clinic, Esslingen, Germany.

Participants.—Study 1 had 36 subjects aged 24 to 88; Study 2 had 22 subjects aged 19 to 86. Locomotor competence in all subjects was assessed using the ability to walk unaided and to perform a tandem stand and tandem walk.

Measurements.—The test battery consisted of timed up and go, freely chosen gait speed, maximum gait speed, chair-rising test, and maximum power in jumping mechanography (Fig 1).

Results.—All subjects performed the jumping mechanography without major problems. Study 1: Of all tests, maximum power in jumping mechanography depicted the smallest intrasubject short-term error (3.6%), the largest intersubject coefficient of variation (45.4%), and the greatest test-retest correlation coefficient ($r = 0.99$). Study 2: The only tests for which the learning effects were confined to the 1% range were the maximum gait speed test and the maximum power in jumping mechanography.

Conclusion.—Assessment of maximum power in jumping mechanography appears to have good test-retest reliability with negligible learning effects. Moreover, it results in a comparatively large intersubject variability, which makes it an interesting method in the assessment of aging effects in middle-aged to older subjects and patients.

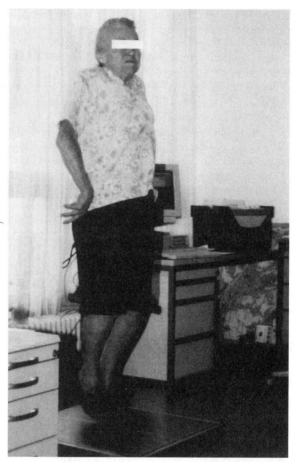

FIGURE 1.—Eighty-eight-year old woman performing jumping mechanography. (Courtesy of Rittweger J, Schiessl H, Felsenberg D, et al: Reproducibility of the jumping mechanography as a test of mechanical power output in physically competent adult and elderly subjects. *J Am Geriatr Soc* 52:128-131, 2004. Reprinted by permission of Blackwell Publishing.)

▶ The use of portable force plates is common in testing anaerobic alactic power output during vertical jump of elite athletes and healthy young subjects. Vertical jumping tests from a force plate to test mechanical power is not often used with elderly subjects. This study tested a sample that consisted of many older subjects who were able to successfully perform the vertical jump test in addition to many other commonly used tests of physical ability. It was suggested that scores on the jump test are closely related to impairment level in the elderly population and may be used for screening for other forms of physical therapy. This technique may prove to be an effective method of assessment of aging effects, although it is not without some risk to the participants when balance is poor or cognitive deficits exist.

M. J. L. Alexander, PhD

Postexercise Protein Metabolism in Older and Younger Men Following Moderate-Intensity Aerobic Exercise
Sheffield-Moore M, Yeckel CW, Volpi E, et al (Univ of Texas, Galveston)
Am J Physiol Endocrinol Metab 287:E513-E522, 2004   8–38

Introduction.—Regular aerobic exercise strongly influences muscle metabolism in elderly and young; however, the acute effects of aerobic exercise on protein metabolism are not fully understood. We investigated the effect of a single bout of moderate walking (45 min at ~40% of peak O_2 consumption) on postexercise (POST-EX) muscle metabolism and synthesis of plasma proteins [albumin (ALB) and fibrinogen (FIB)] in untrained older ($n = 6$) and younger ($n = 6$) men. We measured muscle phenylalanine (Phe) kinetics before (REST) and POST-EX (10, 60, and 180 min) using l-[*ring*-$^2H_5$]phenylalanine infusion, femoral arteriovenous blood samples, and muscle biopsies. All data are presented as the difference from REST (at 10, 60, and 180 min POST-EX). Mixed muscle fractional synthesis rate (FSR) increased significantly at 10 min POST-EX in both the younger (0.0363%/h) and older men (0.0830%/h), with the younger men staying elevated through 60 min POST-EX (0.0253%/h). ALB FSR increased at 10 min POST-EX in the younger men only (2.30%/day), whereas FIB FSR was elevated in both groups through 180 min POST-EX (younger men = 4.149, older men = 4.107%/day). Muscle protein turnover was also increased, with increases in synthesis and breakdown in younger and older men. Phe rate of disappearance (synthesis) was increased in both groups at 10 min POST-EX and remained elevated through 60 min POST-EX in the older men. A bout of moderate-intensity aerobic exercise induces short-term increases in muscle and plasma protein synthesis in both younger and older men. Aging per se does not diminish the protein metabolic capacity of the elderly to respond to acute aerobic exercise.

▶ This is the first study to compare mixed muscle protein synthesis after a 45-minute treadmill walk in younger and older men. The results indicate that walking induces short-term increases in muscle protein synthesis and breakdown (ie, muscle protein turnover) in younger and older men. The authors speculated that "it is possible that increases in muscle protein turnover are the metabolic basis for cellular repair and maintenance in aging skeletal muscle."

D. C. Nieman, DrPH

Influence of Age and Physical Activity on the Primary In Vivo Antibody and T Cell-Mediated Responses in Men
Smith TP, Kennedy SL, Fleshner M (Univ of Colorado at Boulder)
J Appl Physiol 97:491-498, 2004   8–39

Introduction.—The aging immune system is characterized by a progressive reduction in responsiveness to exogenous antigens. This decline is a risk factor for increased incidence of infectious disease. It may be that regular moderate exercise training (cardiovascular training) may offset some of the immune function abnormalities seen in healthy older populations. The relationship between aging and physical activity on the primary antibody and T-cell response to the novel protein antigen keyhole-limpet hemocyanin (KLH) was examined in 46 physically active and sedentary, young (20-35 years) and older (60-79 years) men.

Methods.—Research subjects were immunized IM using 100 μg of KLH. Blood samples were obtained at days 0, 7, 14, 21, and 28. Samples were examined for anti-KLH, immunoglobulin (Ig) M, IgG, IgG1, and IgG2 via

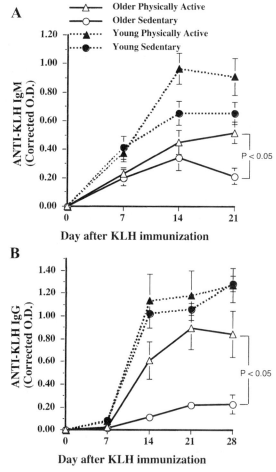

FIGURE 2.—Serum concentrations of anti–keyhole-limpet hemocyanin (*KLH*) immunoglobulin (*Ig*) M (**A**) and IgG (**B**) were assessed in younger and older physically active and sedentary men after KLH immunization. Physically active men had a robust antibody response that was similar to that of the younger groups and significantly greater than that of the older sedentary group. (Courtesy of Smith TP, Kennedy SL, Fleshner M: Influence of age and physical activity on the primary in vivo antibody and T cell-mediated response in men. *J Appl Physiol* 97:491-498, 2004. Copyright The American Physiological Society.)

enzyme-linked immunosorbent assay. On day 21, after IM KLH administration, participants received an intradermal injection with 1 µg of KLH of inflammation documented at 24, 48, 72, 96, and 120 hours to evaluate anti-KLH delayed-type hypersensitivity response.

Results.—There was a significant decrease in all anti-KLH measures with aging, except for anti-KLH IgG2. The physically active older group had significantly higher anti-KLH IgM, IgG1, and delayed-type hypersensitivity responses, excluding IgG2, compared with the sedentary older group (Fig 2).

Conclusion.—Regular physical activity in older men is linked with a more robust immune response to novel antigenic challenge.

▶ These cross-sectional data indicate that physically active older men (aged 65-79) had a more robust immune response to a novel antigen (KLM). Specifically, the physically active compared to inactive older men had an elevated generation of antigen-specific T-cell–dependent antibody and delayed-type hypersensitivity skin response (Fig 2). In an earlier study, my research team had shown that highly physically active older women compared to their sedentary peers had improved mitogen-induced lymphocyte proliferation and natural killer cell activity.[1]

However, when the sedentary older women walked briskly 5 d/wk for 12 weeks, no improvement was seen in various measures of immune function compared to randomized controls. Thus, the improved immune function in physically active older adults may be due to several factors including hereditary background, regular physical activity over many years, body composition, diet, and other lifestyle factors.

D. C. Nieman, DrPH

Reference

1. Nieman DC, Henson DA, Gusewitch G, et al: Physical activity and immune function in elderly women. *Med Sci Sports Exerc* 25:823-831, 1993.

Influence of Physical Activity on Serum IL-6 and IL-10 Levels in Healthy Older Men

Jankord R, Jemiolo B (Ball State Univ, Muncie, Ind)
Med Sci Sports Exerc 36:960-964, 2004
8–40

Background.—Immunosenescence has been proposed as a factor in the age-related decline in physical function. Some diseases that are characterized by chronic inflammation and high levels of interleuken-6 (IL-6) cause a reduction in muscle strength and muscle mass that is often associated with physical disability in old and very old persons. However, it is not known whether functional disability precedes or follows increases in IL-6 levels. It has also been hypothesized that anti-inflammatory cytokines might be involved in successful aging and longevity. Recent studies have suggested that IL-10, a key cytokine that can suppress cell-mediated immunity and maturation of dendritic cells, is increased in healthy elderly persons but declines in frail elderly persons along with dendritic cell antigen-presenting function. The effects of regular physical activity, independent of disease and disability, on the levels of proinflammatory and anti-inflammatory cytokines were assessed in men, 65 to 74 years old.

Methods.—The study participants were screened for inclusion on the basis of the SENIEUR protocol. Participants were also selected on the basis of their weekly volume of aerobic exercise. Twelve healthy SENIEUR males (6 very active and 6 less active) completed the study. Serum concentration of MIP-1α, IL-1ra, IL-1β, IL-6, IL-10, and C-reactive protein (CRP) were measured by enzyme-linked immunosorbent assay.

Results.—Subjects in the very active group showed significantly decreased levels of IL-6 and significantly increased levels of IL-10 compared with those in the less-active group.

Conclusions.—A higher volume of regular physical activity was associated with decreased IL-6 levels and increased IL-10 levels in healthy older men. Exercise may therefore play a vital role in the control of inflammatory markers during the aging process.

▶ These cross-sectional data indicate that physically active elderly men compared to inactive elderly men have lower serum concentrations of IL-6 and higher concentrations of IL-10. Although these data are interesting, they must be considered preliminary, given the small subject numbers and the cross-sectional nature of the research design. Nonetheless, these results give direction for future exercise training studies of elderly individuals to indicate whether health-related benefits occur through an immune mechanism.

D. C. Nieman, DrPH

Functional-Task Exercise Versus Resistance Strength Exercise to Improve Daily Function in Older Women: A Randomized, Controlled Trial
de Vreede PL, Samson MM, van Meeteren NLU, et al (Univ Med Ctr, Utrecht, The Netherlands)
J Am Geriatr Soc 53:2-10, 2005   8–41

Objectives.—To determine whether a functional-task exercise program and a resistance exercise program have different effects on the ability of community-living older people to perform daily tasks.

Design.—A randomized, controlled, single-blind trial.

Setting.—Community leisure center in Utrecht, the Netherlands.

Participants.—Ninety-eight healthy women aged 70 and older were randomly assigned to the functional-task exercise program (function group, n = 33), a resistance exercise program (resistance group, n = 34), or a control group (n = 31). Participants attended exercise classes three times a week for 12 weeks.

Measurements.—Functional task performance (Assessment of Daily Activity Performance (ADAP)), isometric knee extensor strength (IKES), handgrip strength, isometric elbow flexor strength (IEFS), and leg extension power were measured at baseline, at the end of training (at 3 months), and 6 months after the end of training (at 9 months).

Results.—The ADAP total score of the function group (mean change 6.8, 95% confidence interval (CI) = 5.2–8.4) increased significantly more than that of the resistance group (3.2, 95% CI = 1.3–5.0; P=.007) or the control group (0.3, 95% CI = -1.3–1.9; P<.001). Moreover, the ADAP total score of the resistance group did not change significantly compared with that of the control group. In contrast, IKES and IEFS increased significantly in the resistance group (12.5%, 95% CI = 3.8–21.3 and 8.6%, 95% CI = 3.1–14.1, respectively) compared with the function group (-2.1%, 95% CI = -5.4–1.3; P=.003 and 0.3%, 95% CI = -3.6–4.2; P=.03, respectively) and the control group (-2.7%, 95% CI = -8.6–3.2, P=.003 and 0.6%, 95% CI = -3.4–4.6; P=.04, respectively). Six months after the end of training, the increase in ADAP scores was sustained in the function group (P=.002).

Conclusion.—Functional-task exercises are more effective than resistance exercises at improving functional task performance in healthy elderly women and may have an important role in helping them maintain an independent lifestyle.

▶ A sedentary lifestyle is one of the most important factors that can contribute to a loss of independent living among the elderly. Exercise programs have been shown to have a positive effect, such as improvements in strength, aerobic capacity, and balance. The short-term and longer-lasting impact of exercise programs on daily activity performances is relatively unclear. The purpose of this study was to determine the differences between 2 different types of exercise programs on strength, but also on activities of daily living. Elderly women (N = 98; 70 years and older) were randomly assigned to 1 of 3 groups: resistance, functional, or control. Exercises were performed at a local community center 3 times per week in 1-hour sessions for 12 weeks. The functional-task exercise program consisted of strength exercises with weights or weighted vests that were adapted to daily living activities such as climbing stairs or lifting and carrying objects. The authors offered to provide details of the functional exercises upon request. The resistance exercise program was the standard strength-training prescription for older adults outlined by the American College of Sports Medicine and Fit for Your Life. Attendance (90%) and compliance were high for both exercise programs (83% functional group; 74% resistance group). The excellent adherence was due to the design of the exercise interventions. Both programs were performed in small groups (6-12 participants) with training partners and 2 instructors supervising each session. The short-term strength gains of the resistance exercise program were not maintained after 6 months of detraining. However, persons in the functional-task exercise group sustained their gains in functional daily living tasks even after a half year of no formalized, supervised exercise sessions. Future research is needed to determine the ability of elderly adults to transfer exercises conducted in a supervised program to their own environment. It would appear from these findings that exercise programs should focus on incorporating daily living tasks into the prescription.

C. F. Sanborn, PhD

Footwear Style and Risk of Falls in Older Adults
Koepsell TD, Wolf ME, Buchner DM, et al (Univ of Washington, Seattle; Ctrs for Disease Control and Prevention, Atlanta, Ga; Group Health Cooperative, Seattle)
J Am Geriatr Soc 52:1495-1501, 2004   8–42

Objectives.—To determine how the risk of a fall in an older adult varies in relation to style of footwear worn.

Design.—Nested case-control study.

Setting.—Group Health Cooperative, a large health maintenance organization in Washington state.

Participants.—A total of 1,371 adults aged 65 and older were monitored for falls over a 2-year period; 327 qualifying fall cases were compared with 327 controls matched on age and sex.

Measurements.—Standardized in-person examinations before fall occurrence, interviews about fall risk factors after the fall occurred, and direct examination of footwear were conducted. Questions for controls referred to the last time they engaged in an activity broadly similar to what the case was doing at the time of the fall.

Results.—Athletic and canvas shoes (sneakers) were the styles of footwear associated with lowest risk of a fall. Going barefoot or in stocking feet was associated with sharply increased risk, even after controlling for measures of health status (adjusted odds ratio = 11.2, 95% confidence interval (CI) = 2.4–51.8). Relative to athletic/canvas shoes, other footwear was associated with a 1.3-fold increase in the risk of a fall (95% CI = 0.9-1.9), varying somewhat by style.

Conclusion.—Contrary to findings from gait-laboratory studies, athletic shoes were associated with relatively low risk of a fall in older adults during everyday activities. Fall risk was markedly increased when participants were not wearing shoes.

▶ Prevent the fall, prevent the hip fracture. Over 80% of hip fractures are caused by a traumatic fall and not by spontaneous fractures in women with osteoporosis. Extrinsic factors, such as footwear, have been identified that can be modified to help reduce the risk of falls for elderly adults. The researchers conducted a carefully designed study to determine which type of shoe was worn at the time of falls in older adults (≥65 years of age). A fall was defined as an unintentional fall to the ground. Of the 327 falls, 65% of the injuries were contusions or lacerations, but there were 15 fractures (4 hip, 5 hand/wrist, 6 other). Contrary to some laboratory research findings, athletic/canvas shoes were associated with the lowest risk of falls, and the highest risk of falling was related to going shoeless (barefoot or wearing stockings or socks). These findings, although simple, could make a profound difference among the elderly and should become a standard recommendation.

C. F. Sanborn, PhD

The Effectiveness of a Community-Based Program for Reducing the Incidence of Falls in the Elderly: A Randomized Trial
Clemson L, Cumming RG, Kendig H, et al (Univ of Sydney, Australia; Concord Hosp, Sydney, Australia; Central Sydney Area Health Service, Australia)
J Am Geriatr Soc 52:1487-1494, 2004   8–43

Objectives.—To test whether Stepping On, a multifaceted community-based program using a small-group learning environment, is effective in reducing falls in at-risk people living at home.

Design.—A randomized trial with subjects followed for 14 months.

Setting.—The interventions were conducted in community venues, with a follow-up home visit.

Participants.—Three hundred ten community residents aged 70 and older who had had a fall in the previous 12 months or were concerned about falling.

Intervention.—The Stepping On program aims to improve fall self-efficacy, encourage behavioral change, and reduce falls. Key aspects of the program are improving lower-limb balance and strength, improving home and community environmental and behavioral safety, encouraging regular visual screening, making adaptations to low vision, and encouraging medication review. Two-hour sessions were conducted weekly for 7 weeks, with a follow-up occupational therapy home visit.

Measurements.—The primary outcome measure was falls, ascertained using a monthly calendar mailed by each participant.

Results.—The intervention group experienced a 31% reduction in falls (relative risk (RR) = 0.69, 95% confidence interval (CI) = 0.50–0.96; P = .025). This was a clinically meaningful result demonstrating that the Stepping On program was effective for community-residing elderly people. Secondary analysis of subgroups showed that it was particularly effective for men (n = 80; RR = 0.32, 95% CI = 0.17–0.59).

Conclusion.—The results of this study renew attention to the idea that cognitive-behavioral learning in a small-group environment can reduce falls. Stepping On offers a successful fall-prevention option.

▶ Prevent the fall, prevent the osteoporotic hip fracture. The uniqueness of this educational program for the elderly was that the intervention was conducted by social workers with the focus on encouraging behavior changes. The Stepping On program included seven 2-hour sessions on the following topics: risk appraisal; exercises and moving about safely; home hazards; community safety and footwear; vision and falls, vitamin D, and hip protectors; medication management and mobility mastery experiences; and review and plan ahead. The small group educational program was successful in reducing falls. An interesting observation was that the intervention appeared to have a greater impact in the men versus the women. The researchers conjecture that the explanation for the gender differences may be that men have been shown to be less active in health activities and in seeking health knowledge than women. Educational programs to reduce fall prevention can be viable if the behavioral change message promotes personal control and problem-solving activities.

C. F. Sanborn, PhD

Resistance Training in the Early Postoperative Phase Reduces Hospitalization and Leads to Muscle Hypertrophy in Elderly Hip Surgery Patients: A Controlled, Randomized Study

Suetta C, Magnusson SP, Rosted A, et al (Univ of Copenhagen)
J Am Geriatr Soc 52:2016-2022, 2004   8–44

Objectives.—To better understand how immobilization and surgery affect muscle size and function in the elderly and to identify effective training regimes.

Design.—A prospective randomized, controlled study.

Setting.—Bispebjerg University Hospital, Copenhagen, Denmark.

Participants.—Thirty-six patients (aged 60-86) scheduled for unilateral hip replacement due to primary hip osteoarthrosis.

Intervention.—Patients were randomized to standard home-based rehabilitation (1 h/d x 12 weeks), unilateral neuromuscular electrical stimulation of the operated side (1 h/d $\times$ 12 weeks), or unilateral resistance training of the operated side (3/wk $\times$ 12 weeks).

Measurements.—Hospital length of stay (LOS), quadriceps muscle cross-sectional area (CSA), isokinetic muscle strength, and functional performance. Patients were tested presurgery and 5 and 12 weeks postsurgery.

Results.—Mean ± standard error LOS was shorter for the resistance training group (10.0 ± 2.4 days, $P<.05$) than for the standard rehabilitation group (16.0 ± 7.2 days). Resistance training, but not electrical stimulation or standard rehabilitation, resulted in increased CSA (12%, $P<.05$) and muscle strength (22–28%, $P<.05$). Functional muscle performance increased after resistance training (30%, $P<.001$) and electrical stimulation (15%, $P<.05$) but not after standard rehabilitation.

Conclusion.—Postoperative resistance training effectively increased maximal muscle strength, muscle mass, and muscle function more than a standard rehabilitation regime. Furthermore, it markedly reduced LOS in elderly postoperative patients.

▶ Effective exercise interventions are needed following immobilization after surgery. Muscle strength declines approximately 4% per day in patients immediately after immobilization. Further, a significant deficit in muscle strength can persist in the operated leg after hip replacement surgery. The researchers present a very nice study that illustrates the importance of implementing a resistance training program in elderly hip surgical patients in the early postoperative phase. Details are provided in the Methods section regarding the specifics of the resistance training. Briefly, the progressive resistance training program was conducted 3 days per week for 12 weeks beginning with 20 repetition maximums (RMs) at a fairly low intensity (~50% of 1 RM) to avoid injuries, increasing to 8 RMs (~80% of 1 RM). Knee extension exercises were performed on leg press and knee extension machines. Carefully supervised resistance training can be an effective and safe intervention to not only reduce the hospital LOS, but also to increase muscle mass, maximal muscle strength, and functional performance in the elderly.

C. F. Sanborn, PhD

Effects of a Home Program on Strength, Walking Speed, and Function After Total Hip Replacement
Jan M-H, Hung J-Y, Lin JC-H, et al (Natl Taiwan Univ, Taipei; Univ of Southern California, Los Angeles)
Arch Phys Med Rehabil 85:1943-1951, 2004   8–45

Objective.—To assess the efficacy of a home exercise program in increasing hip muscle strength, walking speed, and function in patients more than 1.5 years after total hip replacement (THR).

Design.—Randomized controlled trial.

Setting.—Kinesiology laboratory.

Participants.—Fifty-three patients with unilateral THR were randomly assigned to the training (n=26) and control (n=27) groups. Patients in the training group were further divided into exercise-high (n=13) and exercise-low (n=13) compliance groups according to their practice ratio (high, ≥50%).

Intervention.—The training group underwent a 12-week home program that included hip flexion range of motion exercises for both hip joints; strengthening exercises for bilateral hip flexors, extensors, and abductors; and a 30-minute walk every day. The control group did not receive any training.

Main Outcome Measures.—Strength of bilateral hip muscles, free and fast walking speeds while walking over 3 different terrains, and functional performance were assessed by using a dynamometer, videotape analysis, and the functional activity part of the Harris Hip Score, respectively, before and after the 12-week period.

Results.—Subjects in the exercise-high compliance group showed significantly (P<.05) greater improvement in muscle strength for the operated hip, fast walking speed, and functional score than those in the exercise-low compliance and control groups.

Conclusions.—The designed home program was effective in improving hip muscle strength, walking speed, and function in patients after THR who practiced the program at least 3 times a week, but adherence to this home program may be a problem.

▶ Home exercise programs can be a cost-effective intervention program to increase strength in individuals who have had THR. The unique aspect of this intervention study was that the impact of a home exercise program was examined in patients more than 1.5 years after their THR. The impact of a home-based exercise program obviously hinges on compliance. This study also examined the differences between 2 levels of compliance, an exercise-high compliance group and an exercise-low compliance group, along with a control group. The home-exercise program was a 12-week daily prescription of hip muscle strengthening exercises and 30 minutes of walking at a comfortable pace. The medians (and ranges) of the exercise-high and exercise-low compliance groups were 74% (50%-100%) and 23% (12%-42%), respectively. As expected, the home exercise program was only effective in the high-compliance group. The key point to take home from this study is that anyone implementing a home exercise program must address strategies to increase compliance. The frequency need not be daily, for adherence could be better served with a program that is at least 3 days per week. Also, care should be taken in developing an exercise program that is not too long in duration. This intervention took 50 to 60 minutes per day to complete, which in reflection, was too long. Finally, individuals in the low-compliance group typically led a sedentary lifestyle before THR. Knowing previous physical activity patterns could help identify those at risk for noncompliance and help to tailor appropriate behavior strategies and exercise prescriptions.

C. F. Sanborn, PhD

Group Treatment Improves Trunk Strength and Psychological Status in Older Women With Vertebral Fractures: Results of a Randomized, Clinical Trial
Gold DT, Shipp KM, Pieper CF, et al (Duke Univ, Durham, NC; Veterans Affairs Med Ctr, Durham, NC; Univ of Florida, Gainesville; et al)
J Am Geriatr Soc 52:1471-1478, 2004   8–46

Objectives.—To assess whether group exercise and coping classes reduce physical and psychological impairments and functional disability in older women with prevalent vertebral fractures (VFs).

Design.—Randomized, controlled trial (modified cross-over) with site as unit of assignment; testing at baseline and 3, 6, 9, and 12 months.

Setting.—Nine North Carolina retirement communities.

Participants.—One hundred eighty-five postmenopausal Caucasian women (mean age 81), each with at least one VFs.

Intervention.—The intervention group had 6 months of exercise (3 meetings weekly, 45 minutes each) and coping classes (2 meetings weekly, 45 minutes each) in Phase 1, followed by 6 months of self-maintenance. The control group had 6 months of health education control intervention (1 meeting weekly, 45 minutes) in Phase 1, followed by the intervention described above.

Measurements.—Change in trunk extension strength, change in pain with activities, and change in psychological symptoms.

Results.—Between-group differences in the change in trunk extension strength (10.68 foot pounds, $P<.001$) and psychological symptoms (-0.08, $P=.011$) were significant for Phase 1. Changes in pain with activities did not differ between groups (-0.03, $P=.64$); there was no change in the pain end-point. In Phase 2, controls showed significant changes in trunk strength (15.02 foot pounds, $P<.001$) and psychological symptoms (-0.11, $P=.006$) from baseline. Change in pain with activities was not significant (-0.03, $P=.70$). During self-maintenance, the intervention group did not worsen in psychological symptoms, but improved trunk extension strength was not maintained.

Conclusion.—Weak trunk extension strength and psychological symptoms associated with VFs can be improved in older women using group treatment, and psychological improvements are retained for at least 6 months.

▶ The incidence of mortality and morbidity are high among women who have had osteoporotic hip fractures. However, osteoporotic VFs are more common and are devastating. Pain, trunk weakness, deformity, disability, and impaired psychological functions are associated with VFs. The unique aspects of this program for women with VFs was that the intervention included an exercise component and coping strategies to reduce anxiety, depression, and stress. The exercise program was delivered by physical therapists with the focus on common outcomes of VFs: trunk weakness, reduced trunk extension flexibility, and difficulty with posture. The coping intervention was taught by psychiatric social workers. The intervention was successful in increasing trunk extension and reducing psychological symptoms. Adverse events were minimal (4 of 8000 contact hours) in this sample of women who were at high risk for sustaining another fracture. These findings highlight the importance of qualified licensed health care providers leading the intervention in an at-risk population. Finally, the strength gains were not maintained after the cessation of the intervention. Further studies need to examine strategies for long-term adherence to an exercise regimen.

C. F. Sanborn, PhD

9 Ergogenic Aids, Doping, and Environmental Issues

Erosive Effect of a New Sports Drink on Dental Enamel During Exercise
Venables MC, Shaw L, Jeukendrup AE, et al (Univ of Birmingham, England; GlaxoSmithKline Consumer Healthcare, Coleford, Gloucestershire, England; Univ of Wales, Cardiff)
Med Sci Sports Exerc 37:39-44, 2005   9–1

Purpose.—To compare the potential erosive effect of a prototype carbohydrate-electrolyte drink (PCE) with a neutral control (water) and a commercially available carbohydrate-electrolyte drink (CCE) during exercise.

Methods.—Nineteen healthy adults (male, $N = 16$; female, $N = 3$) took part in this single blind, three-way crossover study. Subjects were given each of the three drinks according to a randomization schedule, approximately balanced for first-order carryover effects. At the beginning of each of the three study periods, the volunteers were fitted with an intraoral appliance containing two human enamel blocks. During each study period, volunteers exercised for 75 $min \cdot d^{-1}$ (5 repetitions of 15 min of exercise, with 5-min rests between exercise repetitions), 5 $d \cdot wk^{-1}$ for 3 wk. Each day, drink aliquots of 200 mL were consumed during a 5-min period before exercise and after every 15-min bout of exercise, followed by a final 400-mL aliquot ingested over a 10-min period: a total of 1400 mL per study day. Dental erosion was measured as tissue loss from the enamel blocks by profilometry at the end of each study period.

Results.—Water, PCE, and CCE produced 0.138 µm (SD 0.090 µm), 0.138 µm (SD 0.038 µm), and 4.238 µm (SD 3.872 µm) of enamel loss, respectively. A Wilcoxon t statistic showed a significant statistical difference between the PCE and CCE drinks ($P < 0.001$), whereas no significant difference could be detected between the PCE drink and water ($P = 0.740$).

Conclusion.—The PCE solution showed minimal erosion compared with the commercially available drink, and was statistically indistinguishable from water under the conditions of this study. Use of CE solutions formulated to minimize erosion during exercise may provide significant dental benefits.

▶ This study showed that adding calcium to a typical sports beverage reduces erosion on dental enamel in subjects who use sports drinks during exercise. The authors admit, however, that the link between consumption of sports drinks and dental enamel erosion in groups of athletes has not been established, and that many other factors within the lifestyle play a role.

D. C. Nieman, DrPH

Carbohydrate Feedings During Team Sport Exercise Preserve Physical and CNS Function
Winnick JJ, David JM, Welsh RS, et al (Univ of South Carolina, Columbia)
Med Sci Sports Exerc 37:306-315, 2005   9–2

Purpose.—This study was designed to examine the effect of carbohydrate (CHO) feedings on physical and central nervous system (CNS) function during intermittent high-intensity exercise with physical demands similar to those of team sports such as basketball.

Methods.—Twenty active men (N = 10) and women (N = 10), with experience competing in team sports, performed three practice sessions before two experimental trials during which they were fed either a 6% CHO solution or a flavored placebo (PBO). Experimental trials consisted of four 15-min quarters of shuttle running with variable intensities ranging from walking (30% $\dot{V}O_{2max}$), to running (120% $\dot{V}O_{2max}$), to maximal sprinting, and 40 jumps at a target hanging at 80% of their maximum vertical jump height. Subjects received 5 mL/kg of fluid before exercise and 3 mL/kg after exercise, in addition to 3 mL/kg over a 5-min span after the first and third quarters, and 8 mL/kg during a 20-min halftime. During each break, the subjects performed a battery of tests measuring peripheral and CNS function, including 20-m sprints, a 60-s maximal jumping test, internal and external mood evaluation, cognitive function, force sensation, tests of motor skills, and target-jumping accuracy.

Results.—Compared with PBO, CHO feedings during exercise resulted in faster 20-m sprint times and higher average jump height in the fourth quarter ($P < 0.05$). CHO feedings also reduced force sensation, enhanced motor skills, and improved mood late in exercise versus PBO ($P < 0.05$).

Conclusion.—These results suggest that CHO feedings during intermittent high-intensity exercise similar to that of team sports benefited both peripheral and CNS function late in exercise compared with a flavored placebo.

▶ I have long maintained (on the basis of simple correlation studies) that the ability to maintain blood sugar levels is important in sports demanding cognitive activity.[1] The article of Winnick and associates lists some of the many aspects of brain function that may be impaired by a decrease in blood glucose levels: mood, motivation, information processing, perceived exertion, and central drive. To this may be added a loss of teamwork, poorer coordination, and difficulty in plotting long-term strategy. Gains of mood state and performance have been described from glucose feeding during tennis[2] and field hockey,[3] but not in one recent report on soccer.[4] It is difficult to conduct a nicely planned experimental trial during the course of a metabolically demanding team sport. The present report is thus based on a combination of running, sprinting, and jumping with a 20-minute rest interval, the whole intended to mimic a typical team game. As expected, observations on those receiving a carbohydrate drink demonstrated benefits in motor skills (jumping and sprinting), force sensation, Profile of Mood State assessments of immediate "vigor" and "fatigue" and the Stroop test (speed reading of words and colors during the fourth "quarter" of the trial. Plainly, team sport players should be encouraged to drink carbohydrate as they are able over the course of a game. The solution provided in this experiment was a 6% carbohydrate/electrolyte mixture, drunk at a rate of 690 mL/h.

R. J. Shephard, MD, PhD, DPE

References

1. Niinimaa V, Wright G, Shephard RJ et al: Characteristics of the successful dinghy sailor. *J Sports Med Phys Fitness* 17:83-96, 1977.
2. Vergauwen L, Brouns F, Hespel P: Carbohydrate supplementation improves stroke performance in tennis. *Med Sci Sports Exerc* 30: 1289-1295, 1998.
3. Kreider RB, Hill D, Horton G, et al: Effects of carbohydrate supplementation during intense training on dietary patterns, psychological status, and performance. *Int J Sports Med* 5:125-135, 1995.
4. Zeederberg C, Leach L, Lambert E, et al: The effect of carbohydrate ingestion on the motor skill proficiency of soccer players. *Int J Sports Nutr* 6:348-355, 1996.

Higher Dietary Carbohydrate Content During Intensified Running Training Results in Better Maintenance of Performance and Mood State
Achten J, Halson SL, Moseley L, et al (Univ of Birmingham, England; Optimal Performance, Bristol, England; QinetiQ, Farnborough, England)
J Appl Physiol 96:1331-1340, 2004   9–3

Introduction.—Overload training is included in most training programs. With insufficient recovery from this overload training, athletes will begin to demonstrate symptoms of short-term overtraining or overreaching. Whether consumption of a diet containing 8.5 g carbohydrate (CHO)/(kg · d) (high CHO; HCHO) compared with a diet containing 5.4 g CHO/(kg · d) (control subjects) during intensified training (IT) would provide better maintenance of physical performance and mood state was determined.

Methods.—Seven male endurance runners (mean maximal O_2 intake [$\dot{V}O_{2max}$], 64.7 ± 2.6 mL/[kg · min]) participated in two 11-day trials in which they consumed either the HCHO or control diet. They participated in IT during the last week in both trials. Their performance was measured with the use of a preloaded 8-km all-out run on the treadmill and 16-km all-out runs outdoors. Substrate utilization was determined via indirect calorimetry and continuous [U-^{13}C]glucose infusion during 30 minutes of running at 58% and 77% $\dot{V}O_{2max}$.

Results.—The time to complete 8 km was negatively affected by IT: the time significantly increased by a mean of 61 seconds and 155 seconds in the HCHO and control groups, respectively. The 16-km times were significantly increased by 8.2% during the control trial only. The Daily Analysis of Life Demands of Athletes questionnaire revealed a significant deterioration in mood states in both trials; a deterioration in global mood scores, as determined by the Profile of Mood States, was more pronounced in the control trial (Fig 5). Scores for fatigue were significantly higher in the control than in the HCHO trial. The CHO oxidation was significantly reduced from 1.7 to 1.2 g/min during the control trial; this was significantly accounted for by a reduction in muscle glycogen oxidation.

Conclusion.—An increase in dietary CHO content from 5.4 to 8.5 g CHO/(kg · d) (41% vs 65% total energy intake, respectively) permitted better maintenance of physical performance and mood state during physical training, thereby diminishing the symptoms of overreaching.

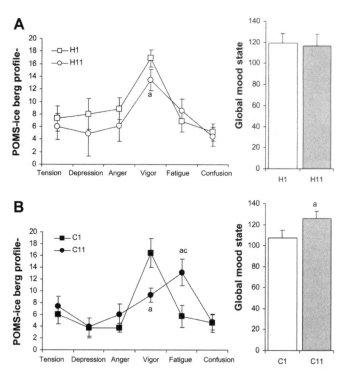

FIGURE 5.—Iceberg profile and global mood state of Profile of Mood States (POMS-65) questionnaire during *day 1* and *day 11* of HCHO trial (H1 and H11, respectively; A) and Con trial (C1 and C11, respectively; B). Values are means ± SE. ^{a}Significantly different from *day 1*; ^{c}significantly different from corresponding day in HCHO trial. (Courtesy of Achten J, Halson SL, Moseley L, et al: Higher dietary carbohydrate content during intensified running training results in better maintenance of performance and mood state. *J Appl Physiol* 98:1331-1340, 2004. Copyright The American Physiological Society.)

▶ Successful training requires an intensity of effort very close to the threshold of overtraining.[1] Such a regimen can lead to a progressive depletion of glycogen stores,[2] and this could make an important contribution to both the decrease in performance and the mood disturbances that are associated with overreaching.[3] The present small cross-over trial supports the idea that muscle glycogen reserves are maintained with a 65% CHO diet but not with a 41% CHO diet.

R. J. Shephard, MD, PhD, DPE

References

1. Fry RW, Morton AR, Keast D: Overtraining in athletes: An update. *Sports Med* 12:32-65, 1991.
2. Costill DL, Bowers R, Branam G, et al: Muscle glycogen utilization during prolonged exercise on successive days. *J Appl Physiol* 31:834-838, 1971.
3. Costill DL, Flynn MG, Kirwan JP, et al: Effects of repeated days of intensified training on muscle glycogen and swimming performance. *Med Sci Sports Exerc* 20:249-254, 1988.

Oxidation of Combined Ingestion of Glucose and Fructose During Exercise

Jentjens RLPG, Moseley L, Waring RH, et al (Univ of Birmingham, England; City Hosp, Birmingham, England)
J Appl Physiol 96:1277-1284, 2004
9–4

Background.—Carbohydrate (CHO) ingestion during prolonged moderate- to high-intensity exercise can postpone fatigue and enhance exercise performance when exercise duration is 45 minutes or longer. Improvements in performance with CHO ingestion help to maintain plasma glucose levels and high rates of CHO oxidation late in exercise, when muscle and liver glycogen concentrations are low. This study examined whether combined ingestion of a large amount of fructose and glucose during cycling results in exogenous carbohydrate oxidation rates exceeding 1 g/min.

Methods.—Eight trained cyclists performed 4 exercise trials of 120 minutes of cycling at 50% maximal power output. Participants received a solution that provided 1.2 g/min glucose (Med-Glu), 1.8 g/min glucose (High Glu), 0.6 g/min fructose plus 1.2 g/min glucose (Fruc + Glu), or water. The trials were assigned in random order. The ingested fructose was labeled with [U-^{13}C] fructose. The ingested glucose was labeled with [U-^{14}C]glucose.

Findings.—Peak exogenous CHO oxidation rates were about 55% higher during the Fruc+Glu trial than during the Med-Glu or High-Glu trials. The mean exogenous CHO oxidation rates during the 60- to 120-minute exercise period were higher during the Fruc + Glu trial compared with the Med-Glu and High-Glu trials. A nonsignificant trend toward a lower endogenous CHO oxidation during the Fruc + Glu trial compared with the other CHO trials was observed (Fig 2).

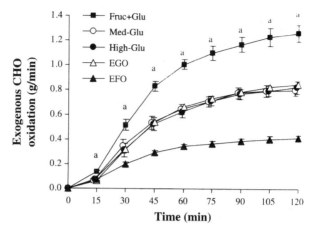

Time (min)

FIGURE 2.—Exogenous carbohydrate (*CHO*) oxidation during exercise with ingestion of Med-Glu, High-Glu, or Fruc+Glu. Values are means ± SE; 8 participants. [a]Significantly different from Med-Glu and High-Glu, *P* < .01. *Abbreviations: Fruc+Glu,* Fructose plus glucose; *Med-Glu,* 1.2 g/min glucose; *High-Glu,* 1.8 g/min glucose; *EGO,* exogenous glucose oxidation in Fruc+Glu; *EFO,* exogenous fructose oxidation in Fruc+Glu. (Courtesy of Jentjens RLPG, Moseley L, Waring RH, et al: Oxidation of combined ingestion of glucose and fructose during exercise. *J Appl Physiol* 96:1277-1284, 2004. Copyright 2004, The American Physiological Society.)

Conclusion.—With ingestion of a glucose-fructose mixture, exogenous CHO oxidation rates during cycle ergometry can exceed 1.1 g/min. Ingesting this mixture results in about 55% higher exogenous CHO oxidation rates compared with ingestion of an isocaloric amount of glucose.

▶ Although the ingestion of exogenous glucose is a useful tactic to augment performance during sustained exercise, particularly when endogenous reserves of CHO have been depleted, the rate of metabolism of such nutritional supplements reaches a ceiling of about 1 g/min, probably because the sodium-dependent glucose transporting mechanism of the intestinal membrane is fully saturated at this rate of ingestion.[1] It is thus logical to seek to boost the intake of CHO supplements by the addition of fructose, a substance that is absorbed from the intestine by a sodium-independent transporter mechanism (GLUT-5).[2]

Sucrose can be added to glucose solutions for a benefit of similar magnitude (see Abstract 9–7). A useful side effect of such treatment is an enhanced absorption of fluid. Gastrointestinal disturbances are one potential objection to the ingestion of CHO other than glucose during vigorous exercise. However, gastrointestinal symptoms do not seem to have been a major cause for concern in the present trial.

R. J. Shephard, MD, PhD, DPE

References

1. Duchman SM, Ryan AJ, Schedl HP, et al: Upper limit for intestinal absorption of a dilute glucose solution in men at rest. *Med Sci Sports Exerc* 29:482-488, 1997.

2. Ferraris RP, Diamond J: Regulation of intestinal sugar transport. *Physiol Rev* 77:257-302, 1997.

High Oxidation Rates From Combined Carbohydrates Ingested During Exercise

Jentjens RLPG, Achten J, Jeukendrup AE (Univ of Birmingham, Edgbaston, England)
Med Sci Sports Exerc 36:1551-1558, 2004   9–5

Introduction.—Studies that have investigated oxidation of a single carbohydrate (CHO) during exercise have reported oxidation rates of up to 1 g/min. Recent studies from our laboratory have shown that a mixture of glucose and sucrose or glucose and fructose ingested at a high rate (1.8 g/min leads to peak oxidation rates of approximately 1.3 g/min and results in approximately 20 to 55% higher exogenous CHO oxidation rates compared with the ingestion of an isocaloric amount of glucose.

Purpose.—The purpose of the present study was to examine whether a mixture of glucose, sucrose and fructose ingested at a high rate would result in even higher exogenous CHO oxidation rates (>1.3 g/min).

Methods.—Eight trained male cyclists ($\dot{V}O_{2max}$: 64 ± 1 mL/kg BM/min cycled on three different occasions for 150 min at 62 ± 1% $\dot{V}O_{2max}$ and consumed either water (WAT) or a CHO solution providing 2.4 g/min of glucose (GLU) or 1.2 g/min of glucose + 0.6 g/min of fructose + 0.6 g/min of sucrose (MIX).

Results.—High peak exogenous CHO oxidation rates were found in the MIX trial (1.70 ± 0.07 g/min, which were approximately 44% higher ($P < 0.01$) compared with the GLU trial (1.18 ± 0.04 g/min. Endogenous CHO oxidation was lower ($P < 0.05$) in MIX compared with GLU (0.76 ± 0.12 and 1.05 ± 0.06 g/min, respectively).

Conclusion.—When glucose, fructose and sucrose are ingested simultaneously at high rates (2.4 g/min during cycling exercise, exogenous CHO oxidation rates can reach peak values of approximately 1.7 g/min and estimated endogenous CHO oxidation is reduced compared with the ingestion of an isocaloric amount of glucose.

▶ Our standard sports nutrition recommendation to endurance athletes has been that the body during exercise can oxidize ingested carbohydrates at a peak rate of about 1 g/min (or about 1 liter of a typical sports drink each hour). This study showed that a glucose, fructose, and sucrose beverage (2:1:1 ratio) providing 2.4 grams of carbohydrate per minute resulted in an exogenous carbohydrate oxidation rate that peaked at about 1.7 g min (the highest rate ever reported in the literature and 44% above the isoenergetic glucose trial). Adding fructose and sucrose to a glucose beverage appears to use additional intestinal transporters, increasing overall carbohydrate absorption. Of practical interest is that the subjects reported fewer gastrointestinal problems with the glucose-fructose-sucrose beverage than the glucose-only beverage.

D. C. Nieman, DrPH

Effects of Ingestion of Bicarbonate, Citrate, Lactate, and Chloride on Sprint Running

van Montfoort MCE, van Dieren L, Hopkins WG, et al (Vrije Universiteit, Amsterdam; Auckland Univ, New Zealand; Univ of Essex, Colchester, England)
Med Sci Sports Exerc 36:1239-1243, 2004   9–6

Purpose.—Ingestion of sodium bicarbonate is known to enhance sprint performance, probably via increased buffering of intracellular acidity. The goal was to compare the effect of ingestion of sodium bicarbonate with that of other potential buffering agents (sodium citrate and sodium lactate) and of a placebo (sodium chloride) on sprinting.

Methods.—In a double-blind randomized crossover trial, 15 competitive male endurance runners performed a run to exhaustion 90 min after ingestion of each of the agents in the same osmolar dose relative to body mass (3.6 $mosmol \cdot kg^{-1}$) on separate days. The agents were packed in gelatin capsules and ingested with 750 mL of water over 90 min. During each treatment we assayed serial finger-prick blood samples for lactate and bicarbonate. A familiarization trial was used to set a treadmill speed for each runner's set of runs. We converted changes in run time between treatments into changes in a time trial of similar duration using the critical-power model, and we estimated likelihood of practical benefit using 0.5% as the smallest worthwhile change in time-trial performance.

Results.—The mean run times to exhaustion for each treatment were: bicarbonate 82.3 s, lactate 80.2 s, citrate 78.2 s, and chloride 77.4 s. Relative to bicarbonate, the effects on equivalent time-trial time were lactate 1.0%, citrate 2.2%, and chloride 2.7% (90% likely limits ± 2.1%). Ingested lactate and citrate both appeared to be converted to bicarbonate before the run. There were no substantial differences in gut discomfort between the buffer treatments.

Conclusion.—Bicarbonate is possibly more beneficial to sprint performance than lactate and probably more beneficial than citrate or chloride. We recommend ingestion of sodium bicarbonate to enhance sprint performance.

▶ High-intensity exercise for 0.5 to 5 minutes is accompanied by a decrease in muscle pH that contributes to fatigue. This study compared 3 pH-buffering agents (sodium bicarbonate, lactate, and citrate) with a placebo (sodium chloride) and found that sodium bicarbonate was superior for sprint performance. Sprint time to exhaustion was about 5 seconds better with sodium bicarbonate compared with placebo. Gastrointestinal distress was low for all pH-buffering agents.

D. C. Nieman, DrPH

Oxidation of Exogenous Glucose, Sucrose, and Maltose During Prolonged Cycling Exercise

Jentjens RLPG, Venables MC, Jeukendrup AE (Univ of Birmingham, England)
J Appl Physiol 96:1285-1291, 2004   9–7

Background.—Glucose in combination with sucrose may result in high rates of carbohydrate (CHO) and water absorption. Whether combined ingestion of a large amount of glucose and sucrose during 2.5 hours of exercise would result in exogenous CHO oxidation rates exceeding 1 g/min was investigated.

Methods.—Nine trained male cyclists participated in 4 exercise trials consisting of 150 minutes of cycle ergometry at 50% maximal power output. By random assignment, participants received a solution providing 1.8 g/min glucose (Glu), 1.2 g/min glucose plus 0.6 g/min sucose (Glu + Suc), 1.2 g/min glucose plus 0.6 g/min maltose (Glu + Mal), or water. The trials were separated by at least 1 week.

Findings.—Peak exogenous CHO oxidation rates were significantly higher during the Glu + Suc trial than during the Glu and Glu + Mal trials. The Glu and Glu + Mal trials did not differ in peak exogenous CHO oxidation rates (Fig 1).

Conclusion.—Ingesting a mixture of glucose and sucrose at high rates during cycle ergometry results in exogenous CHO oxidation rates peaking at about 1.25 g/min. In addition, this mixture resulted in nearly 20% greater exogenous CHO oxidation rates compared with ingestion of an isocaloric amount of glucose.

▶ In the endurance exerciser, exogenous carbohydrate intake and metabolism can be enhanced by ingesting mixtures of glucose and sucrose rather than glucose alone. The response is analogous to that seen when ingesting mixtures of glucose and fructose (see Abstract 9–4).

R. J. Shephard, MD, PhD, DPE

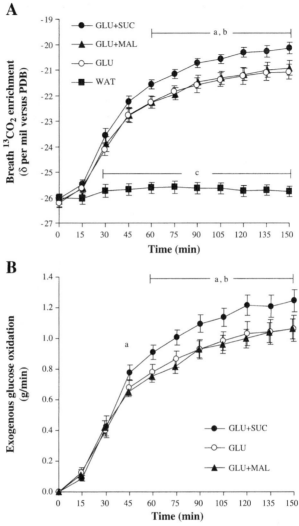

FIGURE 1.—Breath $^{13}CO_2$ enrichment (**A**) and exogenous carbohydrate oxidation (**B**) during exercise without ingestion of carbohydrate (water [*Wat*]) or with ingestion of glucose (*Glu*), glucose and sucrose (*Glu* + *Suc*), or glucose and maltose (*Glu* + *Mal*). Values are means ± SE; 9 participants. Significant differences: [a]Glu + Suc versus Glu + Mal, [b]Glu + Suc versus Glu, [c]Wat versus carbohydrate trials: $P < .05$. *Abbreviation: PDB*, Pee Dee Bellemnitella. (Courtesy of Jentjens RLPG, Venables MC, Jeukendrup AE: Oxidation of exogenous glucose, sucrose, and maltose during prolonged cycling exercise. *J Appl Physiol* 96:1285-1291, 2004. Copyright 2004, The American Physiological Society.)

Combined Ingestion of Protein and Carbohydrate Improves Protein Balance During Ultra-endurance Exercise

Koopman R, Pannemans DLE, Jeukendrup AE, et al (Maastricht Univ, The Netherlands)

Am J Physiol Endocrinol Metab 287:E712-E720, 2004   9–8

Introduction.—The aims of this study were to compare different tracer methods to assess whole body protein turnover during 6 h of prolonged endurance exercise when carbohydrate was ingested throughout the exercise period and to investigate whether addition of protein can improve protein balance. Eight endurance-trained athletes were studied on two different occasions at rest (4 h), during 6 h of exercise at 50% of maximal O_2 uptake (in sequential order: 2.5 h of cycling, 1 h of running, and 2.5 h of cycling), and during subsequent recovery (4 h). Subjects ingested carbohydrate (CHO trial; 0.7 g CHO·kg^{-1}·h^{-1}) or carbohydrate/protein beverages (CHO + PRO trial; 0.7 g CHO·kg^{-1}·h^{-1} and 0.25 g PRO·kg^{-1}·h^{-1}) at 30-min intervals during the entire study. Whole body protein metabolism was determined by infusion of L-[1-^{13}C]leucine, L-[^{2}H$_5$]phenylalanine, and [^{15}N$_2$]urea tracers with sampling of blood and expired breath. Leucine oxidation increased from rest to exercise [27 ± 2.5 vs. 74 ± 8.8 (CHO) and 85 ± 9.5 vs. 200 ± 16.3 mg protein·kg^{-1}·h^{-1} (CHO + PRO), $P < 0.05$], whereas phenylalanine oxidation and urea production did not increase with exercise. Whole body protein balance during exercise with carbohydrate ingestion was negative (-74 ± 8.8, -17 ± 1.1, and -72 ± 5.7 mg protein·kg·$^{-1}$·h^{-1} when L-[1-^{13}C]leucine, L-[^{2}H$_5$]phenylalanine, and [^{15}N$_2$]urea, respectively, were used as tracers. Addition of protein to the carbohydrate drinks resulted in a positive or less-negative protein balance (-32 ± 16.3, 165 ± 4.6, and 151 ± 13.4 mg protein·kg·h^{-1} when L-[1-^{13}C]leucine, L-[^{2}H$_5$]phenylalanine, and [^{15}N$_2$]urea, respectively, were used as tracers. We conclude that, even during 6 h of exhaustive exercise in trained athletes using carbohydrate supplements, net protein oxidation does not increase compared with the resting state and/or postexercise recovery. Combined ingestion of protein and carbohydrate improves net protein balance at rest as well as during exercise and postexercise recovery.

▶ Of all areas in sports nutrition, the influence of exercise on protein metabolism has caused the most confusion and debate. In the 1800s, skeletal muscle protein was thought to be the major source of energy for muscle contractions. Nitrogen balance studies in the 1900s came to the opposite conclusion—prolonged exercise caused no substantial increase in nitrogen loss. The recent use of stable isotope tracers in whole body protein metabolism has caused even more confusion. Studies with ^{13}C-labeled leucine suggested substantial increases in leucine oxidation rates and decreases in protein synthesis during exercise. On the other hand, studies applying [^{15}N$_2$]urea indicated that prolonged endurance exercise was not associated with net protein degradation or oxidation. In this study, athletes exercised for 6 hours on 2 occasions while ingesting carbohydrate or carbohydrate/protein beverages. The most important finding from this study is that even during 6 hours of exercise, net protein oxidation did not increase above the resting state when using data from 3 stable isotope tracers ([^{15}N$_2$]urea, L-[1-^{13}C]leucine, and L-[^{2}H$_5$]phenylalanine. This is a surprising result and contradicts previous (but misleading) studies that only used ^{13}C-labeled leucine. These data, if confirmed, will call into question recent recommendations that elite endurance athletes need 50% more protein than their sedentary peers.

D. C. Nieman, DrPH

Effects of a Carbohydrate-Protein Beverage on Cycling Endurance and Muscle Damage
Saunders MJ, Kane MD, Todd MK (James Madison University, Harrisonburg, Va)
Med Sci Sports Exerc 36:1233-1238, 2004   9–9

Introduction.—It has recently been suggested that the inclusion of small amounts of protein (usually 20% of total calories) in a carbohydrate beverage may provide benefits (ie, increased performance time to fatigue, decreased postexercise muscle damage, and enhanced muscle glycogen repletion) over traditional carbohydrate-only beverages. The effect of consumption of a carbohydrate and protein beverage (CHO+P; 7.3% and 1.8% concentrations, respectively) versus a carbohydrate-only (CHO; 7.3%) beverage on endurance cycling and postexercise muscle damage were examined.

Methods.—Fifteen male cyclists with a mean maximal oxygen intake ($\dot{V}O_{2peak}$) of 52.6 mL/kg/min rode a cycle ergometer at 75% $\dot{V}O_{2peak}$ to volitional exhaustion, followed 12 to 15 hours later by a second ride to exhaustion at 85% $\dot{V}O_{2peak}$. Participants consumed 1.8 mL/kg of randomly assigned CHO or CHO+P beverage every 15 minutes of exercise and 10 mL/kg body mass immediately post exercise. Beverages were matched for carbohydrate content. This resulted in 20% lower total caloric content per administration of CHO beverage. Participants were blinded to treatment beverage and repeated the same protocol 7 to 14 days later with the other beverage.

Results.—During the first ride (75% $\dot{V}O_{2peak}$, participants rode 29% longer ($P < .05$) when consuming the CHO+P versus the CHO beverage (106.3 vs 82.3 minutes). During the second ride (85% $\dot{V}O_{2peak}$), participants performed 40% longer when consuming the CHO+P versus the CHO beverage (43.6 vs 31.2 minutes). Peak postexercise plasma creatine phosphokinase levels, indicative of muscle damage, were 83% lower after the CHO+ P versus the CHO trial (216.3 vs 131.8 U/L). No significant differences were seen between treatments in either trial in exercise levels of $\dot{V}O_2$, ventilation, heart rate, ratings of perceived exertion, blood glucose, or blood lactate.

Conclusion.—A carbohydrate beverage with additional protein calories provided significant improvements in time to fatigue and decreases in muscle damage in endurance athletes.

▶ Should a sports drink include protein? A growing number of studies indicate "Yes" to improve performance, decrease muscle damage, and improve post-exercise protein synthesis.[1] In this study, ingesting about one-half cup of a 4:1 CHO+P beverage improved exercise time to exhaustion by 29% to 40% and reduced plasma creatine phosphokinase levels 12 to 15 hours post exercise by 83% compared to CHO. The authors speculated that muscle damage was diminished with the CHO+P beverage because of increased protein availability within the cell, leading to enhanced protein synthesis and repair. Many other mechanisms may play a role.

D. C. Nieman, DrPH

Reference

1. Borsheim E, Aarsland A, Wolfe RR: Effect of an amino acid, protein, and carbohydrate mixture on net muscle protein balance after resistance exercise. *Int J Sport Nutr Exerc Metab* 14:255-271, 2004.

Caffeine and Ephedrine: Physiological, Metabolic and Performance-Enhancing Effects
Magkos F, Kavouras SA (Harokopio Univ, Athens, Greece)
Sports Med 34:871-889, 2004   9–10

Background.—Sports drinks containing caffeine and ephedrine have become increasingly popular among professional and recreational athletes in recent years as a method for enhancing athletic performance. Evidence is slowly accumulating to suggest that the combination of these 2 drugs may be more efficacious than each drug alone. The current state of knowledge of the physiologic, metabolic, and performance-enhancing effects of caffeine-ephedrine mixtures was reviewed.

Overview.—From a metabolic viewpoint, combined ingestion of caffeine and ephedrine has been observed to increase blood glucose and lactate concentrations during physical exercise, whereas qualitatively similar effects on lipid fuels (free fatty acids, glycerol) are less pronounced. For pulmonary gas exchange during short-term physical exercise, no physiologically significant effects have been reported after ingestion of caffeine, ephedrine, or their combination. However, some sporadic enhancements have been shown in longer or more demanding athletic efforts. Increased heart rate is a relatively consistent cardiovascular effect of the ingestion of a combination of ephedrine and caffeine. It is likely that research in the performance-enhancing effects of caffeine-ephedrine mixtures is hindered by ethical concerns that preclude the administration of potentially hazardous substances to human volunteers. It is true that caffeine and, especially, ephedrine have been associated with several acute adverse effects on health, yet athletes do not seem concerned with these adverse effects so long as they believe their performance will improve.

Conclusions.—Caffeine and ephedrine-containing alkaloids, although not ephedrine specifically, have been removed from the list of banned substances in sport, so it is likely that their use among athletes will increase substantially in the foreseeable future. It remains to be seen whether caffeine-ephedra mixtures will turn out to be one of the most dangerous ergogenic aids in use.

▶ Discussion concerning the possible removal of caffeine from the list of banned substances is surprising. In addition to issues of fair play, there are significant cardiac and psychological concerns associated with excessive doses of caffeine, including occasional deaths.[1] Fortunately, the change in regulations that Magkos and Kavouras predicted on the basis of a newspaper rumor did not take place when the list of prohibited drugs was reviewed by IOC and the World Anti-Doping Agency.

R. J. Shephard, MD, PhD, DPE

Reference

1. Holmgren P, Norden-Petersson L, Ahlner J: Caffeine fatalities. Four case reports. *Forensic Sci Int* 139:71-73, 2004.

Gene Doping in Sports
Unal M, Ozer Unal D (Istanbul Univ, Turkey; Bogazici Univ, Istanbul, Turkey)
Sports Med 34:357-362, 2004   9–11

Background.—"Doping," or the use of forbidden substances or methods to increase physical and/or mental performance, has become a major issue in athletic competitions at the Olympic, professional, and collegiate levels of sport. Gene or cell doping has been defined by the World Anti-Doping Agency (WADA) as "the non-therapeutic use of genes, genetic elements and/or cells that has the capacity to enhance athletic performance." The use of doping to enhance athletic performance has increased in sophistication with advances in technology, and there is no doubt that new research in genetics and genomics will be used not only in the diagnosis and treatment of disease but also in efforts to enhance human performance. The current status of gene doping and candidate performance enhancement genes, the use of gene therapy in sports medicine, and the ethics of genetic enhancement were reviewed.

Overview.—Gene therapies that have been developed for the treatment of diseases such as anemia (the gene for erythropoietin), muscular dystrophy (the gene for insulin-like growth factor-1), and peripheral vascular diseases (the gene for vascular endothelial growth factor) have also been identified as potential doping methods. Several methods exist for the detection of blood doping and erythropoietin use, but athletes who engage in gene doping will avoid detection by injecting themselves with copies of genes that are naturally occurring in the body, such as encoding growth factors or testosterone. As with any gene therapy, the aspect of gene doping that is of greatest concern is the health risks, both known and unknown. At present, it is not possible to discern the likely effects of gene therapy on healthy individuals such as athletes, but it is likely that numerous health problems would ensue. The International Olympic Committee (IOC) and WADA have issued warnings on gene doping that discriminate between gene therapy used in athletes for treatment of legitimate medical conditions and gene therapy used solely for the enhancement of athletic performance. WADA has also called for financial support for research into methods to prevent and detect gene doping among athletes.

Conclusions.—The use of gene transfer technology solely for the enhancement of athletic performance will put the athlete's health at risk. At this time, there is no method for identifying gene doping. Governments and sporting organizations should begin to develop policies with regard to the use of gene therapies by healthy athletes to increase their performance.

▶ The 2004 Olympics has shown that the problem of doping continues to plague high-level athletic competition. As the review of Unal and Unal points out, one of the biggest threats on the current horizon is the modification of genes to enhance performance. The latest IOC protocol specifically prohibits gene manipulation, but, unfortunately, there is yet no practical technique to detect this type of abuse. Already, viruses containing the erythropoietin gene have been used to stimulate production of hemoglobin and muscle growth factors in laboratory animals, and it will not be long before someone is foolhardy enough to try this on an athlete.[1] The IOC is eager to sponsor practical research that will lead to the development of detection methods. One suggestion is to inject athletes with chemical labels that bind to muscle growth factors. If MRI were to detect excessive concentrations of growth factors in muscle, this might be presumptive evidence of genetic manipulation. However, the sophistication of such an analysis precludes its widespread use in athletes.

The available literature is undoubtedly quite limited. However, the review of Unal and Unal would have been enhanced by detailing the search techniques that were used (eg, the database used, the key words chosen, the period surveyed, and reasons for inclusion or exclusion of individual articles).

R. J. Shephard, MD, PhD, DPE

Reference

1. Stikeman A: Deterring gene doping: Officials try to head off abuse by athletes. *Technol Rev* 105:24, 2002.

Mutations in the Hereditary Haemochromatosis Gene HFE in Professional Endurance Athletes
Chicharro JL, Hoyos J, Gómez-Gallego F, et al (Universidad Complutense, Madrid; Asociación Deportiva Banesto, Madrid; Universidad de León, Spain, et al)
Br J Sports Med 38:418-421, 2004 9–12

Introduction.—The autosomal recessive disease, hereditary hemochromatosis, affects several organs. The clinical consequences of iron overload-

TABLE 3.—Comparison of Variables According to the Presence or Absence of HFE Gene Mutations

	Age (Years)	Height (cm)	Mass (kg)	Vo_2MAX (ml/kg/min)	Fe (µmol/l)	Ferritin (µg/l)	Transferrin (g/l)	TSI (%)
HFE mutation	26 (3)	178 (6)	66.1 (6.9)	72.8 (6.5)	18.8 (6.3)	267.2 (151.3)	218.8 (27.6)	36.2 (12.4)
No HFE mutation	26 (3)	178 (6)	67.4 (5.2)	70.8 (6.8)	19.3 (5.7)	224.7 (153.2)	232.4 (26.8)	36.1 (10.8)
Normal ranges					13-32	20-300	24-336	24-45

Note: Values are mean (SD). No significant differences in any of the variables ($P > .05$) were detected among the athlete subgroups.

Abbreviations: Fe, Iron; TSI, transferrin saturation index.

(Courtesy of Chicharro JL, Hoyos J, Gómez-Gallego F, et al: Mutations in the hereditary haemochromatosis gene HFE in professional endurance athletes. *Br J Sports Med* 38:418-421, 2004. Reprinted with permission from the BMJ Publishing Group.)

ing in this disorder can be prevented by an early diagnosis and appropriate treatment. Many elite endurance athletes take iron supplements that may aggravate hereditary hemochromatosis. Substantial evidence exists that mutations in the HFE gene affect blood iron indices. However, genetic evaluations, including screening the general public, are not recommended. Phenotypic analysis based on transferrin saturation continues to be the most economical method for precluding or warranting a more in depth analysis. The prevalence of HFE mutations in elite endurance athletes was assessed and compared with a control group matched by region of origin.

Methods.—Basal concentrations of iron, ferritin, and transferrin and transferrin saturation were ascertained before competition in 65 highly trained athletes. Possible mutations in the HFE gene were assessed by extraction of genomic DNA from peripheral blood. The restriction enzymes *Sna*Bl and *Bcl*l were used to identify mutations 845G→A (C282Y) and 187C→G (H63D).

Results.—The incidence of HFE gene mutation was higher in the elite athletes (49.2%) than in the sedentary control subjects (33.5%). No correlation was seen between mutations and blood iron markers (Table 3).

Conclusion.—A high proportion (49.2%) of these Spanish elite athletes had a mutation in the HFE gene: 29 athletes (44.6%) carried an H63D mutation, and 3 (4.6%) carried a C282Y mutation. Iron stores should be regularly evaluated in elite endurance athletes.

▶ Outstanding athletic performance is being linked to an increasing number of heritable genetic mutations. It has yet to be demonstrated that mutations of the hematochromatosis gene HFE are linked to a high oxygen transport capacity, but it seems clear that the percentage of athletes with H63D heterozygosity is about twice that observed in controls or the general population. Studies of French cyclists have reported conclusions similar to those in this article from Spain.[1] The H63D abnormality seems to be linked to substantially increased body ferritin stores, and the resultant free radical accumulation can accelerate atherogenesis and ischemia–reperfusion damage. The take-home message for the sports physician is that ferritin levels should be checked before prescribing additional amounts of iron for endurance athletes.

R. J. Shephard, MD, PhD, DPE

Reference

1. Deugnier Y, Loréal O, Carré F, et al: Increased body iron stores in elite cyclists. *Med Sci Sports Exerc* 34:876-880, 2002.

Serum sTfR Levels May Indicate Charge Profiling of Urinary r-hEPO in Doping Control

Nissen-Lie G, Birkeland K, Hemmersbach P, et al (Aker Univ, Oslo, Norway)
Med Sci Sports Exerc 36:588-593, 2004   9–13

Background.—Human erythropoietin (EPO), a glycoprotein produced mainly in the kidneys, is the primary regulator of erythropoiesis. A study was undertaken to determine whether changes in the charge pattern of urinary human EPO (u-hEPO) from well-trained athletes before, during, and after controlled administration of recombinant human EPO (r-hEPO) correlate with changes in hemoglobin (Hb), hematocrit (Hct), soluble transferring receptor (sTfR) and maximal oxygen uptake (VO_{2max}).

Methods.—Eight well-trained male athletes participating in a placebo-controlled study of r-hEPO were selected. Five received r-hEPO, 5000 U, and 3 received placebo. Urinary samples were obtained before, during, and after r-hEPO administration. The charge pattern of hEPO was analyzed by isoelectric focusing (IEF).

Findings.—After r-hEPO was initiated, the charge of the u-hEPO variants shifted from an acidic to a more basic pattern. This shift occurred along with increased sTfR levels and appeared before increases in Hb, Hct, and VO_{2max} levels. Up to 3 days after the last injection, IEF profiles were comparable to the charge profile of r-hEPO. After that point, sTfR levels declined, and the charge profiles of the hEPO variants gradually became more acidic. By contrast, Hb, Hct and VO_{2max} levels remained increased for an extended time.

Conclusions.—The relative amount of basic u-hEPO variants correlate significantly with relative levels of sTfR. Thus, the relative levels of sTfR may serve as a marker to select urinary samples for further analysis of r-hEPO by IEF in routine doping control.

▶ Ensuring the fairness of endurance competition has been a challenge since r-hEPO became commercially available. Abuse of this substance has a significant effect on competitive performance,[1,2] and, although banned by the International Olympic Committee, it has been detected in urine collected at competition.[3] Analytic techniques to distinguish r-hEPO from endogenous EPO exploit differences in electric charge and in the sugar part of the molecule.[4,5] Unfortunately, such tests are expensive. A preliminary triage of competitors can be based on hematocrit readings, but such values are also influenced markedly by such tactics as living high/training low. The present report suggests that serum levels of sTfR provide a better screening alternative because serum concentrations of sTfR tend to move in parallel with markers of urinary r-hEPO. Nevertheless, Fig 5 (see original article) shows a substantial scatter in the relationship, and there remains scope for the refining of techniques.

R. J. Shephard, MD, PhD, DPE

References

1. Ekblom B, Berglund B: Effect of erythropoietin administration on maximal aerobic power. *Scand J Med Sci Sports* 1:88-93, 1991.

2. Audran M, Gareau S: Effects of erythropoietin administration in training athletes and possible indirect detection in doping control. *Med Sci Sports Exerc* 31:639-645, 1999.

3. Lasne F, de Ceaurriz J: Recombinant erythropoietin in urine. *Nature* 405:635, 2000.

4. Wide L, Bengtsson C, Berglund B, et al: Detection in blood and urine of recombinant erythropoietin administered to healthy men. *Med Sci Sports Exerc* 27:1569-1576, 1995.

5. Skibeli V, Nissen-Lie G, Trojesen P: Sugar profiling proves that human serum erythropoietin differs from recombinant human erythropoietin. *Blood* 98:3626-3634, 2001.

Norandrosterone and Noretiocholanolone Concentration Before and After Submaximal Standardized Exercise

de Geus B, Delbeke F, Meeusen R, et al (Vrije Universiteit Brussel, Belgium; Universiteit Gent, Merelbeke, Belgium)
Int J Sports Med 25:528-532, 2004   9–14

Background.—Anabolic-androgenic steroids (AASs) have been used for decades for promotion and stimulation of wound healing and recovery. At present, they are used in the treatment of protein deficiency diseases, osteoporosis, and burns. In recent years, there has been a significant increase in the use of AASs as a doping agent to improve muscular strength and performance. The first of these steroids was testosterone, which is quickly metabolized by the liver; as a result, the molecular structure of testosterone was altered to make it more efficacious. The first synthetic AAS was nandrolone, which is a controlled substance according to rules of the International Olympic Committee (IOC). The 2 main urinary indicators used to detect the illegal use of nandrolone are 19-norandrosterone (19-NA) and 19-noretiocholanolone (19-NE). However, recent studies have shown that 19-NA and 19-NE can be endogenously produced in nontreated humans. The concentrations in these studies were close to the IOC threshold of 2 ng/mL for men and appeared to increase after prolonged intense effort. Whether 3 different exercise methods would influence the urinary concentration of 19-NA and 19-NE in healthy young subjects was investigated.

Methods.—A group of 15 amateur hockey players participated in a 30-minute submaximal standardized exercise protocol. The athletes were randomly assigned to 3 different types of exercise, including a cycle ergometer test (cyclic muscle activity), a treadmill test (concentric muscle activity), and a bench-step test (eccentric muscle activity) at a target heart rate corresponding to 65% (±5%) of Karvonen heart rate. Urinary samples were obtained before the test and at 60 minutes and 120 minutes after the end of exercise. The study subjects completed a Likert scale of muscle soreness before exercise and 12 hours after exercise. Concentrations of 19-NA and 19-NE were determined by gas chromatography-tandem mass spectrometry (GC-MS-MS).

Results.—Baseline urinary 19-NA and 19-NE concentrations were under the limit of detection of 0.05 ng/mL, with the exception of one sample, in which no 19-NA or 19-NE was detected after exercise.

Conclusions.—This experiment found no effect of type of exercise on the level of 19-NA or 19-NE excretion. These findings provide confirmation that the current IOC threshold level for nandrolone metabolites is high enough to avoid false-positive cases.

▶ There have been occasional suggestions that an exercise-induced dehydration,[1] or endogenous release of 19-NA or 19-NE[2] could cause urinary concentrations of prohibited androgen metabolites to exceed the limits currently proscribed by international competition. The present relatively small-scale laboratory exercise study on 15 amateur hockey players found that the urinary excretion of nandrolone metabolites remained far below the IOC threshold of 2 ng/mL both during and following activity. However, earlier contrary reports are not necessarily negated by this study, since the exercise was mild (30 minutes at a heart rate <150 beats/min), and the subjects were neither dehydrated nor stimulated by competition.

R. J. Shephard, MD, PhD, DPE

References

1. Le Bizec B, Monteau F, Gaudin I, et al: Evidence for the presence of endogenous 19-norandrosterone in human urine. *J Chromatogr B* 723:157-172, 1999.
2. Kintz P, Cirimele V, Ludes B: Norandrosterone et noretiocholanolone: Les metabolites révélateur. *Acta Clin Belg* 1:68-73, 1999.

Analysis of Non-hormonal Nutritional Supplements for Anabolic-Androgenic Steroids: Results of an International Study
Geyer H, Parr MK, Mareck U, et al (German Sport Univ, Cologne)
Int J Sports Med 25:124-129, 2004   9–15

Background.—Anabolic androgenic steroids, or prohormones, have been available in the United States since 1996. These substances have been advertised as having formidable properties to increase muscle growth and strength. The International Olympic Committee has designated these substances as belonging to the prohibited class of anabolic agents. It has been demonstrated in several studies that the labeling on prohormone supplements is not always reflective of their actual content; in fact, many prohormone products have been found to contain prohormones as well as concentrations different from those stated on the labels. These mislabeling problems are indicative of inadequate surveillance and quality control of the production of dietary supplements, particularly in the prohormone industry. Several recent studies have shown evidence of prohibited prohormones in some nutritional supplements, which were not declared on the label. A broad-based investigation of the international nutritional supplement market was conducted to clarify the extent of the problem.

TABLE 3.—Nutritional Supplements Containing Prohormones, in Relation to the Total Number of Supplements Purchased in Different Countries

Country	No of Products	No. of Positives	Percentage of Positives
Netherlands	31	8	25.8%
Austria	22	5	22.7%
UK	37	7	18.9%
USA	240	45	18.8%
Italy	35	5	14.3%
Spain	29	4	13.8%
Germany	129	15	11.6%
Belgium	30	2	6.7%
France	30	2	6.7%
Norway	30	1	3.3%
Switzerland	13	–	–
Sweden	6	–	–
Hungary	2	–	–
total	634	94	14.8%

(Courtesy of Geyer H, Parr MK, Mareck U, et al: Analysis of non-hormonal nutritional supplements for anabolic-androgenic steroids: Results of an international study. *Int J Sports Med* 25:124-129, 2004. Copyright Georg Thieme Verlag.)

Methods.—From October 2000 to November 2001, 634 nonhormonal nutritional supplements were purchased in 13 countries from 215 different suppliers. The supplements were purchased from suppliers in the United States and in 14 European countries (91.2%) and over the Internet (8.2%).

Results.—Of the 634 samples analyzed, 94 (14.8%) were found to contain anabolic androgenic steroids that were not declared on the label (positive supplements). In relation to the total number of products purchased per country, most of the positive supplements were obtained in The Netherlands (25.8%), in Austria (22.7%), in the United Kingdom (18.8%), and in the United States (18.8%). The labels indicated that all the positive supplements were from companies located in just 5 countries—the United States, The Netherlands, the United Kingdom, Italy, and Germany (Table 3). Of the nutritional supplements obtained from prohormone-selling companies, 21.1% contained anabolic androgenic steroids compared with 9.6% of the supplements from companies not selling prohormones. The positive supplements showed concentrations of anabolic androgenic steroids ranging from 0.01 µg/g to 190 µg/g. The intake of supplements containing nandrolone prohormones adding up to a total uptake of more than 1 µg resulted in positive doping results for norandrosterone for several hours.

Conclusions.—The sports community must become aware of the dangers posed by nutritional supplements that contain anabolic androgenic steroids that are not declared on the supplement label. These findings clearly show that this is an international problem.

▶ In recent years, a growing number of athletes have attempted to explain positive results for anabolic steroids on the basis that they have unwittingly consumed contaminated but otherwise legal nutritional supplements. I was both surprised and disturbed by not only the high percentage of nutritional supplements that contain unlisted steroids but also the implication that cross-contamination appears to have occurred because the same machines were used to prepare different compounds without adequate cleaning of the equipment. There is an urgent need for all countries to insist that those manufacturing nutritional supplements meet the same exacting laboratory standards expected of those producing pharmaceuticals.

R. J. Shephard, MD, PhD, DPE

Relationship Between Diet and Serum Anabolic Hormone Responses to Heavy-Resistance Exercise in Men

Sallinen J, Pakarinen A, Ahtiainen J, et al (Univ of Jyväskylä, Finland)
Int J Sports Med 25:627-633, 2004   9–16

Introduction.—Relationship between dietary intake and serum anabolic hormone concentrations of testosterone (T), free testosterone (FT), and growth hormone were examined at rest as well as after the heavy-resistance exercise (HRE) in 8 strength athletes (SA) and 10 physically active non-athletes (NA). In the first part of the study serum basal anabolic hormone concentrations and dietary intake were examined in the total group of subjects. In the second part of the study a subgroup of 5 SA and 5 NA performed the high volume and high intensity HRE. Dietary intake was registered by dietary diaries for 4 days preceding the loading day. Significant correlations were observed between serum basal T and fat (E%: $r = 0.55$, $p < 0.05$, g/kg: $r = 0.65$, $p < 0.01$) and protein intake (E%: $r = -0.77$, $p < 0.001$, g/kg: $r =$

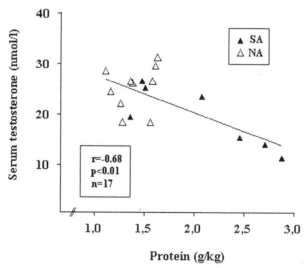

FIGURE 4.—Relationship between serum basal testosterone concentration and grams of protein per kilogram of body weight (protein; g/kg) in a subgroup of five strength athletes (SA) and a subgroup of five non-athletes (NA). (Courtesy of Sallinen J, Pakarinen A, Ahtiainen J, et al: Relationship between diet and serum anabolic hormone responses to heavy-resistance exercise in men. *Int J Sports Med* 25:627-633, 2004. Copyright Georg Thieme Verlag.)

−0.68, p < 0.01) in the total group of subjects (Fig 4). However, when the two groups were examined separately the significant relationships between serum basal T and dietary fat and protein could be noticed in SA only (fat g/kg: SA r = 0.77, p < 0.05; in NA r = 0.44, n.s., protein g/kg: SA r = −0.84, p < 0.05; in NA r = 0.27, n.s.). Both serum T and FT responses to HRE were correlated with fat (E%: r = 0.85, p < 0.01 and r = 0.73, p < 0.05, g/kg: r = 0.72, p < 0.05 and r = 0.77, p < 0.01) and protein (E%: r = −0.81, p < 0.01 and r = −0.69, p < 0.05, g/kg: r = −0.86, p < 0.01 and r = −0.65, p < 0.05). The results suggest the possible role of diet leading to alterations in serum T and FT during prolonged strength training, and that diets with insufficient fat and/or excessive protein may compromise the anabolic hormonal environment over a training program.

▶ Competitors in strength-demanding sports need a larger protein intake than sedentary individuals if they are to develop an appropriate muscle bulk. Commonly the recommended allowance of good quality protein, based on nitrogen balance studies, has been in the range of 1.3 to 2.0 g/kg,[1] as contrasted with the 0.7 to 1.0 g/kg of the RDA for sedentary individuals. Nevertheless, many power athletes substantially exceed the upper limit of the suggested protein intake for athletes, reasoning that if a little meat is good for them, more will be even better. Some physicians have argued that the only adverse effect of an excessive protein intake is the creation of an added demand for the renal excretion of nitrogen. However, the present report, supported by at least 1 earlier study,[2] suggests that a large protein intake is associated with an inhibition of the acute, exercise-induced burst of anabolic hormone secretion that is important to muscle hypertrophy.[3] The average protein intake of the present sample of strength athletes was at the upper limit of earlier recommendations (2g/kg per day). Given the apparent adverse effect upon anabolic hormone secretion, it may be that this ceiling should be reduced. The mechanism of any adverse reaction remains to be determined. The problem may stem from a reduction of fat intake [2] rather than an excess of dietary protein. Interpretation of the present observations is limited by their cross-sectional nature and by a small sample size. Nevertheless, it does seem that there may be a need to examine more closely the diet offered to the strength athlete.

R. J. Shephard, MD, PhD, DPE

References

1. Shephard RJ: *Physiology and Biochemistry of Exercise*, New York, Praeger, 1982.
2. Volek J, Kraemer WJ, Bush JA, et al: Testosterone and cortisol in relationship to dietary nutrients and resistance exercise. *J Appl Physiol* 82:49-54, 1997.
3. Häkkinen K, Pakarinen A: Acute hormonal responses to two different fatiguing heavy-resistance protocols in male athletes. *J Appl Physiol* 74:882-887, 1993.

Are the Cardiac Effects of Anabolic Steroid Abuse in Strength Athletes Reversible?

Urhausen A, Albers T, Kindermann W (Univ of Saarland Saarbruecken, Germany)

Heart 90:496-501, 2004   9–17

Introduction.—The extent to which the effects of anabolic androgenic steroids (AASs) are reversible after discontinuing the use of these agents and the extent to which they leave permanent impairment are controversial. For the first time, the reversibility of adverse cardiovascular effects was evaluated in athletes after long-term abuse of AASs.

Methods.—Doppler echocardiography and cycle ergometry, including measurements of blood pressure at rest and during exercise, were performed in 32 bodybuilders or power lifters; of these, 15 athletes had been taking AASs for at least 12 months (ex-users), and 17 were currently abusing AASs (users). Also evaluated were 15 anabolic-free weight lifters.

Results.—Higher systolic blood pressure was observed in users (mean, 140 mm Hg) than in ex-users (130 mm Hg) ($P < .05$) or weight lifters (125 mm Hg) ($P < .001$). Left ventricular muscle mass related to fat-free body mass and the ratio of mean left ventricular wall thickness to the internal diameter were not significantly higher in users (3.32 g/kg and 42.1%) than in ex-users (3.16 g/kg and 40.3%) and were lower in weight lifters (2.43 g/kg and 36.5% ($P < .001$). Left ventricular wall thickness associated with fat-free body mass was also lower in weight lifters; this did not differ between users and nonusers (Fig 1). Left ventricular wall thickness was associated with a point score estimating AAS abuse in users ($r = 0.49; P < .05$). In all 3 groups, systolic left ventricular functioning was within the normal range. The maximum late transmitral Doppler flow velocity was higher in users (61 cm/s) and ex-users (60 cm/s) than in weight lifters (50 cm/s; $P < .05$ and $P = .054$).

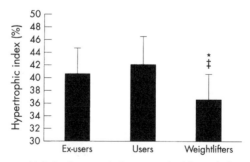

FIGURE 1.—Hypertrophic index (interventricular septum plus left ventricular posterior wall thickness divided by internal diameter). Values are means; *error bars* indicate SD. Ex-users vs weight lifters: *$P < .05$; users vs weight lifters: †$P < .01$. (Courtesy of Urhausen A, Albers T, Kindermann W: Are the cardiac effects of anabolic steroid abuse in strength athletes reversible? *Heart* 90:496-501, 2004. Reprinted with permission from the BMJ Publishing Group.)

Conclusion.—Several years after discontinuation of anabolic steroid abuse, strength athletes continue to exhibit a slight concentric left ventricular hypertrophy compared with AAS-free strength athletes.

▶ In recent years, the abuse of anabolic steroids by power athletes has been linked to an increased risk of various cardiac complications, including cardiac insufficiency, ventricular fibrillation, myocardial infarction, and sudden death.[1-3] It is well recognized that the administration of large doses of such steroids accelerates the atherosclerotic process, and atherosclerotic narrowing of the coronary vessels might seem the likely explanation for such cardiac problems. However, many of the fatalities have occurred either during the course of doping or shortly afterward, which suggests that the cause might lie in an immediate cardiac hypertrophy rather than a more long-term atherosclerotic process—a risk analogous to that noted among nonathletic participants in the Framingham study,[4] who had echocardiographic evidence of large hearts. Investigators are far from unanimous in their agreement that steroid abuse gives rise to a concentric cardiac hypertrophy, but the present study suggests that this is the case. This, in turn, raises the question of the rate of regression of any steroid-induced cardiac hypertrophy. It remains debatable whether the risks seen in nonathletes can be extrapolated to athletes; however, if cardiac hypertrophy is, indeed, a source of cardiac complications for well-trained individuals, it is disquieting to see that much of the hypertrophy persists for at least a year after stopping the doping.

R. J. Shephard, MD, PhD, DPE

References

1. Sullivan ML, Martinez CM, Gennis P, et al: The cardiac toxicity of anabolic steroids. *Prog Cardiovasc Dis* 41:1-15, 1998.
2. Thiblin I, Lindquist O, Rajs J: Cause and manner of death among users of anabolic androgenic steroids. *J Forensic Sci* 45:16-23, 2000.
3. Pärssinen M, Kujala U, Vartiainen E, et al: Increased premature mortality of competitive powerlifters suspected to have used anabolic agents. *Int J Sports Med* 21:225-227, 2000.
4. Levy D, Garrison RJ, Savage DD, et al: Prognostic implications of echocardiographically determined left ventricular mass in the Framingham Heart Study. *N Engl J Med* 322:1561-1566, 1990.

Concomitant Abuse of Anabolic Androgenic Steroids and Human Chorionic Gonadotrophin Impairs Spermatogenesis in Power Athletes
Karila T, Hovatta O, Seppälä T (Univ of Helsinki; Huddinge Univ, Sweden)
Int J Sports Med 25:257-263, 2004   9–18

Background.—Some cases of male infertility with an unknown cause among recreational power athletes as well as competitive athletes may be attributable to abuse of anabolic androgenic steroids (AASs). The nonmedical use of AASs has increased by 50% among male adolescents between 1991 and 1999. Some of these athletes will try to avoid the AAS-induced sper-

TABLE 3.—Characteristics of Anabolic Androgenic Steroid (AAS) Abuse (mean ± SD), Serum Endrocrinologic Parameters (mean ± SD), and Semen Analysis Parameters (mean ± SD) of Minor and Major AAS Users

Parameters	Normal Range and Mean ± SD*	Sample 1		Sample 2		Sample 3		Significance	
		Minor (n = 9)	Major (n = 9)	Minor (n = 9)	Major (n = 7)	Minor (n = 8)	Major (n = 8)	Sample vs Sample P-Value	Minor vs Major P-Value
Lifetime AAS use (years)		4.1 ± 4.8	5.7 ± 3.7						
Duration of the cycle (days)		94 ± 27	188 ± 67						$P \leq 0.01$
Mean daily AAS dose (mg/day)		68 ± 39	127 ± 25						$P \leq 0.01$
Cumulative HCG dose (kIU)		19 ± 9	35 ± 30						
Serum LH (IU/l)	2.0-15.0	0.7 ± 0.9	0.1 ± 0.2‡	1.8 ± 1.9*	0.0 ± 0.1‡	3.4 ± 1.2*	1.5 ± 1.2	$P = 0.035$	$P = 0.24$
Serum FSH (IU/l)	2.0-18.0	0.6 ± 1.0	0.0 ± 0.1‡	1.6 ± 2.6*	0.0 ± 0.0	2.9 ± 1.1*	0.9 ± 1.1	$P = 0.05$	$P = 0.032$
Serum SHBG (nmol/l)	10-60	14 ± 7	13 ± 11	29 ± 15	15 ± 14	28 ± 8	22 ± 22		
Serum testosterone (nmol/l)	9.0-34.0	24.8 ± 35.0	70.7 ± 56.7	9.7 ± 7.2	10.3 ± 5.7*	12.3 ± 5.9†	6.1 ± 3.3*	$P = 0.002$	$P = 0.037$
Serum volume (ml)		3.4 ± 1.9	3.2 ± 2.8	3.0 ± 2.0	3.1 ± 1.3	3.4 ± 2.2	2.4 ± 1.2		
Concentration of spermatozoa ($\times 10^6$/ml)	117 ± 56*	39 ± 66	27 ± 28‡	22 ± 31	39 ± 53‡	82 ± 54	73 ± 86	$P = 0.047$	
Percentage motility (WHO categories a + b)	63 ± 12*	47 ± 18	40 ± 25	58 ± 17	47 ± 28	60 ± 17	46 ± 38		
Normal morphology (% normal spermatozoa)	40 ± 15*	14 ± 12	16 ± 23	21 ± 13	10 ± 20	25 ± 16	23 ± 21		

Note: Sample 1: taken in the end of the cycle; Sample 2: approximately 6 months after the AAS cycle; Sample 3: approximately 1½ months after the AAS cycle. Asterisk indicates mean ± SD in Finnish males. Significance of differences calculated by the use of repeated measures of analysis of variance, and when appropriate, Student's t-test was used to assess the differences between the groups *$P \leq .05$ vs Sample 1; †$P \leq .05$ vs major users; ‡$P \leq .01$ vs Sample 3.

Abbreviations: HCG, Human chorionic gonadotrophin; LH, luteinizing hormone; FSH, follicle-stimulating hormone; SHBG, sex-hormone binding globulin; WHO, World Health Organization.

(Courtesy of Karila T, Hovatta O, Seppälä T: Concomitant abuse of anabolic androgenic steroids and human chorionic gonadotrophin impairs spermatogenesis in power athletes. Int J Sports Med 25:257-263, 2004. Copyright Georg Thieme Verlag.)

matogenesis by combining doses of human chorionic gonadotrophin (HCG) and/or antiestrogens with their AAS abuse. The effects of supraphysiologic doses of AAS on male infertility with or without the concomitant use of HCG were investigated under authentic conditions.

Methods.—The study group was composed of 18 healthy male power athletes using massive doses of AAS. Semen samples were collected during AAS abuse and 1.5 and 6 months after cessation of the abuse. The study participants were also questioned about their reproductive activity 6 years after the study.

Results.—At the end of the AAS cycle, the mean (±SD) sperm count was $33 \pm 49 \times 10^6$/mL, and only 1 study participant had azoospermia. At 1.5 months after cessation of the AAS cycles, the mean sperm concentration was $30 \pm 42 \times 10^6$/mL, and after 6 months the mean concentration was $77 \pm 70 \times 10^6$/mL. Significant differences were noted between the sample drawn 6 months after cessation of the AAS abuse and both samples drawn during and 1.5 months after the abuse. A significant positive correlation was observed between the HCG dose during the cycle and the relative amount of morphologically abnormal spermatozoa (Table 3).

Conclusions.—The concomitant abuse of HCG and supraphysiologic doses of AASs cause transient impairment of the quality of semen in men; nonetheless, spermatogenesis is maintained with this regimen, even with prolonged abuse of massive doses of AASs.

▶ One of the most powerful factors moderating steroid abuse by young athletes is the fear of causing permanent damage to their reproductive systems. As in World Health Organization studies of male contraception,[1] although sperm counts are reduced during periods of steroid abuse, they usually return to normal over 6 months of abstinence. Another disturbing feature is an increase in the proportion of morphologically abnormal sperm during the administration of heavy doses of steroids.[2] Many athletes now take HCG along with steroids. Competitors should be cautioned that HCG does little to protect the steroid abuser against a deterioration in sperm morphological features, although the drop in sperm counts may be reduced by this tactic.

R. J. Shephard, MD, PhD, DPE

References

1. World Health Organization Task Force on Methods for the Regulation of Male Fertility: Contraceptive efficacy of testosterone-induced azoospermia in normal men. *Lancet* 336:955-959, 1990.
2. Torres-Calleja J, Gonzalez-Unzaga M, DeCelis-Carillo R, et al: Effect of androgenic anabolic steroids on sperm quality and serum hormone levels in adult male body builders. *Life Sci* 68:1769-1774, 2001.

Early Fluid Retention and Severe Acute Mountain Sickness

Loeppky JA, Icenogle MV, Maes D, et al (Lovelace Respiratory Research Inst; Univ of New Mexico; Veterans Affairs Med Ctr, Albuquerque, NM; et al)
J Appl Physiol 98:591-597, 2005   9–19

Introduction.—Field studies of acute mountain sickness (AMS) usually include variations in exercise, diet, and environmental conditions over days and development of clinically apparent edemas. The purpose of this study was to clarify fluid status in persons developing AMS vs. those remaining without symptoms during simulated altitude with controlled fluid intake, diet, temperature, and without exercise. Ninety-nine exposures of 51 men and women to reduced barometric pressure (426 mmHg = 16,000 ft. = 4,880 m) were carried out for 8-12 h. AMS was evaluated by Lake Louise

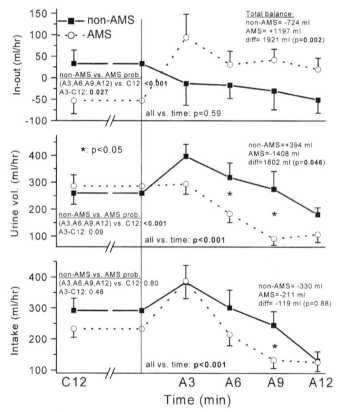

FIGURE 1.—Water balance from fluid intake and urine volume during baseline control and over 12 h at altitude by both groups. Error bars indicate ±1 SE. C12 is the value over a a 3- to 4-h period on the late afternoon-early evening of the control day, and A3, A6, A9, and A12 indicate the end of the 3-h intervals at altitude, ending at about the same time of day as the C12 measurements. Significance is shown for differences (diff) between acute mountain sickness (AMS) and non-AMS for changes in measurements from baseline. *Abbreviations: vol,* Volume; *In-out,* net balance. (Courtesy of Loeppky JA, Icenogle MV, Maes D, et al: Early fluid retention and severe acute mountain sickness. *J Appl Physiol* 98:591-597, 2005. Copyright The American Physiological Society.)

(LL) and AMS-C scores near the end of exposure. Serial measurements included fluid balance, electrolyte excretions, and plasma concentrations, regulating hormones, and free water clearance. Comparison between 16 subjects with the lowest AMS scores near the end of exposure ("non-AMS": mean LL = 1.0, range = 0-2.5) and 16 others with the highest AMS scores ("AMS": mean LL = 7.4, range = 5-11) demonstrated significant fluid retention in AMS beginning within the first 3 h, resulting from reduced urine flow (Fig 1). Plasma Na^+ decreased significantly after 6 h, indicating dilution throughout the total body water. Excretion of Na^+ and K^+ trended downward with time in both groups, being lower in AMS after 6 h, and the urine Na^+-to-K^+ ratio was significantly higher for AMS after 6 h. Renal compensation for respiratory alkalosis, plasma renin activity, aldosterone, and atrial natriuretic peptide were not different between groups, with the latter tending to rise and aldosterone falling with time of exposure. Antidiuretic hormone fell in non-AMS and rose in AMS within 90 min of exposure and continued to rise in AMS, closely associated with severity of symptoms and fluid retention.

▶ There have been many field studies demonstrating a general relationship between fluid retention and the various manifestations of AMS. However, it has been difficult to disentangle the direct effects of hypoxia from the influence of other stressors (severe exercise, exposure to extreme environments, and dietary deficiencies). The present study was conducted under the controlled conditions of a hypobaric chamber. The main weaknesses in applying the findings to mountaineers are that the total period of exposure to hypoxia was relatively short (9 hours), and the subjects were resting throughout. Observations were also cross-sectional in type, fluid balance data being compared between individuals with high and low scores on currently accepted acute mountain-sickness scales. As in earlier reports,[1,2] the data show a marked contrast between the early diuresis seen in those with a "normal" response to hypoxia, and those developing AMS. The cases of AMS show an associated increase in the secretion of antidiuretic hormone. The explanation is uncertain, but it may be related to an early sensation of nausea seen in individuals who are vulnerable to AMS.[3]

R. J. Shephard, MD, PhD, DPE

References

1. Ullmann E: Acute hypoxia and the excretion of water and electrolyte. *J Physiol (Paris)* 155:417-437, 1961.
2. Heyes MP, Farber MO, Manfredi F, et al: Acute effects of hypoxia on renal and endocrine function in normal humans. *Am J Physiol* 243: R265-R270, 1982.

Strenuous Physical Exercise Inhibits Granulocyte Activation Induced by High Altitude

Choukè A, Demetz F, Martignoni A, et al (Ludgwig-Maximilians-Univ, Munich; Southtyrolean Mountain Rescue, Bolzano, Italy)

J Appl Physiol 98:640-647, 2005   9–20

Introduction.—To test the hypothesis of whether strenuous physical exercise inhibits neutrophils that can get activated by hypobaric hypoxia, we analyzed the effects of both high altitude and strenuous exercise alone and in combination on potentially cytotoxic functions of granulocytes in healthy volunteers (n = 12 men; average age 27.6 yr; range 24-38 yr). To this end, a field study was prospectively performed with an open-labeled within-subject design comprising three protocols. *Protocol I* (high altitude) involved a helicopter ascent, overnight stay at 3,196 m, and descent on the following day. *Protocol II* (physical exercise) involved hiking below an altitude of 2,100 m with repetitive ascents amounting to a total ascent to that of *protocol III*. *Protocol III* (combination of physical exercise and high altitude) involved climbing from 1,416 to 3,196 m, stay overnight, and descent on the following day. In *protocol I*, number of granulocytes did not change, but potentially cytotoxic functions of cells (CD18 expression and superoxide production) were early and significantly upregulated. In *protocol II*, subjects

TABLE 3.—$\beta2$-Integrin Expression and Extracellular Superoxide Anion Release by Granulocytes and IL-6 Plasma Concentrations

	Reference Values	Time Point	Protocol I	Protocol II	Protocol III
IB4, rel. fl. units	35-45	T0	42.9 ± 1.3	45.8 ± 2.7	42.2 ± 5.2
		T1	54.1 ± 4.5*‡	40.1 ± 0.9	39.2 ± 1.7
		T2	37.2 ± 1.4	39.2 ± 1.8	44.3 ± 3.7
		T3	39.9 ± 2.07	40.8 ± 2.8	38.3 ± 3.2
Spontaneous, $O_2^- \times 10^6$ PMNL $\times$ 15 min^{-1}	5-15	T0	2.0 ± 0.7	5.3 ± 2.6	3.6 ± 2.2
		T1	12.1 ± 4.1*	0.7 ± 0.5*	2.4 ± 0.8
		T2	2.7 ± 1.4	4.7 ± 1.87	7.9 ± 3.5
		T3	3.1 ± 1.7	8.6 ± 4.0	4.0 ± 2.0
fMLP, $O_2^- \times 10^6$ PMNL $\times$ 15 min^{-1}	20-50	T0	24.9 ± 3.1	30.9 ± 6.3	36.2 ± 4.6
		T1	23.6 ± 5.1	17.7 ± 1.8*	11.1 ± 1.9*
		T2	22.1 ± 5.1	28.7 ± 1.9	32.2 ± 6.2†
		T3	23.1 ± 4.9	32.3 ± 5.7	21.8 ± 3.6†
IL-6, pg/ml	<12.5	T0	7.7 ± 1.9	5.0 ± 3.9	2.7 ± 0.3
		T1	8.1 ± 2.2‡	25.7 ± 6.1*	31.0 ± 8.3*
		T2	12.5 ± 7.4	2.4 ± 1.4†	3.4 ± 0.6†
		T3	1.9 ± 0.7	1.7 ± 0.42†	12.5 ± 2.9*

Note: Values are means ± SE; n = 12 subjects. $\beta2$-Integrin expression (CD18) of resting polymorphonuclear leukocytes were determined by monoclonal antibody IB4 and are expressed as relative fluorescence units (rel. fl. Units). Spontaneous and stimulated ex vivo superoxide anion (O_2^-) production are calculated as the rate of O_2^- generated from 10^6 polymorphonuclear neutrophil leukocytes (PMNL) within 15 min in the absence or presence of the chemoattractant N-formy-methionyl-phenyl-alanine (fMLP) ($O_2^- \times 10^6$ PMNL $\times$ 15 min^{-1}). Reference values derived from the literature. Paired *t* test level of significance corrected according to Bonferoni.

*$P < 0.05$ vs. T0.

†$P < 0.05$ vs. T1.

‡$P < 0.05$ vs. *protocols II* and *III*.

(Courtesy of Choukè A, Demetz F, Martignoni A, et al: Strenuous physical exercise inhibits granulocyte activation induced by high altitude. *J Appl Physiol* 98:640-647, 2005. Copyright The American Physiological Society.)

developed granulocytosis, but functions of cells were inhibited. In *protocol III*, granulocytosis occurred at higher values than those observed under *protocol II* (Table 3). Potentially cytotoxic functions of cells, however, were strongly inhibited again. In conclusion, high altitude alone, even moderate in extent, can activate potentially cytotoxic functions of circulating granulocytes. Strenuous physical exercise strongly inhibits this activation, which may give protection from an otherwise inflammatory injury.

▶ A variety of stressors, including high-altitude exposure, can induce a potentially damaging inflammatory response on the part of the human immune system.[1] Sometimes, moderate exercise compounds the effect of any environmental stressors, but as this report documents, strenuous exercise can cause a transient suppression of immune function. This is best known and recognized by the "window of opportunity" that it apparently offers for respiratory infection.[2] However, it may also serve a biologically useful function, with the immunologic downregulation protecting the body against secondary tissue inflammation. Practical issues for the clinician are whether the person who ascends to altitude by a helicopter or lift is more vulnerable to inflammatory stress than the legitimate climber, and whether such reactions contribute to the inflammation seen in high-altitude pulmonary edema.[3]

R. J. Shephard, MD, PhD, DPE

References

1. Shephard RJ: Immune changes induced by exercise in an adverse environment. *Can J Physiol Pharm* 76:539-546, 1998.
2. Nieman D: Exercise and resistance to infection. *Can J Physiol Pharm* 76:573-580, 1998.
3. Schoene RB, Swenson ER, Pizzo CJ, et al: The lung at high altitude: Bronchoalveolar lavage in acute mountain sickness and pulmonary edema. *J Appl Physiol* 64:2605-2613, 1988.

Sildenafil Increased Exercise Capacity During Hypoxia at Low Altitudes and at Mount Everest Base Camp: A Randomized, Double-blind, Placebo-controlled Crossover Trial

Ghofrani HA, Reichenberger F, Kohstall MG, et al (Univ Hosp Giessen, Germany; Justus-Liebig Univ, Giessen, Germany)
Ann Intern Med 141:169-177, 2004   9–21

Introduction.—Alveolar hypoxia produces pulmonary hypertension and enhanced right ventricular afterloading, which may impair exercise intolerance. Some evidence shows that the phosphodiesterase-5 inhibitor sildenafil causes pulmonary vasodilatation. The effects of sildenafil on exercise capacity were evaluated under conditions of hypoxic pulmonary hypertension in a randomized, double-blind, placebo-controlled, crossover investigation.

Methods.—Fourteen healthy mountaineers and trekkers underwent measurements of systolic pulmonary arterial pressure, cardiac output, and peripheral arterial oxygen saturation at rest and during evaluation of their maximal exercise capacity on a cycle ergometer: (1) while breathing a hypoxic gas mixture with a 10% fraction of inspired oxygen at low altitude (Giessen), and (2) at high altitude (the Mount Everest base camp). Participants were randomly assigned to treatment with 50 mg oral sildenafil or placebo.

Results.—At low altitude, acute hypoxia diminished arterial oxygen saturation to 72.0% at rest (95% CI, 66.5%-77.5%) and 60.8% at maximal exercise capacity (95% CI, 56.0%-64.5%). Systolic pulmonary artery pressure increased from 30.5 mm Hg (95% CI, 26.0-35.0 mm Hg) at rest to 42.9 mm Hg (95% CI, 35.6-53.5 mm Hg) during exercise in participants in the placebo group. Sildenafil (50 mg) significantly increased arterial oxygen saturation during exercise ($P = .005$) and decreased systolic pulmonary arterial pressure at rest ($P < .001$) and during exercise ($P = .031$). Sildenafil increased the maximal power output (172.5 W [95% CI, 147.5-200.0 W] vs 130.6 W [95% CI, 108.8-150.0 W]; $P < .001$) and maximal cardiac output ($P < .001$) compared with placebo. At high altitude, sildenafil had no influence on arterial oxygen saturation at rest and during exercise compared with placebo (Fig 3). Sildenafil decreased systolic pulmonary artery pressure at rest ($P = .003$) and during exercise ($P = .021$) and increased maximal power output ($P = .002$) and cardiac output ($P = .015$). In 2 participants, sildenafil worsened existing headaches at high altitude.

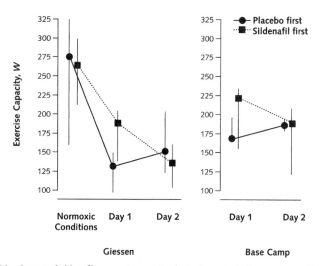

FIGURE 3.—Impact of sildenafil on exercise capacity during hypoxic challenge at low and high altitudes. Maximum exercise levels were assessed at low altitude in Giessen and at the base camp on Mount Everest. At Giessen, participants underwent exercise testing under normoxic conditions at baseline and during hypoxic challenge after receiving placebo or sildenafil in a crossover design on day 1 and day 2. Each group (placebo first and sildenafil first) included 7 participants. Exercise testing was also performed on day 1 and day 2 at the base camp. The placebo-first group had 7 participants, and the sildenafil-first group had 6 participants. *Data points* represent medians; *error bars* represent 95% CIs. (Courtesy of Ghofrani HA, Reichenberger F, Kohstall MG, et al: Sildenafil increased exercise capacity during hypoxia at low altitudes and at Mount Everest Base Camp: A randomized, double-blind, placebo-controlled crossover trial. *Ann Intern Med* 141:169-177, 2004.)

Conclusion.—Sildenafil decreases hypoxic pulmonary hypertension at rest and during exercise while maintaining gas exchange and systemic blood pressure. Sildenafil is the first known drug to increase exercise capacity during severe hypoxia, both at sea level and at high altitude.

► It is an interesting commentary on pharmaceutical research that many of the drugs commonly used by the clinician were originally designed for some entirely different purpose! Sildenafil was developed for the treatment of erectile dysfunction. However, it also appears to induce vasodilatation in well-ventilated alveoli, thus countering pulmonary hypertension without modifying systemic arterial pressure.[1] Pulmonary hypertension is undoubtedly one important manifestation of acute mountain sickness,[2] and the sildenafil-induced correction of pulmonary hypertension and the associated increase of physical work capacity will be helpful to mountaineers. However, it is disappointing that headaches are increased by sildenafil in some people, as this also is often a significant problem for mountaineers.[3] None of the participants involved in the present study were vulnerable to pulmonary edema, and it will be important to make future observations on patients with such vulnerability.

R. J. Shephard, MD, PhD, DPE

References

1. Ghofrani HA, Wiedemann R, Rose F, et al: Sildenafil for treatment of lung fibrosis and pulmonary hypertension: A randomized controlled trial. *Lancet* 360:895-900, 2002.
2. Hackett PH, Roach RC: High altitude illness. *N Engl J Med* 345:107-114, 2001.
3. Lassen NA: Increase of cerebral blood flow at high altitude: Its possible relation to AMS. *Int J Sports Med* 13(Suppl 1):47S-48S, 1992.

Three Year Follow Up of a Self Certification System for the Assessment of Fitness to Dive in Scotland
Glen S (Stirling Royal Infirmary, Livilands, Scotland)
Br J Sports Med 38:754-757, 2004   9–22

Background.—Before March 2000, all divers in the major diving organizations in the United Kingdom were required to have a medical examination to confirm their fitness to dive. At that time, a new system that used a self-administered screening questionnaire was developed to allow divers to be assessed when necessary by physicians with diving medicine experience. The effect of the new medical system on medical referee workload, diver exclusion rates, and diving incident frequency was assessed.

Methods.—All divers in Scotland were required to complete a questionnaire to screen for conditions that might impair their fitness to dive (Table 1). Divers who answered "yes" to any of the questions had their medical background assessed by a diving physician. If necessary, these patients received a clinical examination or investigation. The rate of diver exclusions based on

---

TABLE 1.—UK Sport Diving Medical Committee Self-administered Questionnaire

---

Have you suffered at any time from diseases of the heart and circulation including high blood pressure, angina, chest pains and palpitations?
Have you at any time had chest or heart surgery?
Have you suffered from or had to take medication for asthma?
Have you ever had collapsed lung or pneumothorax?
Have you ever had any other chest or lung disease?
Have you suffered at any time from blackouts, fainting, or recurrent dizziness?
Have you had regular ear problems in the past 10 years?
Do you have an ileostomy, colostomy or ever had repair of a hiatus hernia?
Have you ever had epilepsy or fits?
Have you had recurrent migraines?
Have you ever had any other disease of the brain or nervous system (including strokes or multiple sclerosis)?
Have you ever had any back or spinal surgery?
Have you any history of mental or psychological illness of any kind, fear of small spaces or panic attacks?
Have you any history of alcohol or drug abuse in the past five years?
Do you have diabetes?
Are you currently taking any prescribed medication (except the contraceptive pill)?
Are you currently receiving medical care or have you consulted the doctor in the last year other than for trivial infection or minor surgery?
Have you ever been refused a diving medical certificate or life insurance or been offered special terms?
Have you ever had, or been treated for, decompression illness?

(Courtesy of Glen S: Three year follow up of a self certification system for the assessment of fitness to dive in Scotland. *Br J Sports Med* 38:754-757, 2004. Reprinted with permission from the BMJ Publishing Group.)

---

the questionnaire response was recorded in conjunction with analysis of the incident reports.

Results.—There was an increase from 1.2% to 5.7% in the number of forms requiring review by diving physicians in the year after the introduction of the new medical system. The number of forms requiring review gradually increased to 7.7% in subsequent years. The number of divers who could not be certified as fit to dive increased slightly form 0.7% to 1.0% after 1 year and, subsequently, to 2% after 3 years. Most divers were certified as fit to dive on the basis of the questionnaire alone, and only 0.9% required objective investigation, such as exercise testing or echocardiography. Analysis of the incidents in 3 years of follow-up confirmed that none of the incidents was attributable to an undetected pre-existing medical condition. Two incidents involved divers with hypertension, but both of these divers had received medical examinations on the basis of their responses to the questionnaire.

Conclusions.—The new self-administered questionnaire system implemented in Scotland is an effective screening tool for identification of divers in need of comprehensive evaluation by physicians with experience in diving medicine.

▶ It is now accepted that physicians can use a simple self-administered instrument such as the Physical Activity Readiness Questionnaire (PAR-Q) to make a preliminary triage of their patients' ability to exercise safely.[1] It is thus logical to develop similar but more specialized instruments to allow a preliminary screening of groups such as divers. Where necessary, further assessment can then be undertaken by physicians with diving experience. However, general medical examinations rarely detect significant abnormalities among divers.[2] The present study of Scottish divers as yet lacks the extensive subject base of the PAR-Q, but to date, there is no evidence that diving incidents have arisen because of abnormalities missed during the preliminary triage. Indeed, the only significant incidents involved possible neurological decompression illness in 2 individuals with hypertension; these had, in fact, been screened by physicians rather than the questionnaire.

R. J. Shephard, MD, PhD, DPE

References

1. Thomas S, Reading J, Shephard RJ: Revision of the Physical Activity Readiness Questionnaire (PAR-Q). *Can J Sport Sci* 17:338-345, 1992.
2. Glen S, White S, Douglas J: Medical supervision of sport diving in Scotland: Reassessing the need for medical examination. *Br J Sports Med* 34:375-378, 2000.

Facial Baroparesis Secondary to Middle-Ear Over-Pressure: A Rare Complication of Scuba Diving
Hyams AF, Toynton SC, Jaramillo M, et al (Univ of Bristol, England)
J Laryngol Otol 118:721-723, 2004   9–23

Introduction.—A facial nerve palsy, as a result of middle-ear high pressure, is a rare complication of sub-aqua diving. It may occur as a result of an acute pressure change in the middle ear during ascent in those patients who have experienced difficulty equalizing their middle-ear pressure during the prior descent. We present the case history of this occurring in a 21-year-old diver (Fig 1) and discuss the pathophysiology, management and the previous

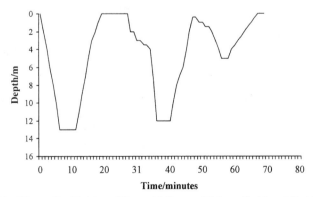

FIGURE 1.—Dive profile. (Courtesy of Hyams AF, Toynton SC, Jaramillo M, et al: Facial baroparesis secondary to middle-ear over-pressure: A rare complication of scuba diving. *J Laryngol Otol* 118:721-723, 2004.)

literature. The correct diagnosis of this condition is important if unnecessary, and potentially hazardous, recompression treatment is to be avoided.

▶ Although a rare condition among divers, there have been previous reports of facial nerve paresis subsequent to submersion.[1] The cause is thought to be a compression of the vascular supply of the nerve, secondary to failure of pressure-equalization and a tearing of tissues in the Fallopian canal.[2] The problem is best prevented by taking care to equalize middle-ear pressures during a dive. However, the paresis usually resolves once middle-ear pressure has equalized. Correct diagnosis can avoid the complication of unnecessary treatment in a hyperbaric chamber.

R. J. Shephard, MD, PhD, DPE

References

1. Molvaer OI, Eidsvik S: Facial baroparesis: A review. *Undersea Biomed Res* 14:277-293, 1987.
2. Nagai H, Nakashima T, Suzuki T, et al: Effect of middle ear pressure on blood flow to the middle ear, inner ear, and facial nerve in guinea pigs. *Acta Otolaryngol (Stock)* 116:439-442, 1996.

Risk of Decompression Illness Among 230 Divers in Relation to the Presence and Size of Patent Foramen Ovale
Torti SR, Billinger M, Schwerzmann M, et al (Univ Hosp, Bern, Switzerland)
Eur Heart J 25:1014-1020, 2004
9–24

Background.—The risk of decompression illness (DCI) developing in divers with a patent foramen ovale (PFO) is not clear. This study determined the absolute and relative odds of DCI events with and without subsequent treatment in a decompression chamber in relation to the presence and size of a PFO.

Methods.—Two hundred thirty scuba divers (mean age, 39 years) participated in the study. Contrast transesophageal echocardiography was performed to detect a PFO and grade the size on a scale of 0 to 3. Before transesophageal echocardiography, participants completed a questionnaire regarding their health, diving habits, and diving accidents. Inclusion criteria required 200 dives or more and strict adherence to decompression tables.

Findings.—Twenty-seven percent of the divers had a PFO. The overall absolute risk of a DCI event was 2.5 per 10^4 dives. One or more major DCI events was documented for 18 divers with a PFO and 10 divers without a PFO. Among divers with a PFO, the incidence per 10^4 dives of a major DCI was 5.1; of a DCI lasting longer than 24 hours, it was 1.9; and of being treated in a decompression chamber, it was 3.6. These incidences were 4.8- to 12.9-fold greater than for divers with no PFO. As the PFO size increased, so did the risk of a major DCI, of a DCI lasting more than 24 hours, and of being treated by recompression (Fig 3).

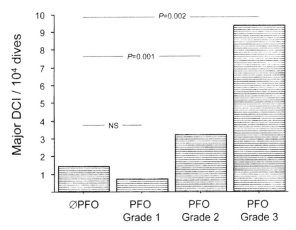

FIGURE 3.—Mean number of decompression illness (*DCI*) events per 10^4 dives (*vertical axis*) in relation to different sizes of patent foramen ovale (*PFO*). No PFO (Ø) = grade 0). (Reprinted from Torti SR, Billinger M, Schwerzmann M, et al: Risk of decompression illness among 230 divers in relation to the presence and size of patent foramen ovale. *Eur Heart J* 25:1014-1020, 2004. Copyright 2004, with permission from the RCOG.)

Conclusion.—The presence of a PFO is associated with a low absolute risk of 5 major DCI events per 10^4 dives. The odds of this happening are 5 times greater than for divers without a PFO. The risk of experiencing a major DCI parallels PFO size.

► In people with a normal circulation, any bubbles that form during decompression tend to be filtered out in the pulmonary capillaries. However, if there is a large PFO, bubbles can move into the left side of the circulation, potentially causing problems from various types of systemic embolus.

The present study suggests that if there is a patent foramen (irrespective of size), the risk of major decompression events is increased 5-fold. Nevertheless, in the short term, the absolute rate of major DCI events is still sufficiently low that there is no major contra-indication to scuba diving. Of greater concern is the possibility of long-term neurologic damage from asymptomatic episodes of cerebral ischemia.[1]

Until this issue has been resolved, Torti et al recommend against scuba diving in those with large (second or third degree) patencies of the foramen ovale. In those with smaller openings in the foramen, the risks of diving can be reduced by careful adherence to decompression tables, use of nitrox rather than compressed air, limitation of dives to a depth of 25 to 30 m, prohibition of repetitive diving, avoidance of Valsalva maneuvers during ascent, and avoidance of vigorous exercise soon after leaving the water.[2]

R. J. Shephard, MD, PhD, DPE

References

1. Schwerzmann M, Seiler C, Lipp E, et al: Relation between directly detected patent foramen ovale and ischemic brain lesions in sport divers. *Ann Intern Med* 134:21-24, 2001.
2. Schwerzmann M, Seiler C: Recreational scuba diving, patent foramen ovale and their associated risks. *Swiss Med Wkly* 131:365-374, 2001.

Serum Electrolyte Concentrations and Hydration Status Are Not Associated With Exercise Associated Muscle Cramping (EAMC) in Distance Runners

Schwellnus MP, Nicol J, Laubscher R, et al (Univ of Cape Town, Newlands, South Africa; Med Research Council, Parow, South Africa)
Br J Sports Med 38:488-492, 2004   9–25

Introduction.—Data are lacking concerning the correlation between exercise-associated muscle cramping (EAMC), dehydration, and serum electrolyte status. The association between the development of EAMC in ultradistance runners and concomitant changes in serum electrolyte concentrations and hydration status was prospectively evaluated at the Two Oceans Ultra-marathon, a 56-km road race held yearly in Cape Town, South Africa.

Methods.—Seventy-two runners were followed up for development of EAMC. All participants were weighed before and immediately after the racing event. Blood samples were obtained before the race, immediately after, and 60 minutes after the race and were evaluated for glucose, protein, potassium, calcium, and magnesium concentrations, serum osmolality, hemoglobin, and packed cell volume. Twenty-one runners had a history of severe EAMC during racing (cramp group), and 22 runners had no history of EAMC during racing (control subjects).

Results.—No significant between-group differences were found in prerace versus postrace body mass, percent change in body mass, blood volume, plasma volume, or red cell volume. The immediate postrace serum sodium concentration was significantly lower (139.8 vs 142.3 mmol/L; $P = .004$) in the cramp group than in the control subjects. The immediate postrace serum magnesium concentration was significantly higher in the cramp group than in control subjects (0.73 vs 0.67 mmol/L; $P = .03$) (Table 3).

Conclusion.—No clinically important associations were found between changes in serum electrolyte concentrations or hydration status and the development of EAMC in ultradistance runners before or immediately after a race or during the clinical recovery from EAMC.

▶ Clinicians have reached a general consensus that muscle cramping reflects an electrolyte imbalance, particularly an imbalance of calcium and magnesium ions.[1] On this basis, many athletic drinks now offer substantial quantities of magnesium to runners. The present article offers a comparison of serum electrolyte concentrations between athletes who develop cramps and those who

TABLE 3.—Values for Pre-Race, Immediate Post-Race, and 60 Minute Post-Race Serum Sodium, Potassium, Total Calcium, and Total Magnesium Concentrations, Serum Osmolality, Plasma Glucose Concentration, Plasma Proteins, Packed Cell Volume, and Hemoglobin Results for the Cramping and Control Groups, Expressed as Mean (SD) and Mean (1st and 3rd Quartiles)

Variable	Pre-race		Immediate Post-race		60 Min Post-race	
	Cramp (n = 21)	Control (n = 22)	Cramp (n = 21)	Control (n = 21)	Cramp (n = 13)	Control (n = 16)
Mean (SD)						
Sodium (mmol/l)	139.2 (2.1)	139.3 (2.0)	139.8 (3.1)*	142.3 (2.1)*	140.3 (1.9)	141.7 (1.7)
Potassium (mmol/l)	4.5 (0.4)	4.4 (0.4)	4.9 (0.6)	4.7 (0.5)	4.7 (0.5)	4.6 (0.5)
Calcium (mmol/l)	2.2 (0.1)	2.2 (0.1)	2.3 (0.2)	2.3 (0.1)	2.2 (0.3)	2.2 (0.2)
Magnesium (mmol/l)	0.81 (0.1)	0.83 (0.1)	0.73 (0.1)*	0.67 (0.1)*	0.75 (0.1)	0.73 (0.1)
Osmolality (mmol/kg)	284 (5)	282 (4)	280 (6)	284 (10)	284 (7)	283 (8)
Glucose (mmol/l)	6.3 (3.1)	6.1 (1.1)	6.8 (1.9)	6.5 (2.0)	6.3 (1.0)	6.5 (1.1)
Plasma proteins (g/l)	73.3 (5.3)	72.7 (3.9)	76.4 (5.2)	73.7 (15.5)		
PCV (%)	40.0 (4.0)	42.0 (4.0)	40.0 (3.0)	40.0 (3.0)		
Haemoglobin (g/dl)	15.5 (1.1)	15.5 (0.8)	15.7 (1.0)	15.5 (3.2)		
Median (1st and 3rd quartiles)						
Sodium (mmol/l)	139 (138, 140)	139 (138, 141)	140 (139, 142)*	143 (141, 144)*	141 (138, 141)	142 (141, 143)
Potassium (mmol/l)	4.5 (4.2, 4.6)	4.3 (4.2, 4.5)	4.9 (4.5, 5.4)	4.7 (4.5, 5.0)	4.8 (4.2, 5.0)	4.6 (4.3, 4.9)
Calcium (mmol/l)	2.2 (2.1, 2.2)	2.2 (2.1, 2.2)	2.3 (2.2, 2.4)	2.3 (2.2, 2.4)	2.3 (2.0, 2.4)	2.2 (2.1, 2.3)
Magnesium (mmol/l)	0.8 (0.8, 0.9)	0.8 (0.8, 0.9)	0.8 (0.7, 0.8)*	0.7 (0.6, 0.7)*	0.8 (0.7, 0.8)	0.7 (0.7, 0.8)
Osmolality (mmol/kg)	284 (280, 285)	282 (280, 286)	280 (277, 286)	283 (279, 291)	284 (279, 286)	285 (282, 287)
Glucose (mmol/l)	5.3 (4.7, 6.7)	5.8 (5.6, 7.1)	6.5 (5.6, 7.6)	6.7 (5.8, 8.1)	6.3 (5.9, 7.0)	6.6 (5.5, 7.4)
Plasma proteins (g/l)	71.9 (69.6, 74.3)	72.7 (71.1, 75.4)	75.0 (73.3, 78.8)	76.2 (75.0, 80.6)		
PCV (%)	40 (40, 40)	40 (40, 40)	40 (40, 40)	40 (40, 40)		
Haemoglobin (g/dl)	15.4 (14.6, 16.1)	15.7 (14.9, 16.1)	15.6 (15.2, 16.2)	16.2 (15.6, 16.9)		

*Significant difference in the immediate post-race values between the cramp and control groups ($P < .05$).

Abbreviation: PCV, Packed cell volume.

(Courtesy of Schwellnus MP, Nicol J, Laubscher R, et al: Serum electrolyte concentrations and hydration status are not associated with exercise associated muscle cramping (EAMC) in distance runners. *Br J Sports Med* 38:488-492, 2004. Reprinted with permission from the BMJ Publishing Group.)

do not. The authors reach the somewhat controversial conclusion that changes in electrolyte balance are not responsible for the observed symptoms, despite data that show a significant difference in serum magnesium concentrations between those competitors who developed cramps and those who did not. The investigators argue that the intergroup difference in mineral concentrations is small and not of clinical significance. I certainly applaud the attempt to distinguish between the statistical significance and the clinical significance of laboratory findings. On the other hand, both subject groups did show a substantial drop in serum magnesium concentrations during competition, and it seems quite possible that the additional mineral loss in the symptomatic group may have been just sufficient to push them to the cramping threshold.

R. J. Shephard, MD, PhD, DPE

Reference

1. McGee SR: Muscle cramps. *Arch Intern Med* 150:511-518, 1990.

The Effects of Continuous Hot Weather Training on Risk of Exertional Heat Illness

Wallace RF, Kriebel D, Punnett L, et al (US Army Research Inst of Environmental Medicine, Natick, Mass; Univ of Massachusetts, Lowell; Uniformed Services Univ of the Health Sciences, Bethesda, Md)
Med Sci Sports Exerc 37:84-90, 2005   9–26

Background.—The United States military first implemented heat illness prevention guidelines on the basis of the hourly wet-bulb globe temperature (WBGT) index in the 1950s after experiencing a high rate of heat illness at one basic training base. The training guidelines currently being used by the Marine Corps state that continued exercise is permitted with a WBGT index from 80° to 84.9°F. At temperatures of 90°F and above, all activity is to be stopped. However, one study has reported that many episodes of exertional heat illness (EHI) occurred with WBGT values well below the safe range of 80° to 84.9°F. It was also reported that a majority of the EHI cases in this study were exposed to a WBGT above 80°F on the day before becoming a case. Thus, it is possible that there is a cumulative exposure effect that continues to the next day of training. Whether a cumulative daily average WBGT index over 1 or 2 preceding days is a better measure for prediction of EHI than is the current daily average WBGT was investigated.

Methods.—This case-crossover study was conducted in male and female recruits who were undergoing basic training at one Marine Corps recruit depot. Weather measurements were obtained for 2069 cases of EHI during 1979 to 1997 and for randomly selected control periods before and after each EHI episode.

Results.—The risk of EHI increased with WBGT. EHI risk was associated not only with the WBGT at the time of the event but also with the average

WBGT on the previous day. Alternative combinations of WBGT components were identified that were better predictors of risk for EHI.

Conclusions.—There is evidence of a cumulative effect of the previous day's heat exposure on the risk of EHI in Marine Corps recruits undergoing basic training. A simple index for use in predicting risk of EHI is presented. This index utilizes the dry-bulb temperature and the relative humidity.

▶ This study is important in showing that exercise-induced heat illness can develop when temperatures remain within the traditional "green label" safe temperature zone, a finding previously noted by Kark and his associates.[1] One factor contributing to adverse events, despite relatively moderate temperatures, seems to be a cumulative effect of previous heat exposures. In the circumstances of the present experiments, the likelihood of heat illness was predicted better when account was taken of heat exposure on the previous day, but predictions were not improved further by looking at preceding days. Caution must be shown in applying the reported findings to athletes. The subjects of these experiments were military personnel. Patterns of exercise and clothing are explained rather sketchily, but are presumably typical of a military training exercise rather than athletic competition. Claims are made for the development of improved indices of heat stress, but it is important that the new prediction formulae have yet to be tested on an independent group of subjects.

R. J. Shephard, MD, PhD, DPE

Reference

1. Kark JA, Burr PQ, Wenger CB, et al: Exertional heat illness in Marine Corps recruit training. *Aviat Space Environ Med* 67:354-360, 1996.

Cooling Vest Worn During Active Warm-Up Improves 5-km Run Performance in the Heat
Arngrímsson SÁ, Petitt DS, Stueck MG, et al (Univ of Georgia, Athens)
J Appl Physiol 96:1867-1874, 2004   9–27

Background.—It has been well established that a high ambient temperature has an adverse effect on performance in endurance activities such as distance running. Laboratory studies have shown that lowering the core temperature before exercise (precooling) can delay the fatigue that occurs in constant-rate exercise, such as distance running, or can increase the work performed in a given period of time. However, although there is considerable research to suggest that precooling is effective in improving performance in moderately prolonged exercise, there is little evidence that precooling could be used to improve the performance of athletes in competition. Whether a cooling vest worn during an active warm-up would improve an athlete's 5-km run time in the setting of high ambient temperature was determined.

Methods.—The study group was composed of 17 competitive runners (9 men and 8 women) who completed 2 simulated 5-km runs on a treadmill

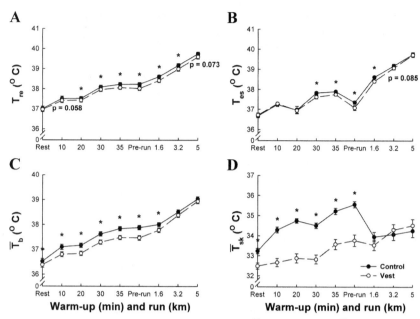

FIGURE 1.—Rectal (T_{re}; A), esophageal (T_{es}; B), mean body ($\overline{T}_b$; C), and mean skin ($\overline{T}_{sk}$; D) temperatures during the warm-up and the simulated 5-km run. Values are means ± SE. Vest, experimental condition in which subjects wore a cooling vest with ice packs during warm-up. Control, condition in which subjects wore a regular T-shirt during warm-up. *Significant difference between conditions, $P <.05$. (Courtesy of Arngrímsson SÁ, Petitt DS, Stueck MG, et al: Cooling vest worn during active warm-up improves 5-km run performance in the heat. *J Appl Physiol* 96:1867-1874, 2004. Copyright The American Physiological Society.)

after a 38-minute active warm-up during which they wore either a T-shirt (control) or a vest filled with ice (vest) in a hot, humid environment.

Results.—Wearing the cooling vest during the warm-up significantly blunted increases in body temperature, heart rate, and the perception of thermal discomfort during warm-up compared with the control condition (Fig 1). Most of the differences between the control and vest groups at the start of the 5-km run were eliminated in the first 3.2 km of the run, and no statistically significant differences were found between the 2 groups in terms of body temperature, heart rate, and the perception of thermal discomfort at the end of the run. However, the 5-km run time was significantly faster for runners in the vest group, and a faster pace was most evident in the last 2 thirds of the run.

Conclusions.—The wearing of a cooling vest during active warm-up by track athletes can improve an athlete's performance in a 5-km run in the heat. The reduced thermal and cardiovascular strain and reduced thermal discomfort early in the run seems to allow runners to maintain a faster pace later in the run.

▶ The idea of precooling someone who is to compete in a hot climate is rather controversial. Cooling would counter the athlete's warm-up; thus, it might be expected to worsen performance. However, possibly, a benefit may be derived if the use of a vest restricts cooling to the body core and the limb temperature is maintained by a simultaneous active warm-up. The data of Arngrímsson and associates support this idea, at least when study participants are running over a distance of 5 km. Most of the thermal benefit relative to the control run (ie, lower core temperatures and reduced thermal sensations) had disappeared after running 3 km, so a greater relative benefit might be observed over a distance somewhat shorter than 5 km. Both of the reported trials were run on a laboratory treadmill, without air movement or radiant heating. The observations should, thus, be repeated under normal track conditions.

R. J. Shephard, MD, PhD, DPE

Heat Stroke: A Review of Cooling Methods
Hadad E, Rav-Acha M, Heled Y, et al (Heller Inst of Med Research, Tel Hashomer, Israel; Tel Aviv Univ, Israel)
Sports Med 34:501-511, 2004   9–28

Introduction.—The prognosis of heat stroke is directly associated with the extent of hyperthermia and its duration. Thus, the most important component in the treatment of heat stroke is rapid cooling.

Cooling Methods.—Several methods for cooling have been reported, including immersion in water at various temperatures, evaporative cooling ice pack applications, pharmacologic treatment, and invasive techniques. A literature review showed a large diversity in the model investigated, in the preliminary clinical stage, and in the method applied. The cooling methods evaluated were water immersion and evaporative cooling. Most data, based on experimental models or healthy research subjects, indicate that evaporative cooling is the method of choice. However, water immersion was also found to have advantages when used on patients with heat stroke. In the field, when administration of immediate cooling measures is crucial, splashing copious amounts of water (1-16°C) over the individual, along with fanning, is strongly recommended. On arrival at a clinical facility, treatment should be matched to the patient's age and clinical background. Young patients may be able to tolerate aggressive treatment with ice water (1-5°C), whereas older patients and those with cardiovascular illness should not be exposed to unnecessary risks; tepid water (12-16°C) and fans should be used in these populations.

Conclusion.—Current knowledge does not support the superiority of evaporative cooling over water immersion. Wider randomized controlled trials need to be performed on patients with heat stroke to compare the various cooling techniques before a determination can be made of the cooling method of choice.

▶ Heat stroke is potentially one of the most serious complications of prolonged endurance exercise.[1] If a competitor is exposed to the radiant energy from bright sunlight, heat stroke can develop at disarmingly low environmental temperatures. The extent of injury and the risk of death depend on the length of time for which an excessive core temperature is maintained. In an emergency tent, immediate spraying with water, fanning, and evaporative cooling may be the only therapeutic options. However, if available, water immersion ensures more rapid cooling of the body. In young adults, the water temperature can safely be as low as 1°C to 5°C. It remains unclear whether such low temperatures are dangerous to older people. One study of a heat wave in Kansas City[2] found a mortality rate of 18% in elderly patients who were treated by ice-water immersion. However, this may have reflected the effects of the initial heat exposure rather than an adverse response to very cold water. Other laboratory options such as the use of the muscle relaxant dantrolene and peritoneal or gastric lavage remain controversial.

R. J. Shephard, MD, PhD, DPE

References

1. Bouchama A, Knoichel JP: Heat stroke. *N Engl J Med* 346:1978-1988, 2002.
2. Tucker LE, Stanford J, Graves B, et al: Classical heatstroke: Clinical and laboratory assessment. *South Med J* 78:20-25, 1985.

The Impact of Prolonged Exercise in a Cold Environment Upon Cardiac Function
Shave R, Dawson E, Whyte G, et al (Brunel Univ, Uxbridge, Middlesex, England; Rigshospitalet, Copenhagen; Olympic Med Inst, London; et al)
Med Sci Sports Exerc 36:1522-1527, 2004   9–29

Purpose.—The purpose of the present study was to examine the impact of cold exposure coupled with prolonged exercise upon postexercise left ventricular (LV) function and markers of myocardial damage.

Methods.—Eight highly trained male athletes (mean ± SD; age: 28.2 ± 8.8 yr; height: 1.78 ± 0.07 m; body mass: 74.9 ± 7.6 kg; $\dot{V}O_{2max}$: 65.6 ± 7.0 mL·kg^{-1}·min^{-1}) performed two 100-mile cycle trials, the first in an ambient temperature of 0°C, the second in an ambient temperature of 19°C. Echocardiographic assessment was completed and blood samples drawn before, immediately postexercise, and 24-h postexercise. Left ventricular systolic (stroke volume [SV], ejection fraction [EF], and systolic blood pressure/end systolic volume ratio [SBP/ESV]) and diastolic (early [E] to late [A] filling ratio [E:A]) parameters were calculated. Serum was analyzed for creatine kinase isoenzyme MB (CK-MB$_{mass}$) and cardiac troponin T (cTnT). cTnT was analyzed descriptively whereas other variables were assessed using two-way repeated-measures ANOVA.

Results.—No significant change was observed in systolic function across time or between trials. A significant difference between trials was observed in E:A immediately after exercise (1.4 ± 0.4 [19°C] vs 1.8 ± 0.3 [0°C]) ($P < 0.05$). CK-MB$_{mass}$ was significantly elevated immediately after exercise in both trials ($P < 0.05$). Positive cTnT concentrations were observed in two subjects immediately after the 19°C trial (0.012 µg·L^{-1} and 0.034 µg·L^{-1}).

Conclusions.—Cycling 100 miles in an ambient temperature of 19°C is associated with an acute change in diastolic filling that is not observed after prolonged exercise at 0°C. Prolonged exercise is associated with minimal cardiac damage in some individuals; it appears that this is a separate phenomenon to the change in diastolic filling.

▶ Exercise-induced cardiac fatigue (EICF) and exercise-induced cardiac damage are well reported phenomena related to prolonged or endurance exercise. The relationship between the 2 conditions is as yet unclear. It has been proposed that EICF may be related to exercise performed in hostile environmental conditions (hot and cold temperature, high humidity, and moderate to high altitudes). This study systematically examines the effect of prolonged exercise (100-mile cycle trials) in trained subjects participating in cold (0°C) conditions versus warm (19°C) conditions. No significant difference was observed in cardiac function between these 2 environmental states. However, it was noted that the cardiac muscle enzyme CK-MB was significantly elevated in both groups, suggesting that minimal cardiac damage occurs in some individuals. The answer to the intriguing conundrum of EICF remains open.

P. McCrory, PhD

Hypercapnia Increases Core Temperature Cooling Rate During Snow Burial
Grissom CK, Radwin MI, Scholand MB, et al (LDS Hosp, Salt Lake City, Utah; Univ of Utah, Salt Lake City; Sorenson Genomics, Salt Lake City, Utah; et al)
J Appl Physiol 96:1365-1370, 2004   9–30

Background.—The international triage and treatment recommendations for avalanche burial victims have assumed an average core body temperature cooling rate of 3°C per hour during an avalanche burial. This assumption has been based on previous retrospective studies. Hypothermia is a major medical problem that requires treatment in individuals who survive an avalanche burial, but asphyxiation is the major cause of death in an avalanche burial. Hypercapnia occurs in an avalanche burial as a result of breathing expired air, and the effect of hypercapnia on hypothermia is unknown. Previous studies have shown that the development of hypercapnia and hypoxemia during an avalanche burial is delayed by the presence of an air pocket in the snow for breathing or by the use of an artificial breathing device that diverts expired air away from inspired air drawn from the snowpack. The core-temperature cooling rate during snow burial under normocapnic and hypercapnic conditions was determined.

Methods.—The rectal core body temperature was measured in 12 research subjects buried in compacted snow that simulated avalanche burial conditions. The research subjects wore a lightweight clothing insulation system during 2 different study burials. In the first burial, the research subjects breathed with a device that resulted in hypercapnia over 30 to 60 minutes. In

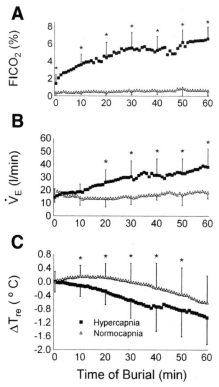

FIGURE 4.—Mean fraction of inspired carbon dioxide (FI_{CO_2}; A), $\dot{V}E$ (B), and rectal core body temperature (T_{re}; C) during burial in dense snow for up to 60 minutes during the hypercapnic and normocapnic studies (n = 12). Five of the subjects in the hypercapnic study did not complete the full 60 minutes of burial (studies terminated at 26, 30, 35, 38, and 42 minutes). T_{re} data are presented as difference from values at time 0 of burial (ΔT_{re}). Values are means ± SD. *Significant difference between the hypercapnic and the normocapnic study ($P < .05$). (Courtesy of Grissom CK, Radwin MI, Scholand MB, et al: Hypercapnia increases core temperature cooling rate during snow burial. *J Appl Physiol* 96:1365-1370, 2004. Copyright The American Physiological Society.)

the second burial, the research subjects were buried under identical conditions with a modified breathing device that maintained normocapnia.

Results.—The rate of the decrease in the core temperature was greater with hypercapnia than with normocapnia. In the hypercapnic study, the fraction of inspired carbon dioxide increased from 1.4 ± 1.0% to 7.0 ± 1.4%, minute ventilation increased from 15 ± 7 to 40 ± 12 L/min, and oxygen saturation decreased from 97 ± 1% to 90 ± 6% (Fig 4). The variables were unchanged during the normocapnic study.

Conclusions.—The cooling rate during snow burial was found to be less than has previously been reported and was increased by hypercapnia. These findings may have important implications for the prehospital treatment of victims of an avalanche burial.

▶ Many avalanche victims die of asphyxia; however, if a rescue occurs, then the treatment of hypothermia is often an urgent necessity. Currently, it is assumed that the core temperatures of avalanche victims decrease by 3°C/h,[1] but Grissom and colleagues point out that accumulation of carbon dioxide in an air pocket beneath an avalanche can cause hyperventilation, thus accelerating the cooling process. The experimental study involved the somewhat forbidding protocol of burying study participants alive in carefully standardized snow packs; not surprisingly, it was necessary to pay volunteers. The carbon dioxide levels rose to 6%, which is about the concentration at which maximal stimulation of breathing occurs, and as the figure illustrates, the decrease in rectal temperature during hypercapnia was approximately doubled relative to normocapnic conditions. Unfortunately, the comparison is weakened because the order of testing was not randomized. In an actual avalanche, other variables influencing the cooling rate would include the type of clothing that is worn, any trauma that has been sustained, and the use of safety equipment such as the AvaLung. It is important to note that in some victims, cardiac arrest can occur in as little as 10 minutes.[1] At the other extreme, 1 healthy young man is known to have survived 20 hours of burial, at the end of which his core temperature had dropped to 25.6°C.[2]

R. J. Shephard, MD, PhD, DPE

References

1. Locher T, Walpoth BH: Differential diagnosis of circulatory failure in hypothermic avalanche victims: Retrospective analysis of 32 avalanche accidents. *Schweiz Rundsch Med Prax* 85:1275-1282, 1996.
2. Spiegel RW: Rescuing an avalanche victim alive after 20 hours, in *AIRMED 2002 Lectures* (CD ROM). Zurich, Switzerland, Swiss Air Rescue, 2002.

Subject Index

A

Abdominal cramps
  in female athletes, evaluation of small
    bowel and colonic transit time
    using pH telemetry, 259
Acetabular tear
  in soccer players, long-term outcome,
    83
Achilles tendinopathy
  vs. patellar tendinopathy,
    histopathological comparison, 119
Achilles tendon
  immediate response after strength
    training evaluated by MRI, 138
ACL injuries (*see* Anterior cruciate
    ligament [ACL] injuries)
Active Script Program
  for promotion of physical activity, 1
Acute mountain sickness
  early fluid retention and, 380
Adipose tissue
  interindividual variation, influence of
    measurement site, 247
Adolescent(s)
  cardiovascular fitness and exercise as
    determinants of insulin resistance in
    females, 326
  energy costs of physical activities, 323
  exercise behavior in, effect of
    office-based physicians' advice, 324
  growth spurts in female gymnasts, 327
  high-intensity intermittent anaerobic
    exercise in, recovery from, 328
  interaction between calcium intake and
    menarcheal age on bone mass gain
    in, 307
  lifestyle factors and development of
    bone mass and bone strength in,
    306
  thermoregulation during rest and
    exercise in the cold, 330
Aging
  (*see also* Older adults; Women,
    postmenopausal)
  jumping mechanography reproducibility
    in physically competent adult and
    elderly subjects, 339
  physical activity and serum IL-6 and
    IL-10 levels in healthy older men,
    343
  on primary in vivo antibody and T
    cell-mediated responses in men,
    341

protein metabolism in older and
    younger men following
    moderate-intensity aerobic exercise,
    341
Airway cells
  composition at rest and after an all-out
    test in competitive rowers, 241
Airway hyperresponsiveness
  field exercise vs. laboratory eucapnic
    voluntary hyperventilation for
    identification in elite cold weather
    athletes, 239
Altitude (*see* High altitude)
Amenorrhea
  in athletes, cardiovascular effects, 312
Anabolic-androgenic steroids
  analysis of non-hormonal nutritional
    supplements for presence of, 372
  endogenous norandrosterone and
    noretiocholanolone concentration
    before and after submaximal
    standardized exercise, 371
  relationship between diet and serum
    anabolic hormone responses to
    heavy-resistance exercise in men,
    374
  reversibility of cardiac effects in
    strength athletes, 376
  with and without human chorionic
    gonadotropin, spermatogenesis in
    power athletes and, 377
Ankle
  chronic instability, effect on dynamic
    postural control, 140
  injuries
    high sprains, diagnosis, treatment,
      and recovery time, 142
    identification of a fibular fracture in
      an intercollegiate football player in
      a physical therapy setting, 134
    inversion, acute peroneal
      compartment syndrome following,
      131
    risk factors in volleyball, 34
    shoe rim and shoe buckle
      pseudotumor in elite and
      professional figure skaters and
      snowboarders, 144
    syndesmosis sprains in professional
      hockey players, 145
    warm-up program for prevention in
      young athletes, 46
  lateral ligament anesthesia and
    single-leg stance ability, 198

Author Index